Y0-BQG-535

SpringerWienNewYork

Otto-Michael Lesch
Henriette Walter
Christian Wetschka
Michie Hesselbrock
Victor Hesselbrock

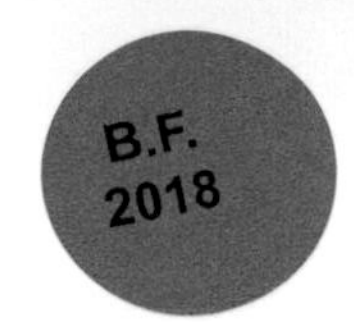

Alcohol and Tobacco

Medical and Sociological Aspects of Use, Abuse and Addiction

SpringerWienNewYork

Otto Michael Lesch, MD
Henriette Walter, MD
Medical University of Vienna, Austria

Christian Wetschka, PhD
Vienna, Austria

Michie N. Hesselbrock, PhD
Victor Hesselbrock, PhD
University of Connecticut, Farmington, CT, USA

Printed in Germany

SpringerWienNewYork is part of
Springer Science+Business Media
springer.at

Copy editing: Claire Speringer, 1030 Vienna, Austria
Typesetting: PTP-Berlin Protago-TEX-Production GmbH, 10779 Berlin, Germany
Printing: Strauss GmbH, 69509 Mörlenbach, Germany

Printed on acid-free and chlorine-free bleached paper
SPIN: 12610372

With 122 Figures

Library of Congress Control Number: 2010935024

ISBN 978-3-7091-0145-2 SpringerWienNewYork

Acknowledgements

After more than 30 years working with psychiatric patients especially with addicted patients I thank many friends, experts and researchers. At the beginning of my work in 1972 Berner P., Mader R. and Strotzka H. supported my education and they made it possible to organize in a catchment area a social psychiatric network. In this network a long term treatment (chain: outpatient-inpatient-outpatient) could be developed. There it was possible to investigate the long term course of psychiatric, especially of alcohol addicted patients. After 4 years of work the first results could be published. In this ongoing research an international discussion process started. Boening J., Pelc I., Tabakoff B., Platz W. and DeWitte P. have always drawn my attention to the fact, that in addictive processes psychosocial factors have the same importance than biological vulnerabilities. These experts but also a lot of others from many countries helped me to publish the most important results and invited me to many international conferences to discuss our data. My research team produced many new results and I have to thank them for many interesting hours bringing in new and important research ideas. Especially I would like to thank H. Poltnig, who died much to early, for producing the first LAT-documentation. Henriette Walter helped to produce the first German manuscript, Christian Wetschka brought in his social therapeutic expertise and Michie and Victor Hesselbrock included their knowledge about the subgroups of alcohol dependence used in the United States.

Last but not least I have to thank my family, especially my wife Elisabeth, because they had to miss me many weekends in the last 30 years. They formed a climate to be able to relax and also made clear that beside working with addicted patients many other much more exiting sites in life exist.

Otto Lesch

Assistant: Josefine Kalenda
Translation: Miriam Mahler

Foreword

It is a pleasure to write this foreword for the text by Professor Otto-Michael Lesch and colleagues dealing with the important topics of alcohol and tobacco. The thoughts offered from this broad based book are likely to be applicable to readers with interests in a wide range of substances of abuse. An earlier version of this text, published in German, has stood the test of time, and the updated chapters in this edition were developed in consultation with eminent clinicians and researchers from sociology (Christian Wetschka), social work (Michie Hesselbrock), and psychology (Victor Hesselbrock) – contributions that complement the approaches offered by Professor Lesch.

The content reflects the wealth of experience of the authors, including the more than 30 years in the field expended by Professor Lesch. The information offered here includes observations on the history of relevant diagnoses; descriptions of the importance to societies of alcohol and tobacco use and problems; theories of factors that contribute to discussions of the diagnostic approaches of the American Psychiatric Association's DSM, as well as those generated by the World Health Organization; along with expansions of these criteria to detecting substance related problems in clinical practice. An important part of the material deals with the sequelae of alcohol and tobacco use, including comorbidity with psychiatric syndromes. The emphasis on comorbidities is an essential component for a clinically oriented text dealing with alcohol and tobacco as psychiatric symptoms, especially anxiety and depression, can both increase the risk for substance dependence and reflect important consequences of their clinical course.

A special strength of this book, not surprisingly, is a sophisticated description of a broad range of possible typologies of alcohol and tobacco dependence. While much emphasis is placed on the approach developed by Professor Lesch and his colleagues, the text is careful to discuss additional approaches, including those related to genetic predispositions.

Underscoring the clinical usefulness of the information offered is the breadth of the discussion of treatments. These include combinations of sociological and psychological approaches, as well as a presentation of potentially useful pharmacological therapies. The book also recognizes the interest that clinicians are likely to have in preventing alcohol- and nicotine-related disorders.

In closing, this updated English version of a well established text has much to offer a wide range of clinicians.

The book should be considered as potentially important reading for students entering our field as well as for well established practitioners.

Marc A. Schuckit, MD,
Distinguished Professor of Psychiatry
Department of Psychiatry
University of California, San Diego
Editor, *Journal of Studies on Alcohol and Drugs*
NIAAA's Jack Mendelson Honorary Award, NIAAA Keller Honorary Award, Middleton Award for the best research within the VA system, American Psychiatric Association's Hofheimer Prize (now the APA Award for Research), Society for Biological Psychiatry's Gold Medal Award for lifetime achievement, Research Society on Alcoholism's Distinguished Scientist and Seixas Awards, James B. Isaacson Memorial Award, Jellinek Award.

Foreword

Alcoholism and smoking are the most frequent causes of addiction in our century. The extent to which alcohol is associated with health problems is remarkable, with Europe sadly adopting a leading role. 55 million adult Europeans use alcohol irresponsibly and 23 million can be categorized as alcohol dependent. The costs of treating the medical sequelae of alcohol abuse and related occupational deficits, which are paid by the health systems, are tremendous, e. g. Germany has reported costs of 20 billion Euros per annum. Besides the dependence itself, a myriad of alcohol related sequelae ranging from accidents to suicide, as well as social and occupational problems (family problems, unemployment), need to be examined. A particular cause for concern is the permanently declining age of initiation for alcohol use, which in the meantime has dropped to the age of 13–14. In view of the early onset of chronic alcohol consumption, an increase in the number of alcohol dependents and severe alcohol related sequelae, e. g. liver cirrhosis, have to be expected in the future.

Most alcohol dependents also smoke and, in fact, there are hardly any who do not. The effects of smoking are similarly health damaging and a German study has shown that around 110,000 people die each year from tobacco-related causes (cancer, cardiovascular disease and respiratory diseases). Alcohol and tobacco dependence has remarkably wide-ranging effects on almost all organs of the human body. For this reason, it is very important that not only psychiatrists and addiction experts tackle this subject, but that physicians, regardless of their specialisation, are also aware of the problem and are able to diagnose and choose adequate and timely interventions.

With his book, "Alcohol and Tobacco: Medical and Sociological Aspects of Use, Abuse and Addiction", Professor Otto-Michael Lesch, a psychiatrist of the highest international reputation, with over 40 years of experience in treating dependents, has not only explored all of the major issues, but has also managed to consider most aspects of dependence (prevention, diagnostics, sequelae, therapy). Despite the comprehensive scope of his book, the authors have successfully managed to discuss certain aspects in more depth without losing sight of the whole picture. In this book, both theory-based researchers as well as professionals in practice will find the information they are looking for. Especially interesting are a number of case studies from practice which have been included in the book. Here, the authors have put special emphasis on the typology of alcohol dependence which Lesch himself developed. Lesch's typology of alcohol dependence has received wide acceptance internationally and has recently been re-evaluated and structured by a research group, directed by Lesch. The reason why this typology is so important is because it can be used as a tool to predict both the assessment for prognoses, and therapeutic responses to different therapies.

With his work, Otto-Michael Lesch continues the classical tradition of German-speaking psychiatrists in the domain of alcohol research and treatment. In this respect, he sets new standards in almost all areas by introducing modern viewpoints and new scientific results. As President of the European Society for Biomedical Research on Alcoholism (ESBRA), I would like to congratulate Otto-Michael Lesch and his colleagues on this work and also thank him sincerely. The English version is now available for many interested readers in the European Community and I hope it helps to increase the quality of life of dependent patients.

Helmut K. Seitz, MD, PhD, AGAF
Distinguished Professor
of Internal Medicine,
Gastroenterology and Alcohol Research,
University of Heidelberg, Germany
Honorary Professor, Huazhong
University, Wuhan, P. R. China
Director, Salem Medical Center,
Heidelberg, Germany
Head, Department of Medicine and
Center of Alcohol Research
Liver Disease and Nutrition, Salem
Medical Center, Heidelberg,
Germany President of European
Society for Biomedical Reseach
on Alcoholism
(ESBRA)

Statement

In as far as this book uses personal terms and definitions, they apply equally to women and men; for the sake of clarity, and without any intention to discriminate, only one gender-specific denomination has been used.

Table of contents

1

2

3

10

1

Information about the origination of this book

As alcohol and tobacco consumption often occur concomitantly, scientific and therapeutic interest in both substances has significantly increased over the past years. The concomitant use has clearly more damaging effects than alcohol or tobacco use by itself. In practice, patients have often mentioned that they were able to quit the consumption of one substance without difficulty, but at the same increased the consumption of the other (e.g. if the patients managed to quit smoking, their alcohol consumption significantly increased). Our knowledge about dependencies is permanently expanding and basic research keeps improving explainations of the functioning of specific brain circuits. Therefore it is very important for us to deliver findings that clinical practitioners can apply in therapy or during consultations with tobacco and alcohol dependents. A differentiation between phenomena like the reward system, dependence memory, withdrawal symptoms or the craving for tobacco and alcohol is needed in order to carry out objective therapy and consultation. Very old concepts can still be found in the literature today (Bleuler M. 1983; Forel A. 1930, 1935; Haller R. 2007), which are formulated into general rules for the therapy of dependents. Yet, often, these authors use values which are unacceptable today. Relapse is always viewed as something negative and the negative stigma of the "dependence" diagnosis still remains a problem. This book will try to deliver objective information which shows that a dependence has nothing to do with faults or personal weakness. Practitioners have divorced themselves from these general therapy guidelines and now use "individual therapy for every patient". These therapies are "therapy according to dimensions", "resource-oriented therapy" or therapy which accepts unchangeable variables and seeks to influence changeable variables. Although we principally agree with these modern approaches, this book will nevertheless outline factors with global validity, which have been shown to be effective in the therapy of dependent patients. Scientific findings about subgroups according to Lesch's typology form the basis of therapy, but often need to be modified according to the individual. Classifications according to subgroups that suggest that dependencies are exclusively caused by the effects of a substance, can often be found in the literature. In this book, we will outline different interactions between personality, environment and the effects of the substance.

1.1 Aims of this book

Today we know that dependence is a disease that covers the individual in its entirety and which is linked to brain dysfunctions, making the consumption of addictive drugs often only a complicating factor. Therefore in this books chapters on prevention, diagnostic procedures, motivation and therapy (chapters 4, 5 and 9) we will put particular emphasis on factors, that help those who are affected, and less on measures influencing tobacco- and alcohol availability. According to the EU-resolution on addiction prevention 2005–2008, the prior prevention measure is to reduce the demand for addictive drugs. The reduction of substance availability is surely needed, but often only leads to a change in substances used. All other measures, like bans and rules, influence substance abuse, but in no way impact the number of dependences. There is a 7 % lifetime prevalence of dependences, remaining the same across different cultures, with the only difference being in terms of the choice of substance. Yet smoking significantly contributes towards dependences in almost all cultures. In chapter 3.5 we will outline the influence of smoking on the development of dependence, in particular alcohol dependence.

Chapter 5 will predominantly focus on dependence, abuse, withdrawal and sequelae, by employing ICD-10 and DSM-IV criteria. The current diagnostics approach is in the form of "top-down diagnoses" (first the diagnosis of dependence is made and severity and treatability are rated). All therapists and researchers with a clinical occupation are discontent with this overly simple diagnostic approach, which defines groups of diseases overly heterogenically. Therefore subgroups like typologies have been developed which, depending on the clinical problem, are based on sufficient scientific data which are relevant for therapy and research, e.g. Fagerstroem positive vs. negative or the alcohol typology according to Cloninger, Babor, Hesselbrock or Lesch. Since 1999, large international bodies have been working towards improving this diagnostic and the DSM-V is planned to be available in 2011 and the ICD-11 in 2014 (Fig. 1).

These diagnostic instruments measure individual categories straightforwardly and according to severity. At the moment, there is discussion about whether to include a "bottom-up diagnosis", so that, depending on the clinical problem, a focus, stemming from different categories, can be set within the diagnosis. Animal studies and basis research use very specific diagnostic categories, e.g. withdrawal animal models or genetic animal models. When these results are transferred to research with humans, this model transferred 1:1 to the diagnosis dependence according to DMS-IV and ICD-10, it becomes clear that the corresponding symptoms of these models need to be considered as well (e.g. if animal models have used a withdrawal model, patients with acute withdrawal symptoms are consequently included in this study).

As these different categories reflect different biological vulnerabilities, internal circuits, which can be linked to clinical problems, will be described in chapter 7.3.2.2. These theoretical aspects lead to a recommendation for different medication for withdrawal, relapse prophylaxis and treatment.

Many authors have emphasised that dependence is based on a psycho-

Fig. 1 DSM-V Timeline Overview

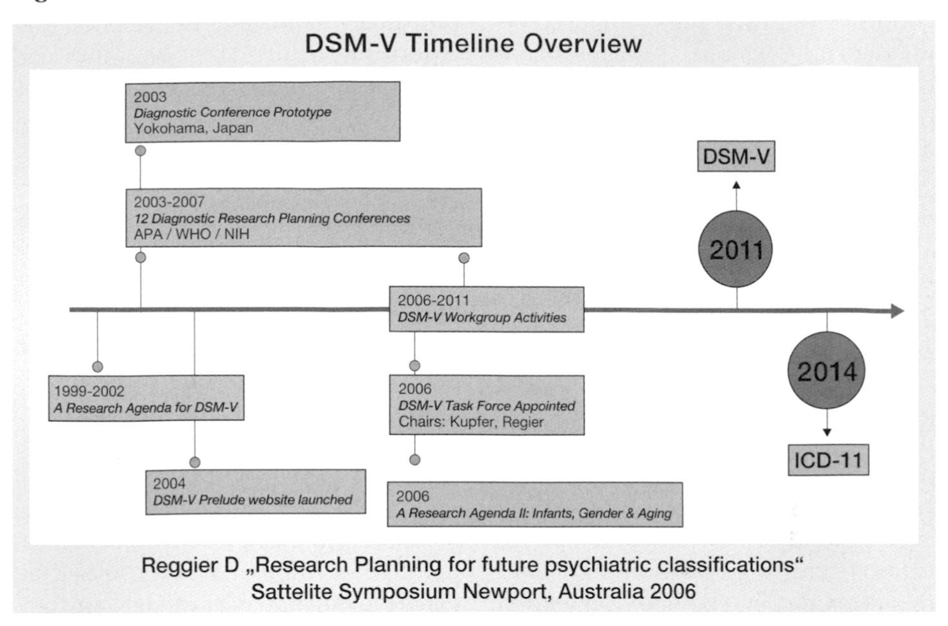

socio-biological development. As I am not aware of any disease which does not show any psycho-socio-biological factors in its development, we will try to describe subgroups which illustrate the different weighting of these three aetiologies. Psychological theories about the development of dependence will be outlined in chapter 3.2, although these theories were shown to be therapeutically relevant in behavioural therapy, systemic therapy and hypnotherapeutic concepts only. As dependencies are more prevalent in marginal groups and can be linked to poverty, chapter 10 focuses extensively on socio-therapeutic approaches. This chapter will introduce case studies which show that social integration improves drinking behaviour and quality of life even in severely deprived dependents (e.g. homeless or dependent individuals in prisons could be re-socialised).

1.2 Personal reasons for the first author writing this book

By writing this book, I have sought to present scientific findings from the past 30 years in such a way that they can be integrated into daily practice of consultation and treatment. Of course, I am well aware that this aim cannot be fully realised and I would like to apologize to all readers in advance because I am sure that there are very important topics which have not been sufficiently tackled. Following the publication of the German standard text, "Alcoholism – abuse and dependence. Genesis – consequences-therapy", which significantly influenced my clinical practice in 1975, several great textbooks in English have been published (e.g. Johnson B et al. 2003: "Handbook of Clinical Alcoholism Treatment"; Rommelspacher H. and Schuckit M. 1996: "Drugs of Abuse") as well as literature in German-speaking countries (Batra A. 2005: "Tobacco dependence. Scientific principles and treatment"; Wiesbeck GA. 2007: "Alcoholism-research – current knowledge, future perspectives"). Following 32 years of collaborative work between many of these authors and my research group, I would like now to summarize in this book both our scientific findings and our reflections on international research.

Alongside my scientific work, my practical work with patients is something which I have always wanted to maintain. Many patients have been very grateful and have kept in touch over the years. However, in the past ten years, I have noticed more and more that smoking has not been sufficiently considered in the past. Smoking behaviour is extremely important in regards to life expectancy in long-term abstinence and dependence experts should focus more on smoking. Blood vessels previously damaged by alcohol and chronically irritated mucosa, often lead to life-shortening diseases, caused by tobacco ingredients. This is why I want to outline the importance of both addictive drugs in this book. The combination with illicit drugs, which is of increasing importance, will only be discussed briefly, as it is beyond the scope of this book. Most chapters include original quotations from international texts and from publications of our research group. As this book is intended to be a practical document for practitioners, I have only made citations if they seem very important. The complete literature can be found in the appendix. As I don't consider myself an expert on sociological models, my colleague, Christian Wetschka, who has had many years of sociotherapeutic experience, has written the chapter on sociotherapy.

2

Addiction – a short overview of a widespread disease

2.1 Introduction

Many addictive drugs are primarily made up of herbal substances and are certainly older than humanity. Other addictive drugs are derived from fermented fruits or distilled grains. Addictive drugs are pharmacologically effective substances and therefore comply with the accepted pharmacological rules. They have been applied by mankind for thousands of years and a range of diseases have been treated with addictive drugs. It has been known for more than 2000 years that viruses can be driven away by using smoke (fire or tobacco smoke) and alcohol. Only 150 years ago, contaminated water in Europe caused severe bodily discomfort (sometimes even with lethal consequences). Yet, these adverse health effects were in no case observable when alcohol was consumed in small amounts. Alcohol is still used as a desinfectant agent and, even today, Shamans of the Upper Amazonas still use alcohol and smoke to blow off viruses. The psychopharmacological effects of alcohol have always been known and in virtually every culture there were distinct rules stating at which doses, at what time and on which occasions alcohol and tobacco were allowed to be consumed, and even enjoyed (Indian Rituals [e. g. calumet] or mandatory carousals in the Mexican culture). However, outside of its prescribed use in these rituals, alcohol and tobacco consumption was always severely punished, sometimes even to the point of death.

Already in the 3rd century B.C., distinct rules regarding the consumption of alcohol were recognized by Plato and Plinius the Elder (who lived from 23–79 A.D.) who specified these rules more precisely in the chapter "Medicine and Pharmacology" of his opus "Naturalis Historiae" (Plinius Secundus G. 1669). In one of his writings, he defined "abuse" and outlined several therapeutic recommendations regarding the treatment of addictions.

These rules for the use of addictive drugs are as valid today as they were over 2000 years ago. For instance, Plato suggested that one shouldn't car-

Fig. 2 666th letter by Plato

- No alcohol should be consumed until the age of 18, so that not even more fire is added to existing fire and so that the exuberant feelings of the adolescents won't get out of control.
- Between age 19 and 42 low amounts should be consumed at times and in a controlled fashion, but in no case before consultations, treatments or when meeting a woman.
- After age 43 the name of Dionysus should be called and excessive amounts of alcohol should be consumed sporadically, so that the troubles of aging can be endured and the soul stays euthymic.

ry out treatment or political consultations while intoxicated. Plato also highlighted the various ways in which an unborn child could be damaged by its mother's alcohol consumption. Of course, in our times the age limit has clearly shifted (43 years then is the equivalent to 70 years today).

2.2 Prevention

Within the field of prevention, measures that are taken to reduce the demand for addictive drugs (primary prevention) are distinguished from early interventions ("to look closely at the problem and recognize it instead of turning away "), which start before the drug is actually abused or in the very early stages of abuse (secondary prevention), and strategies which treat abusers and addicts (tertiary prevention). The best prevention results are achieved when the problem is recognized and addressed early. Furthermore, sufficient interventions should be offered to help those that are affected and these should be more precisely tailored to suit specific homogeneous risk groups (EU Report 2007).

An important way to combine prevention and intervention methods is through counselling provided by abstinent addicts to high-risk youth. Teenagers learn from role models and abstinent addicts act as deterrents to their alcohol abuse (Lesch OM. 2007).

2.3 The Diagnosis addiction

Specific to their relevant addictive drug, abuse, addiction and withdrawal symptoms are defined in all classifications (e.g. DSM-IV, ICD-10). Yet, secondary disorders are mainly caused by the addictive drug itself, combined with the effects of tobacco and alcohol, leading to a variety of secondary disorders (e.g. tobacco causes pulmonary disease or alcohol causes liver disease). Conventional classification systems like the ICD-10 and the DSM-IV each have their own very different history and have been conceptualized for very different reasons. The world health organisation (WHO) has introduced the international classification system foremost because it has sought to achieve a higher comparability of diseases and their frequency in a wide range of countries. With this increased comparability, criteria, which lead to an improvement of the medical care system in specific countries, were to be developed. In the case of a multiple diagnosis for one and the same patient, the different diagnoses should be coded and, if possible, the type of therapeutic setting should be pinned down for each of the coded diseases (e.g. abstinence in an in-patient or outpatient setting). ICD-10 classification has proven itself suitable for the recording of a wide range of addictions in different countries. In numerous countries this has lead to public health insurance sponsoring the therapies of addicts, but it has also resulted in very general therapies being offered, some of which employ all sorts of methods (ranging from Shamanism in Brazil to electric cerebral stimulation in Russia). These forms of therapy are often entirely inadequate methods of treatment and this generalized way of diagnosing an addiction is not diagnostically conclusive enough for therapy.

Consequently, many definitions of subgroups have since been developed which can be used for diverse purposes (e.g. genetic studies, therapy studies, aetiology studies). The American Psychiatric Society has developed the fourth version of its classification system (DSM-IV), in which the diagnoses are clearly narrower than in the ICD-10. The DSM-IV already includes subgroups and these diagnostic classifications should be employed especially for research purposes so that research results become more internationally comparable (Widinger TA. et al. 1994). The DSM-IV Source Book indicates why specific criteria were incorporated in the diagnostic of addiction and suggests research approaches that should be continued (administration of research). Today there is still dissatisfaction with both sets of criterion and both the WHO and the American Psychiatric Association are working towards new and revised criteria (see chapter 5). (Lesch OM 2009, Addiction in DSM V and ICD-11 State of the Art), Fig. 1.

2.4 Aetiology of addiction

As already pointed out, the aetiology of abuse and addiction lies in the vulnerability of individuals and not in the effects of various drug substances.

We would like to explain this by using the aetiology of "Diabetes Mellitus" as an example. Diabetes Mellitus is a disease of the glucose metabolism and other vulnerabilities (e.g. insulin metabolism). Diabetes mellitus has been divided into two subgroups. In one group, genetic vulnerabilities are the prime factors (glucose metabolism, insulin sensitivity), whereas in the other group, environmental factors, psychological problems and the metabolic syndrome affect symptomatology. Here, the body can't convert sugar that is taken in high doses accordingly. Sugar is a substance that can be harmful to the health of both groups. Depending on dosage and frequency of intake, it can even be fatal. Likewise, a rapid withdrawal of sugar intake leads to severe bodily dysfunctions in Diabetes Mellitus patients, which can even lead to death (diabetic coma, Grand Mal seizures, vegetative symptoms and "Symptomatic transitory psychotic syndrome" according to Wieck H., 1956, Berner P., 1986). This concept is mainly used in German speaking countries. Any disturbances of the brain lead to cognitive impairments. Independent of the cause of these disturbances, the location in the brain and the speed of the development of the "brain trauma" influences the depth of unconscious states, the level of cognitive impairment and the severity of psychiatric symptoms. If the developmental time is short, the person reacts with different stages of unconsciousness. If the developmental time is longer, e. g. chronic alcohol intoxication, different degrees of cognitive impairment occurs stepwise with different psychiatric symptoms. As shown in Fig. 3, transitional cognitive impairments produce step by step these syndromes. During recovery, psychiatric syndromes lessen in severity. For example, a Delirium Tremens changes to delusional states and then to affective mood disturbances and so on.

Many addicts show a primary vulnerability that may be genetic in origin, or a vulnerability resulting from physical or psychiatric damage in the early years, often while in the womb during the first weeks of pregnancy (e.g. as a result of mothers who smoke and/or drink). Severe psychological trauma can combine with genetic vulnerabilities (i.e., gene-environment interac-

Fig. 3 Transitional Organic Impairment – psychiatric syndromes: steps of development and recovery (Wieck H. 1956).

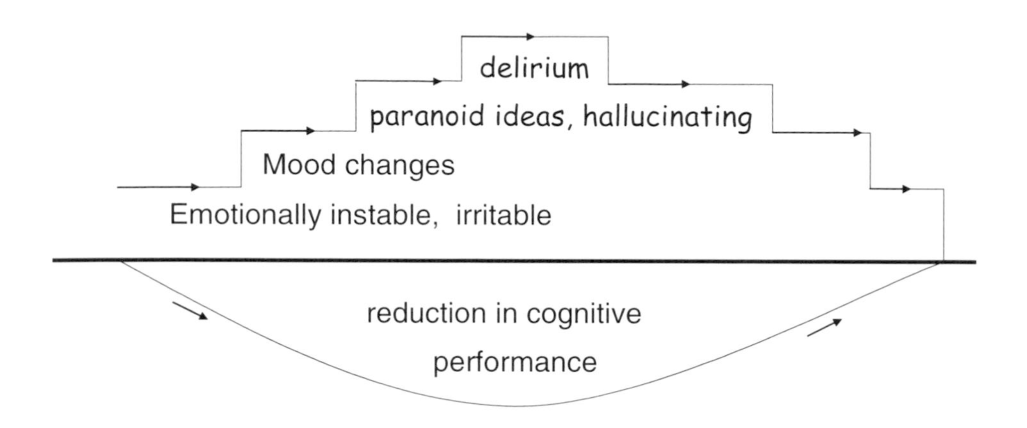

tion), and this combination can be as important for the aetiology as the primary genetic vulnerabilities. Often, the addictive substance is consequently used as a strategy to cope with the difficulties of everyday life. The psychological aetiology model of addiction, which has been developed according to psychotherapeutic schools of thought, only explains subaspects of development but has not led to an identification of specific psychotherapeutic procedures.

Methods of behavioral therapy (e. g. Brenda Method), family therapy as well as hypnotherapeutic treatments are based upon scientific data which suggest effectiveness. Nevertheless, there are both positive as well as negative studies in this area (Hester RK and Miller WR, 2003; Volpicelli JR et al. 2001). Tobacco and alcohol are easily accessible everywhere. Therefore they can easily be used of by individuals with various psychiatric problems. Smoking obviously has a different function for patients coming from a schizophrenic spectrum than for patients with an obsessive compulsive behaviour pattern or an impulse control disorder (see chapter 3.6).

2.5 Secondary disorders and addiction

Tobacco- and alcohol abuse as well as addiction can damage most parts of the somatic system. Diseases that range from changes in the vascular system to pre-cancerous and malignant tumours lead patients to various outpatient treatment centres, clinics and hospitals, e. g. departments for internal medicine, surgery, acute medicine, psychiatry and to the general practitioner/primary care provider. Secondary disorders of this kind are caused not only by the consumption behaviour, but also by infectious diseases, maladaptive diet and a primary sensitivity of all kinds of organs. Every individual has his own unique organ system and when it is exposed to unfavourable conditions, illness can result. In chapter 7 important somatic illnesses are introduced to highlight the medical significance of tobacco and alcohol, whilst at the end of this chapter the importance of the interaction between alcohol and medicine taken for somatic diseases will be highlighted. These interactions change the effects and toxicity of most medicines. In many cases, these interactions explain why medical treatment does not result in improvement or leads, in some cases, to an exacerbation of symptoms. This relationship between somatic changes and addictive substances can sometimes be examined using biological markers so that the alcohol/drug consumption behaviour can be appropriately judged both cross-sectionally and in the longterm course (chapter 8.2).

2.6 Secondary diseases and brain functions

Primary and secondary changes in central nervous system functioning and the influence of addictive drugs on all neurotransmitter systems are one of the basics understanding the psychological consequences of heavy use and the mechanisms leading to the genesis and maintenance of dependent behaviour. The biology of the reward system as well as the biological mechanisms of the drug addiction memory are functions which are important for addiction therapy ("Symptomatic transitory psychotic syndrome" according to Wieck") and the different craving mechanisms also need to be recognized too.

2.7 Subgroups of addicts

The clinical heterogeneity of tobacco and alcohol addiction is undisputed, with over 100 alcohol typologies having been developed worldwide. Today there is some consensus that a four-group typology will capture and identify the majority of patients. When comparing different typologies from different authors it becomes apparent that there is considerable concordance across different classification systems. Results from the general population and clinical samples indicate that subgroup categorization is relatively stable over at least 5 years (see chapter 6). In our own research group (Lesch & Walter), we have developed a typology of alcoholism that has been tested internationally by using physiological, biological, therapeutic and genetic studies. This typology seems quite suitable for testing a variety of clinical questions. These studies also confirm that the identified alcoholic subgroups are relevant for therapeutic considerations and prognosis (see chapter 6.3). For example, even though nicotine addiction and smoking behaviour are different from alcohol dependence, using Lesch's typology we were able to identify therapy relevant subgroups of dependent smokers who certainly need different therapies (Lesch OM. et al. 2004, 2007, 2010).

2.8 Motivation of addicts

An important aspect of every addiction is the fact that these patients are seldom motivated to change their consumption behaviour. This amotivational behaviour is an important diagnostic criterion of addiction. The patient should be made aware that there is an interest in him as a person and that he is being consulted. It is imperative that the patient has the freedom to define independently the goals of therapy. Often the first goal of the therapy is that the patient seeks contact more frequently with the therapy centre and asks for information about the therapy planned and the prognosis. In line with these conversations and, apart from psycho education, a "motivation" process should be initiated. This process should lead to a decline in consumption behaviour and maybe even to abstinence. Prochaska and DiClemente have fittingly described the phases of motivation, and one should be aware of the patient's current phase of motivation in order to start the motivation process (Prochaska. J. and DiClemente C. 1992). The fundamental elements of motivation are to begin the process in the patient's present phase and to be patient during the therapeutic process in order to achieve the goals of treatment. (see also Miller WR. and Rollnick S. 2002: Motivational interviewing: Preparing people for change).

The goals should be clearly formulated, realistic and achievable within a short time. It is important that both patient and therapist have mutually agreed upon a therapy goal. The manner in which the motivation activities are conducted depends upon the patient's personality and the specific social setting. Secondary diseases or self-harming behaviour often enforce an adherence to the crisis concept. Within this context, actions must be carried out to ensure the survival of the affected (e.g., in-patient psychiatric admittance in case of suicidal behaviour or esophageal bleeding may lead to admission on to a surgery unit).

2.9 The path from motivation to therapy

In the case of addiction, a therapeutic process can be effective since many affected individuals need long-term support. Acute detoxification therapies are only recommended in combination with adequate medical management which leads to a minimization of withdrawal symptoms and reduces risk of seizures or other possible complications. In many cases, it is better to slowly reduce the addictive substance instead of abruptly discontinuing the drug use (Pharmacological extinction method according to Sinclair JD, 2001). In the majority of cases, in-patient therapies should be kept as short as possible and afterwards an adequate outpatient/ambulatory setting should be offered. Depending on the drug of addiction and patient typology, a plethora of measures is necessary. These measures are outlined in chapter 9. Assistance carried out with respect for the patient's dignity is the goal of every therapy. Relapses are to be accepted. They are part of the life course of addiction; the patient can perceive his drinking behaviour as a relapse only after he himself has accepted "abstinence" as a therapy goal (Schmidt G. 1992).

2.10 Addiction and relapse

Today relapse is still seen as something negative, in spite of addiction research being able to show that for patients in

Fig. 4 Old and new thinking about relapse

Old thinking	New thinking
• Relapses are expressions of poor therapy and personal failure • A relapse means that the entire therapy was useless • Relapses are catastrophes • Relapses are further step into self-destruction • Relapses are autonomous processes, "there is nothing one can do about it" • Relapses end in a lingering illness • Relapses are an expression of a definite decision to keep on drinking • The primal cause for a relapse is the craving for alcohol • The first glass ends in a loss of control	• Relapses can actually show that something incrusted is being overcome • Relapses are chances for development • Relapses are to be respected as attempts to cope with one's own problems • Relapses should be valued as forms of resistance • Relapses are attempts of self-healing (e.g. Maintenance of self-esteem), they don't appear from nowhere • Relapses are integral to every development • Abstinence is not the central indicator for judging a therapy • The path out of addiction requires time • Relapses is not equal relapse

(see STAR-Training according to Koerkel and Schnidler)

a therapeutic process it is sometimes necessary and even beneficial to experience relapse. There are subgroups of addicts whose primary therapy goal is to reduce the severity of their relapses. New and old thinking about a relapse is illustrated in Fig. 4 (see chapter 9.6).

2.11 Specific groups of addicts

2.11.1 Co-morbidity of tobacco and alcohol-addiction

Co-morbidity with other psychiatric disorders needs to be considered for tobacco/nicotine dependence as well as for alcohol addiction. Co-morbidity often influences the therapeutic process and is an important consideration for prognosis. Anxiety and depression symptoms are almost always observed during both alcohol intoxication and withdrawal. They usually subside within two to three weeks of absolute abstinence, even without any therapy, and only require an antidepressant medication when the symptoms continue after three weeks. During abstinence, tranquilizers and hypnotics should only be administered in exceptional cases for this group of patients with affective disturbance.

2.11.2 Overweight, eating disorders

The problems of being overweight, smoking and drinking to much alcohol, show an obvious concordance in genesis and aetiopathology. Post-menopausal women who smoke to control their weight represent an even more specific patient group of smokers. About 20% of addicts have an eating disorder before the onset of addiction. As new scientific information becomes available about these phenomena, new therapeutic strategies also need to be considered.

2.11.3 Gender

Today we know more than 50 considerable gender differences which need to be considered in research and therapy of addicts. These differences are so important that results which have been obtained in research with men, cannot be transferred to women. Most studies don't include enough women to be able to make valid conclusions about women. These gender differences don't only manifest in alcohol metabolism, but also in regard to coping strategies (coping with stress situations) in addiction symptoms. Women already develop severe bodily dysfunctions after five years of alcohol abuse whilst in men these dysfunction do not become apparent until twelve years later. Addicted women are left by their husbands, whilst addicted men are usually still cared for by their wives, although their husbands may treat them very offensively (verbally as well as physically).

2.12 Addiction and the homeless

In regard to the development process according to Lesch, addiction leads to severe social deprivation, in particular in type IV, but also in type III. This is why a whole chapter (10) tackles the social therapy of these marginal groups. The chapter shows the massive deficits of the medical system in respect of this "disease group" (which is often affected by homelessness), and demonstrates how it is possible to get very good results using addiction therapy (Platz W. 2007).

Despite their social deprivations, these patients often have a very high individual potential. In a theatre group, we were able to show that homeless individuals were able to make very good artistic contributions and when their potential was utilized, the quality of the results was often astonishing (see chapter 10). The football competition for the homeless which takes place every year shows that homeless individuals can be good athletes and are able to play, e.g. football despite their physical disadvantages.

2.13 Polytoxicomania

In the US as well as in some European countries like Portugal or Netherlands, the chaotic consumption of alcohol, tobacco and illegal drugs is rather a norm. German-speaking regions and rural wine-growing districts also show this combination of alcohol and tobacco, but this is rarely combined with the consumption of illegal drugs. Often in the USA, it is merely possible to differ between addicts with rare or frequent cocaine consumption. In France the concomitant use of Benzodiazepines in addicts is rather the norm than the exception.

This topic is exceedingly extensive and goes beyond the scope of this book. This disease group might have been well examined from a sociological perspective, but from a medical-psychiatric perspective, the literature can only be judged as modest (see for example Johnson BA et al. 2003; Rommelsbacher H and Schuckit MA. 1996). In 2007, a Portuguese research group published an article on subgroups of addicts, in which they provided support for the theory that polytoxicomanic subgroups of adolescent addicts could be distinguished from all other groups, as defined for example by the NETER typology or typology according to Lesch, and therefore should be treated with a different therapy (Pombo S et al. 2007). Lesch's types III and IV could also be defined in opiate dependent patients using a large sample of opiate addicts (n = 930). These opiate addicts, separated into types III, IV and others, showed many differences in the degree of severity of their psychosocial disturbances, chose different maintenance medication and needed significantly different duration of admission (Hermann P. and Wallner Ch. in preparation).

2.14 Non-substance dependence

These pathological behaviour patterns (pathological gambling, work addiction, religious addiction etc.) affect a great number of people and have been coded in the ICD-10 and DSM-IV into the categories "behavioural disorders" and "impulse control disorders". From our psychiatric knowledge, these behaviours should be combined as reactions caused by different psychiatric disorders (in the German literature, the so called "monomanias").

Eating disorders seem to have specific biological and psychological aetiologies and should therefore comprise a group in itself. The extent to which all of these disorders can be summarized as impulse control disorders is being discussed around the world. Some of these forms of behaviour and experiences meet the criteria for delusional elements, as described in the novel "The Gambler" by F. M. Dostojewskij. The gambler knows that in Roulette, e.g., number 13 will show. He is absolutely certain that his interpretation is correct and is unshaken in his conviction, thereby meeting Jasper's criteria for a delusion. Since as far as therapy and the progress of "monomanias" are concerned, little depends on behaviour but much on the *function* of the "monomanias", no specific therapy recommendation can be made for non-substance dependences. For this reason, we shall not be addressing this patient group in this book. It was a difficult process to get substance caused dependence accepted as a medical condition so that its treatment can be financed by medical insurance. Too few paid therapies are available for tobacco dependents with high biological dependence (Fagerstroem score ≥ 5). From a psychiatric perspective, the dilution of the term "dependence" is absolutely counterproductive. Today it is very modern to define new disorders (ranging from work to sex addiction), with each behaviour pattern being defined as a separate disorder.

Here one needs to bear in mind that these "new disorders" and their definitions represent for many groups a means of earning money or gaining other advantages. These new definitions don't actually help those affected, but only serve to overburden the medical system. As a consequence, the funds are lacking for the therapy of severely ill psychiatric patients (e.g. there are no comprehensive intensive care facilities, not enough psychiatric liaison provisions in the medical and social care systems, and too few hospital places for psychiatric patients. As a result, we can only help these patients to a minimal degree because we have no effective therapy methods at our disposal). The realization of effective and specific therapies according to subgroups of disorders would on the other hand save costs and thus relieve our medical system.

3

Aetiology of addiction

3.1 The psycho-socio-biological model

Psychological, social, biological and genetic causes are assumed to play a role in all psychological disorders but only little of this aetiological thinking has led to practical approaches that can be realized in therapy. This has also been the case in the field of addiction where the need to define psychological, biological, sociological and aetiological factors has repeatedly been posited.

The indisputable heterogeneity of addictions is tackled in chapter 5 and 6. Of course, the addiction sub-groupings draw on psychological, biological, sociological and aetiological factors as well, but the weighting and the importance of the particular factors are each very different, depending on the subgroup. Alcohol and tobacco dependents who regularly try to reduce withdrawal symptoms by administering alcohol or tobacco, but otherwise don't show any abnormalities in personality or in their social environment, aetiologically differ from alcohol and tobacco addicts, who use alcohol and tobacco in specific situations to cope with stress and have no or only mild withdrawal symptoms.

Following a description of individual aetiological theories, a model with a psychological, sociological and biological perspective will be introduced in chapter 6 which is suitable for the patient as it has psycho-educative as well as motivational aspects. The model also explains the dynamic process of addiction as an interplay of cause and effect in relation to the addictive drug, substance withdrawal and the consequences.

3.2 Psychological theories

There are numerous psychological theories and virtually every psychological school of thought has developed a model to explain the aetiopathogenesis of addiction (Springer-Kremser M. and Ekstein R. 1987). Many of these are limited in their significance; others again have proven to be valuable in therapy. For many years, moral models have obstructed the perception of the causes of addictions, but during the last decades, opinion has tended towards the rejection of moral models. As religious groups still make considerable contribution to the care of substance dependents, moral perspectives should still not be underestimated. The "point of no return" as a central characteristic for the diagnosis of addiction shows that a lack of motivation to change one's lifestyle, or to live without tobacco and alcohol, is an essential part of addiction. During intoxication and withdrawal, a state which virtually always goes hand in hand with a symptomatic transitory psychotic syndrome, motivation is only minimally subject to the patient's acts of free will.

Psychological theories which are today being discussed in connection with the causes of addiction and which are, according to Lesch's typology, used in psychotherapy as relapse prophylaxis, are outlined in the following paragraphs.

3.2.1 Behavioural approaches

In behavioural explanation models, questions regarding the functionality of alcohol and mechanisms of consumption, which describe the prevention and the risk factors of the addiction process, are predominant. Consumption is understood as a learned behaviour which is affected by the respective life situation and individual variables. In 1943, Hull CL already formulated his tension reduction theory, based on Pavlov's classic conditioning model, which indicated that individuals learn specific reactions to stimuli that lead to a reduction of states of tension in the body (Hull CL. et al. 1943). According to this theory, alcohol and tobacco addiction are behaviours that are learned through reinforcement and which lead to a reduction of tension (often anxiety). However, the consumption behaviour leads in turn to an increase in tension with the result that higher intake of alcohol and nicotine is needed in order to produce the same effect i. e. to relieve the feelings of stress. This cycle is drawn upon as an aetiological factor in the development of addictions. In Skinner BF.'s model (transactional model of operant conditioning), it is also emphasized that positive and negative stimuli can strengthen or weaken the consumption behaviour (Skinner BF. et al. 1938). The fact that the effects of nicotine and alcohol are immediate is perceived as a positive stimulus, and this stimulus acts in turn as an incentive to smoke or drink. To sum up briefly, environmental and individual stimuli affect consumption behaviour, and the immediate experienced effect is in itself seen as a positive stimulus to further consumption. Withdrawal symptoms, which do not occur until later, are perceived as punishment and have a weak influence on the consumption behaviour as a result of the time lag (Schmitz JM. and DeLaune 2003). In expectation theory, it is postulated that the activating stimulus, consumption behaviour and consequences can lead to an expectation which can constrain or promote intake anew. Six expectations can be defined in regards to alcohol consumption:

1. the expectation that the addictive drug makes a perspective more positive and enjoyable
2. the expectation that the addictive drug enhances individual and social well-being
3. the expectation that the addictive drug positively influences sexuality
4. the expectation that the addictive drug enhances power and aggression
5. the expectation that the addictive drug enhances social assertiveness
6. the expectation that the addictive drug reduces and even removes tensions

This interplay between expectations and the pharmacological effect of alcohol and tobacco is also displayed biologically and permits behavioural pharmacological thinking which is also of therapeutic relevance.

85 % of the population drink alcohol and, depending on age, 50 % of 18 year olds and 30 % of 50 year olds smoke. Adolescents learn on the basis of a model and, early in their life, they learn that almost all festive occasions are connected with alcohol. This social learning also allows us to define places and situations in which people smoke and drink and which are today described as "hot spots" (restaurant, party etc.). In the same manner, we can define places and situations where people neither smoke nor drink as so called "cool spots" (e. g. sports and other activities).

The greater an individual's access to "cool spots", and the more coping strategies he has, the lower the risk of his developing an addiction. Individuals, who live their lives mainly in "hot spots", and have a lower number of other coping options, have a higher risk of developing an addiction and it is more difficult for them to "free" themselves from an addiction. Behavioural therapeutic concepts are based especially on theoretic learning models. In pharmacological studies, behavioural therapy is likely to be standardized and in these studies of addicts, the behavioural therapeutic method has established itself in the form of a standardized interview (Method according to BRENDA: B = Biopsychosocial evaluation, R = Report [Report for the patient], E = Empathy, N = Need [Evaluation of needs], D = Direct advice, A = Evaluation of reaction; according to Volpicelli JR et al. 2001).

In practice, this behavioural therapeutic approach is highly relevant for type I and type IV patients according to Lesch.

3.2.2 Models of depth psychology

These models predominantly present pre-morbid personality disorders. Childhood development is a process that can be disrupted at certain points and abnormal developments might occur that can lead to a disposition to develop an addiction. Zingerle (1994) emphasised three central functions of addiction in the light of depth psychology, which are, firstly, addiction as a means of satisfaction, secondly, addiction as a means of defence (e. g. depression and anxiety) and thirdly, addiction as a means of compensating e. g. for a sense of inferiority (Zingerle H. 1994). In this regard, we have postulated in our work that the defence mechanisms of type III according to Lesch must be attended to, while for type II according to Lesch the compensation mechanisms in regard to low self-esteem are to be prioritized. Developmental and therapy studies about these concepts, which could connect Lesch's typology with depth psychological models, are still lacking. In a three-month in-patient, depth-psychological group concept, we formed groups with type I and type II patients according to Lesch and then measured what kind of changes took place in patients and also in the therapists after three months. In groups with type II patients, the analytic group work was described as particularly interesting, challenging and also effective by both patients and therapists. In groups with type I patients, both patients and therapists perceived the regular group meetings as especially tedious and to a certain extent even extremely boring

(Platz W. and Lesch OM., unpublished data).

3.2.3 Depth psychological approach

Strotzka H. already formulated in 1982 that addiction can be viewed as a fixation in the oral development stage (Strotzka H. 1982). The daily satisfaction of drives by smoking and drinking demonstrates the effort to solve drive conflicts, while the drive is uncontrolled and unsublimated. Freud stressed the oral-erotic components and explained this by a deprivation of affection and by emotional dysfunctions in early childhood, with the delay of maturation being a central aspect. According to Freud, changes in affects and the handling of emotions which is based on underlying and unrealised insecurity, anger and guilt are fundamental criteria for the development of an addiction. When intoxicated, an adult regresses, and inhibitions and defensive behaviour are removed and therefore repressed sources of pleasure are accessible again. The addictive drug enables the individual to step back from the principle of reality to the child's principle of pleasure and therefore to escape reality (Freud S. 1905; Innerhofer P. et al.; Vogler E. and Revenstorf D. 1978). For Freud, masturbation is the prototype of addiction and Rado even speaks of a "pharmaceutical orgasm" (Rado S. 1926, 1975). One of the motives of consumption behaviour is the urge to unleash one's potential for pleasure. Fenichel O sees the causes of increased alcohol consumption in frustration and internal inhibitions, the weak ego is exposed to the rivalling impulses of the "super-ego" and the "id" and it is unable to satisfy needs and desires for pleasure meaningfully (Fenichel O 2006). Thus, alcohol helps to liberate the ego that is restricted by the super-ego, which results in a reduction of tension and anxiety and hence an increase of pleasure. Strotzka also describes the oral character as decisive for depression: "A patient with a severe depression is an orally dependent individual who is deprived of vital supplies." (Strotzka H 1982). In our work group it was therefore pointed out that these aetiological suggestions are extremely important for Lesch's type III and thus should be included in the therapeutic process. The common psychological causes of addiction and depression can then be treated.

3.2.4 Ego-psychological approaches

Dysfunctions in the ego organisation lead to dysfunctions in perception, which results in a lack of differentiation of emotions and their meaning, dysfunctions in object relationships, which are often connected to primitive defence mechanisms, frustration intolerance, affective and impulse control dysfunctions, dysfunctions of judgement, especially in anticipating the effect of one's own behaviour on others, and dependence conflicts between symbiotic requirements and autonomy tendencies. Feuerlein W sees the consumption of addictive drugs as a possible way of strengthening the ego that is weakened in its structure (type II according to Lesch). Furthermore, Knight RP sees alcoholism as an attempt to solve emotional conflicts which emerge from heightened expectations regarding drive satisfaction, aggression, guilt, regression and the tendency to punish oneself (Knight RP 1937). De Vito RA sees excessive alcohol abuse as a protection against various threatening emotions, e. g. strong and hostile affect states (De Vito RA 1970).

At the same time, inhibitions are removed and the venting of these emotions becomes possible.

Alcohol protects and stabilises the weak ego by regulating affect and constraints and here alcohol functions like the defence mechanisms of a healthy individual (Feuerlein W. 1981, 1989).

Today we would like to discuss the weakness to control impulses in type I according to Lesch and the problem of subject-object-relationship in Lesch's type III, as well as ego weakness in type II. The link between weakness of impulse and compulsion, as measured by Anton RF's obsessive-compulsive scale, is the cause for the drinking behaviour in type IV patients, but further research is still needed in this area (Anton RF et al. 1995).

3.2.5 The psychological model of object relations

Melanie Klein points out the important function of the mother for development, where the nurturing, protecting and good mother is compared with the frustrated, harmful and bad mother (Klein M 1972). If the internalisation of the good mother doesn't work out, a primitive and immature object relationship is developed (Balint M 1970). The differentiation of self and object representations has failed and thus there is no stable balance between these two object relationships. These persons need external objects, often social attachment figures, who should be available at any time to satisfy needs. If these external objects fail in these functions, the primitive defence collapses. The "grandiose self" that has been maintained by external support, collapses into an insecure ego and addictive drugs are then used to regulate this loss of self-worth (type II according to Lesch; Heigl-Evers A et al. 1981; Heigl-Evers A and Standke G 1991; Heigl FS and Heigl-Evers A 1991). In this development, gender differences need to be considered (Kernberg OF 1979). A number of representatives of the object relations' psychological approach emphasise the auto destructive tendencies of addiction. For example, Menninger KA sees self-destruction as a fundamental characteristic of addiction, whereas he views alcoholisms as a special form of self-punishment, which corresponds to a slow and chronic suicide (type III according to Lesch; Heigl FS and Heigl-Evers A 1991, Menninger KA 1974).

3.2.6 Theoretical approach of Narcissism

Traumata in an early development stage, in which a child can't regulate its self-worth adequately, can cause addiction. A weak and inadequately integrated self and a deficiency of conceptions and inner images lead to a strong sensitivity towards narcissistic insults and addictive drugs are supposed to compensate for this effect but in fact, merely support the generally shallow feeling of grandiosity (Menninger KA. 1974) and reduce the ability to be critical about one's own behaviour. In 1979, Kemberg described how alcohol is abused by narcissistic individuals in order to protect their pathologically large ego and to fend off the environment which is perceived as hostile and frustrating (Adams JW. 1978; Kernberg OF. 1979; Kernberg OF. et al. 2000; Passett P. 1981; von Scheidt J. 1976).

3.2.7 Explanation models according to family psychotherapy

From a systemic perspective, addictions are not only related to the individual, but also are a result of the dysfunction of an entire ecological system in which the individual lives. A human being lives in balance between the individual, behaviour and the environment. Changes in this system and dysfunctions of this balance demand an adaptation of the perception and behaviour of the individual. If the individual is not able to stabilise this balance, addictive drugs are used to influence these disordered cycles. Alcohol, for example, becomes the central principle for organising the interaction with the partner and its main function is the maintenance or restoration of the balanced state (Schmid C. 1993). Systemic problems in type I alcohol addicts are to be seen as secondary problems which are mainly caused by chronic intoxication and should be respected especially at the beginning of the therapy. The powerful and assertive partner of type II according to Lesch is an important aetiological and therapeutic factor in regard to the self-esteem of the addict. In type III according to Lesch, missing closeness between partners and between the patient and the social environment is often an important aetiological and therapeutic factor, with the patient feeling extremely powerful. In type IV according to Lesch, there is often no partner or a partner who also drinks and the entire environment is perceived as negative and hostile. Only during intoxication, are patients able to mirror their aggression and these interactions then lead to those processes which make the consumption behaviour so difficult to break. Relatives or partners of all addicts go through the process of co-addiction. In the beginning, the relative or partner might admire the addict for being able to drink such large amounts of alcohol. After the first excesses, the consumption behaviour becomes noticeable to the relative and the addict promises to reduce his drinking; then control mechanisms are established and when these are not effective, the relative assumes the "role of a judge" and starts to make judgements about the "morally wrong behaviour" (for more information on the topic Co-addiction see: Beiglboeck W. et al. 2006).

3.3 Social explanation approaches

Epidemiological studies have shown that smoking and drinking behaviour depends on social conditions. Countries with a permissive alcohol climate have considerably higher rates of alcohol use and abuse than countries in which drinking alcohol is an undesired behaviour (e.g. Christian countries vs. Muslim countries). Countries with social security, guaranteed education and a secure workplace have a lower drug problem than countries with insecurities and insecure education. Addictive drug consumption is conditioned in families and is related to biological factors, which will be described later (see chapter 3.4). Social learning, on the basis of the model of the beloved parents, certainly plays a significant role. The socialisation of gender is very different, depending on culture, and certainly influences smoking-and drinking behaviour. There is extensive literature substantiating the fact that values taught adolescents by their families, and which dominate the peer groups to which they belong, significantly influence behaviour. "Peer group" research could clearly show that the group's attitude towards addictive drugs and behaviour is more important than individual attitudes towards substance abuse. The group decides whether its members smoke or drink. Social developments in a society, which provides adolescents with no freedom or space to experiment, but only offers bans and rules, support alcohol consumption behaviour. Adolescents need to have time and room to live out their youth appropriately. Rules that are too rigid and are not accepted as rules by adolescents, promote the consumption behaviour. The world of grown-ups doesn't observe rules or rituals anymore, but nevertheless tries to prescribe these rituals to adolescents. This double standard promotes substance abuse. Changes in family structures (e.g. almost 60% divorce rate in Vienna, patchwork families, 40% single mums, life lived at the poverty level etc.) lead to developmental dysfunctions, which in turn promote abuse (Jessor SL and Jessor R 1978; Lazarus RS and Launier R 1978). The greater the discrepancy in earning capacity in a country, the higher the incidence of substance abuse is. Gender differences in salaries, but also in socialisation (e.g. powerful, money earning male vs. dependant women or vice versa) promote substance abuse. McClelland DC et al. show that for example men use alcohol to be able to better act out their power and strength (McClelland DC et al. 1972). Yet, the extent to which the sociological aetiologies depend on culture and social wealth needs to be described in a way which is more clearly differentiated and could be examined in more detail by experts on sociological questions (Cahalan D 1970; Eisenmann G 1973; Engel U and Hurrelmann K 1993; Niderberger JM 1987; Quensel S 2004; Reinhardt JD 2005; Schulz W. 1976; Springer A 1995; Vogler E 1978; Zander M et al. 2006).

Addictions are more or less equally common in all western societies. It is assumed that around 7% of the population in every culture develops the criteria of an addiction. However, the choice of substance depends on social conditions, availability and the image of the addictive drug. Social developments and pressures which over time negatively impact an individual's psychological state and rob him of perspectives for the future, lead to significantly more psychiatric symptoms.

The more often these appear, the more likely it is that an addictive drug is used as a psychotropic. In the chapter on prevention (4), factors are extracted which need to be supported in order to reduce the development of addictions. Principally, such measures should be aimed at the individual according to his/her system (the principle is to "to look at the problem and help" instead of "looking away and making rules"). The reduction in demand for the addictive drug is the goal of every method of prevention. Reduction in the availability of an addictive drug usually leads to a shift to another addiction process and does not prevent a single addiction. In Russia, it was shown that despite fierce control and poverty that makes the purchasing of addictive drugs financially difficult, adolescents reach for the cheapest drugs (for example inhaling white gas) or breathe into a plastic bag until they suffer from an intoxication or symptomatic transitory psychotic syndrome. Cases of death when breathing into a plastic bag aren't rare and have been observed in Western Europe as well. Furthermore, the era of prohibition in the US did not result in a decline in the prevalence of alcohol addiction, but instead there was an increase in criminality, primarily associated with an increase in illegal trafficking.

3.4 Biological theories about the aetiology of tobacco and alcohol addiction

Basic research literature on both alcohol and tobacco is very extensive and therefore only selected studies will be outlined in this book. This extensive literature focuses not only on diseases like "addiction", but also on associated phenomena like the effects of addictive drugs, withdrawal symptoms, craving or sequelae in both humans and animals. Information on biological addiction theories can be derived mainly from neuronal models, animal experiments, cell cultures, genetic data but also from developmental, clinical, and twin/family studies in humans. The potentially damaging effects which tobacco and alcohol have on a young individual, and especially on brain development, is an important aetiological factor in the development of increased susceptibility to addiction throughout childhood and adolescence.

3.4.1 Important findings about tobacco and alcohol use from basic research

Alcohol and tobacco consumption are closely linked and often individuals who consume alcohol in high amounts are also heavy smokers (Bien TH and Burge R 1990; Collins AC 1990; Zacny JP 1990). It has been suggested that tobacco amplifies the "to-feel-better" effect of alcohol, and this effect can be explained by the impact on mesolimbic dopaminergic receptors, located in the nucleus accumbens (Koob GF. et al. 1998; Koob GF. 2006). The complex behaviour of smoking and drinking has more recently been conceptualized as an interplay between genetic factors and environmental influences. Heath AC et al. state that the heritability of alcohol dependence is about 64 % (Heath AC et al. 1997). Similar studies on nicotine addiction show a heritability of approximately 60 % (True WR et al. 1997). The genetic basis of smoking and drinking has been supported by twin and family studies. In a study of tobacco and alcohol addicts, True et al. found a genetic correlation of 0.68 %, supporting the notion that there may be common genetic vulnerabilities underlying both alcohol and tobacco addiction (True WR et al. 1999). The occurrence of both forms of addiction in families is however not entirely genetic, but could also be partially explained by intoxication during pregnancy (a drinking and/or smoking mother). Linkage and genome-wide association studies have examined the human genome, but the different loci identified to date have not yet been replicated. However, almost all of the specified loci appear to impact the regulation of the dopamine system. Furthermore, there are other findings implicating the noradrenalin system, the serotonergic system and the nicotine acetylcholine receptor. Wodarz N et al. illustrated the role of the serotonergic systems in relationship to drinking and smoking behaviour (Wodarz N et al. 2004). In both alcohol and nicotine addiction deficits of serotonin were found. Here, especially Cloninger type II alcoholism, an anti-social personality and symptoms like aggression, suicidal tendencies, fire starting and pathological gambling were assosiated with serotonergic deficits (Bailer UF et al. 2004, 2005, 2007; Brown GL and Linnoila MI 1990; Cloninger CR 1987; Frank GK et al. 2005; Kruesi MJ et al. 1992, Virkunnen M et al. 1994). Pettinati HM et al. showed that both inhibitory as well as activating serotonergic functions play a role by suggesting that an imbalance in the serotonergic system is crucial in the development of addiction (Pettinati HM et al. 2003). Chronic biological aspects of the serotonergic system should not be underestimated (Praschak Rieder N et al. 2008). Lallemand F et al. showed that changes in the glutamate-GABA systems can be observed with different chronological onsets in addiction and nicotine withdrawal (Lallemand F et al. 2006. 2007). The imbalance sometimes ceases to exist after an extended period of time. For those patients who have severe withdrawal symptoms (Lesch type I) during abstinence, and who suffer from strong alcohol cravings, medications to restore this balance are recommended (Acramprosate).

Previously, the opiate system, which plays a modulating role in the dopaminergic system, has been discussed with increased interest. Results from animal studies, which showed that opiate receptor blockers reduce drinking behaviour, have been replicated in humans by O'Malley SS et al. 2002 and Volpicelli JR et al. 1997 (see chapter 9.2.1). Alcohol aggravates the release of dopamine and this indirectly activates the dopamine system.

The cholinergic system is of central interest, especially in regard to the interaction of smoking and alcohol. Ethanol affects and activates acetylcholine nicotine receptors. This activation of the nicotine receptors on dopamine neurons could help explain the interaction of tobacco and alcohol addiction (Cardoso RA et al. 1999; Mann K 2004; Soederpalm B et al. 2000). Damage to the cholinergic neurons in the basal cortex has been found and this damage could lead to a degradation of cholinergic functions. Further, neuroimaging studies have shown that activity in the hippocampus is reduced and thus these deficits in the cholinergic system could be responsible for the cognitive dysfunction frequently seen in alcohol dependent individuals. (Arendt F 1994).

Furthermore, the CB1-recepor is also assumed to have an indirect dopamine agonistic effect, although the exact mechanism of this action is still unknown. Cannabionid receptor type 1 (CB1) receptors are thought to be the most widely expressed G-protein coupled receptors in the brain. It is supposed that CB1-receptor antagonists influence tobacco and alcohol consumption behaviour (Soyka M et al. 2008).

3.4.2 Aspects of alcohol and tobacco metabolism

Tobacco consists of about 4.800 different ingredients which can have varying effects on biological systems depending upon their combination. Nicotine seems to be the most important ingredient for affecting brain metabolism, while carbon monoxide, acetaldehyde, methanol and other tobacco ingredi-

Fig. 5 Methanol content (mg/l) in alcoholic beverages

Methanol content (mg/l) in alcoholic beverages

Beer 4–50	Sliwowitz 1500–4000
White wine 15–45	Rum 6–70
Red wine 70–130	Scotch 100–130
Brandy 200–350	Irish 10–110
Cognac 180–370	Bourbon 200–300
Cherry brandy 1900–2500	Aquavit 5–650
Plum brandy 3000–4500	Gin 10–1350
Liqueur 10–560	Vodka 5–170

Bonte W 1987

ents have only received little attention. Changes in the nicotine acetylcholine receptor and effects on the monoamineoxidase system (MAO) are very important factors in the development of tobacco addictions. In addition to ethanol, alcoholic beverages also contain methanol and other multiple chained alcohols. Metabolic products like acetaldehyde (Fig. 5) from alcohol, and formaldehyde from methanol may also contribute to the development of addiction.

The metabolism of ethanol and methanol clearly varies especially among alcohol dependent subjects compared to a healthy control sample. Here, genetic variations in alcohol metabolism (aldehyde dehydrogenase) may be crucial aetiological factors. For example, both ethanol and methanol metabolism differ in the subgroups defined by the Lesch typology. The elimination rates in this typology were examined in 61 intoxicated alcoholics. In type I subjects, both ethanol and methanol are rapidly eliminated, although an ethanol level of over 0, 2 mg/l still remains in the blood. On the other hand, the elimination of ethanol and metha-

Fig. 6 Methanolelimination in regard to Lesch's typology

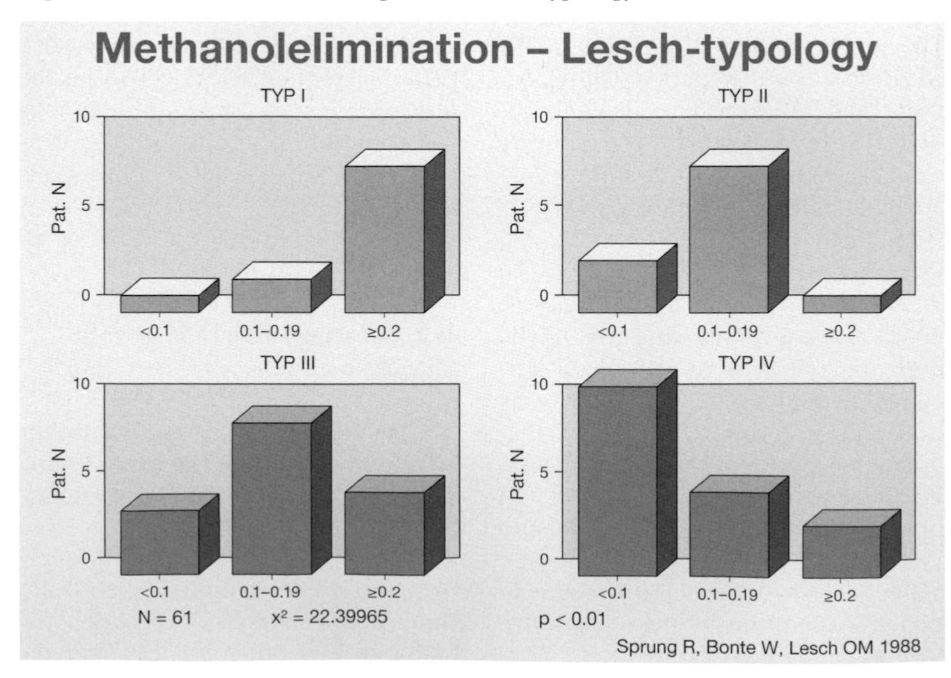

nol in type IV occurred at a considerably slower rate. (Sprung R et al. 1988).

It is hypothesized that many of the damaging effects of heavy alcohol consumption are primarily generated by aldehydes with the peripheral damage caused by alcohol itself. Aldehydes, together with dopamine, condense into TIQ's (tetrahydroisoquinlines) and indolamines condense into beta-carbolines. These beta-carbolines (norharmanes in particular) not only result from alcohol but from ingredients in tobacco as well.

3.4.3 Maternal tobacco and alcohol use during pregnancy: a risk factor for the offspring?

A potentially important precondition for the development of a biological addiction is the potential damage to the developing foetal brain through maternal use of addictive drugs. Smoking and alcohol during pregnancy can lead to significant changes in the offspring's brain functioning. Maternal drinking behaviour is a common cause of foetal brain damage. Further, not only the mother's smoking but also passive smoke can be extremely damaging. In lower socio-economic classes, families often live in very small cramped apartments or houses. With many family members smoking, the mother can be exposed to high levels of passive tobacco smoke.

3.4.3.1 Smoking during pregnancy

Numerous studies have shown that smoking during pregnancy has profound negative effects on the unborn child (Chantenoud L et al. 1998; Haustein KO 2000; Kries RV 2001; Ledermair O 1988; Salafia C and Shiverick K 1999). For instance, new born infants of smoking women have a three times higher risk of dying from "sudden infant death syndrome" (SIDS) during the first year of age (Jorch G 2001, Wisborg K et al. 2000).

Carcinogenic substances have been found in the urine of newborns whose mothers' smoked actively or were exposed to passive smoking thereby increasing the children's risk of cancer. The children of mothers who smoked during pregnancy also show reduced pulmonary function during the first years of life and are more likely to develop acute respiratory disease (ARDS) (Mutius Ev 2001; Trager JB and Hanrahan JP 1995).

The children of smoking mothers often show delays in their psychological development (Naeye RL and Peters ED 1984), possibly because smoking influences brain development in the unborn (Roy TS. and Sabherwal U 1994). For instance, learning difficulties (Aramakis VB et al. 2000; Butler R and Goldstein H 1973; Fabian-Fine R et al. 2001), attention deficits (McCartney JS and Fried PA 1994) and behavioural problems at elementary school age can all be ascribed to the negative effects of maternal and paternal tobacco consumption on the child's central nervous system (Makin J. and Fried PA. 1991; Wakschlag LS et al. 1997).

Childhood diabetes and an almost two-fold risk for being severely overweight at elementary school age can be ascribed to an abnormality in metabolic programming caused by foetal malnutrition. The foetus' body has prenatally adjusted in order to be born into an environment with poor nutritional conditions. A lifelong insulin insufficiency then develops along with an increased tendency to store fat (Montgomery SM and Ekborn A 2002).

3.4.3.2 Alcohol use during pregnancy

Chronic alcohol consumption during pregnancy is one of the main causes of fetal abnormalities. One of the most severe forms of abnormalities, described for the first time by the French paediatrician Paul Lemoine in 1968, is the "fetal alcohol syndrome" (FAS or Alcohol embryopathy). FAS is a differentially developed combination of diverse abnormalities and developmental problems in children of alcoholic mothers. The frequency of occurrence of FAS in western industrial nations is approximately 3 in 1000 newborn babies, but it is higher in certain ethnic groups and in underdeveloped countries.

Although children with the "fetal alcohol effect" (FAE) were exposed "in utero" to ethanol, they do not show all of the symptoms of FAS. Nevertheless, these children bear the consequences of the mother's alcohol consumption during pregnancy, including learning difficulties, impaired language development etc. It has been estimated that there are twice as many children with FAE than children with FAS (up to 10 of 1000 new born children). Alcoholic mothers are often very reluctant to provide information about their alcohol use or addiction and therefore, in these cases, research can only depend on estimations. The combination of alcohol use and smoking during pregnancy is particularly damaging to the unborn. The dopaminergic systems damaged by alcohol and smoking during their development and cell positioning in the fetal brain, are of particular interest. Neuroimaging studies show that several brain regions are especially affected.

- The corpus callosum is reduced in size and these reductions are also found in children with "Attention Deficit Hyperactivity Disorder" (ADHD) where the frontal area is particularly affected. These hyperactive children with attention deficits are at increased risk for developing an addiction in later life.
- The basal ganglia structures are not only important for motor functioning, but also for cognitive functioning, including affective memory. MRI studies show the nucleus caudate to be most affected.
- The cerebellum, where cognitive and autonomous motor functions are located, is also affected. Here the dysfunction leads to clumsiness and difficulty in appraising and negotiating new situations.

Animal studies (Crew's FT and Obernier's JA research groups) indicate that after exposure to high doses of alcohol over a few days, young and genetically predisposed rats showed significant morphological changes in different areas of the brain. During complete abstinent episodes, these same animals then showed cognitive deficits, including difficulty generating new solutions to certain tasks (Crews FT et al. 2000; Crews FT and Braun CJ 2003; Obernier JA et al. 2002). These findings are supported by a control study where young rats had considerable difficulties exiting a water barrel, following exposure to ethanol (Obernier JA et al. 2002).

In this study rats learned to escape the cold water by using an exit

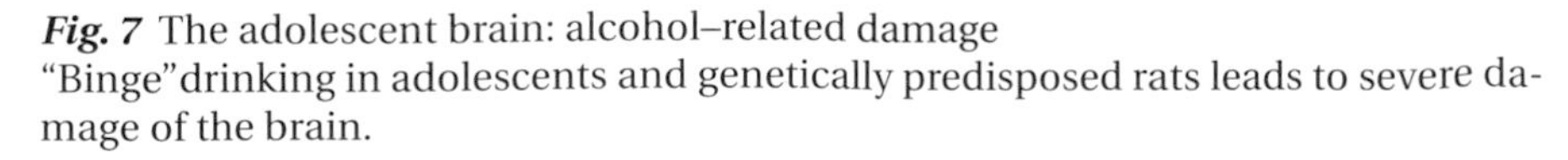
Fig. 7 The adolescent brain: alcohol–related damage
"Binge"drinking in adolescents and genetically predisposed rats leads to severe damage of the brain.

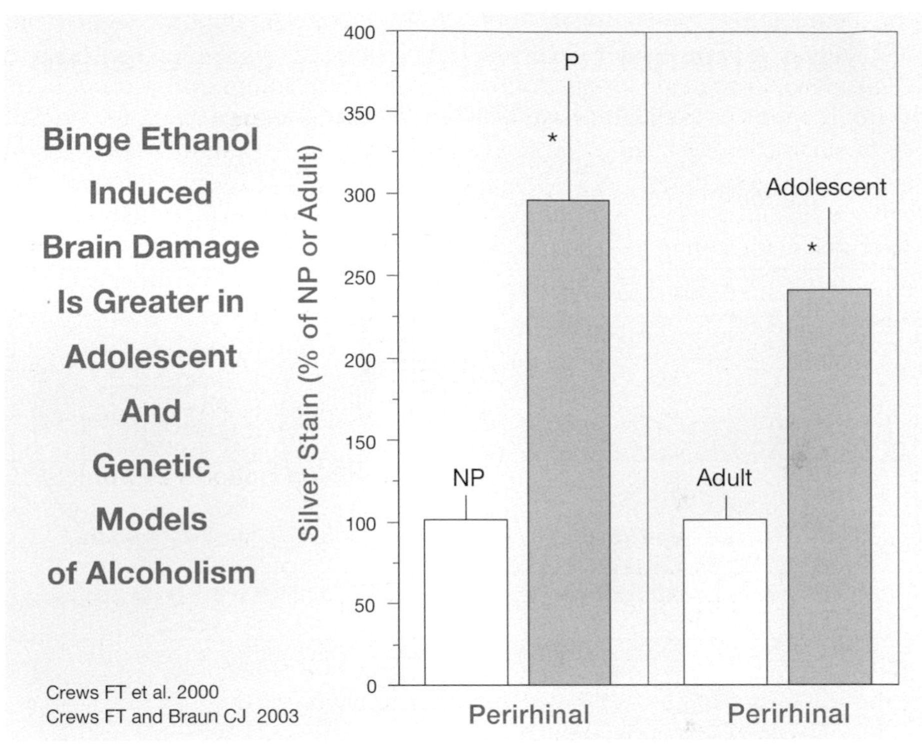

(platform). After learning this task, the rats were exposed to a "binge-drinking" experiment. Following three weeks of complete abstinence this group of "binge-drinkers" was compared with a control group. Following relocation of the platform to another quadrant of the test chamber and after a "binge-drinking" episode, the rats were not able to find their way to the red spot again (Figs. 7 and 8).

Both alcohol and its Aldehyde metabolites can enter the placenta and affect fetal cells. During the first twelve weeks of pregnancy (organ formation in the embryo), there is a high sensitivity to potentially damaging influences and agents. During this period, all of the body cells can be damaged as a result of inadequate tissue development.

Since the liver of the fetus is developing, it is not able to metabolise ethanol like the liver of an adult. Alcohol accumulates in the infant liver and damages the organism. Furthermore, other fetal health consequences can be observed in pregnant addicts. A deficiency of minerals, vitamins, zinc, magnesium and calcium certainly has a negative effect on the growth and development of the child.

Embryonic damages that are caused by alcohol range from slight cognitive deficits, difficult to detect, to the

Fig. 8 Alcohol and Problem solving strategies
Short-term intoxicated rats in the relearning Morris Water Maze Test

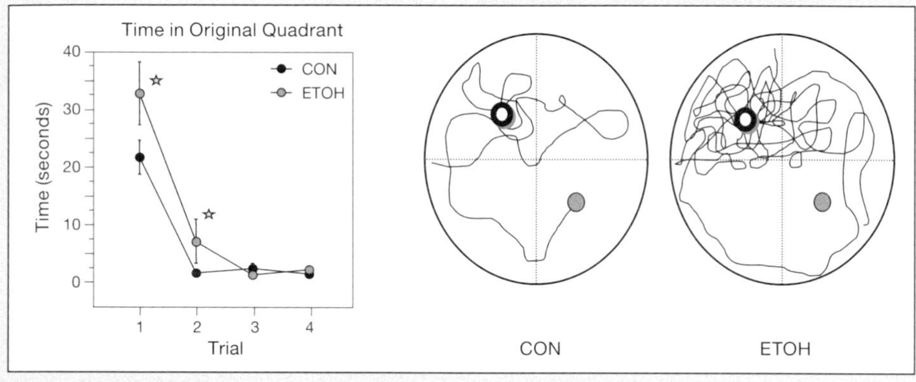

most severe physical disabilities and dysmorphology. We distinguish between the effects of alcohol on the fetus on the one hand, and alcohol related embryopathy on the other, as summarized by Majewski F, Streissgut AP and Loeser (Loeser H 1995; Majewski F 1987; Streissguth AP et al. 1990).

These lesser sequelae of alcohol, which typically manifest in learning and behaviour difficulties, are often viewed as minor dysfunctions, although they may have considerable influence on the life development of those affected. Problems at school, low educational attainment and sometimes even criminal activities are more frequently observed in FAE patients than in the normal population. These poor outcomes combined with social deficits can then, in turn, lead to addiction. The fact that alcoholism runs in families, could, next to genetic factors and the modelling of alcohol use behaviour by family members, be a result of these early dysfunctions. Apart from alcohol intoxication, tobacco and its ingredients can also lead to damage of the unborn child, including disruption of neuronal circuits. Alcohol and smoking increase the amount of free radicals, e. g. acetaldehyde found in the unborn.

When these changes lead to manifested damages of the organs, we speak of "alcoholembryopathy". Virtually all organs can be affected, although there is still not enough research data regarding the contribution of maternal smok-

Fig. 9 Fetal Alcohol Syndrome (FAS) Diagnostic Criteria

The criteria for the diagnosis of fetal alcohol syndrome, after excluding other diagnoses, are:

A. **Evidence of prenatal or postnatal growth impairment, as in at least 1 of the following:**
a. Birth weight or birth length at or below the 10th percentile for gestational age.
b. Height or weight at or below the 10th percentile for age.
c. Disproportionately low weight-to-height ratio (= 10th percentile).

B. **Simultaneous presentation of all 3 of the following facial anomalies at any age:**
a. Short palpebral fissure length (2 or more standard deviations below the mean).
b. Smooth or flattened philtrum (rank 4 or 5 on the lip-philtrum guide).
c. Thin upper lip (rank 4 or 5 on the lip-philtrum guide).

C. **Evidence of impairment in 3 or more of the following central nervous system domains:** hard and soft neurologic signs; brain structure; cognition; communication; academic achievement; memory; executive functioning and abstract reasoning; attention deficit/hyperactivity; adaptive behaviour, social skills, social communication.

D. **Confirmed (or unconfirmed) maternal alcohol exposure.**

Fig. 10 Diagnostic criteria for the partial fetal alcohol syndrome and for alcohol related neurodevelopmental disorder and for the term alcohol-related birth defects

The diagnostic criteria for partial fetal alcohol syndrome, after excluding other diagnoses, are:
A. Simultaneous presentation of 2 of the following facial anomalies at any age:
a. Short palpebral fissure length (2 or more standard deviations below the mean).
b. Smooth or flattened philtrum (rank 4 or 5 on the lip-philtrum guide).
c. Thin upper lip (rank 4 or 5 on the lip-philtrum guide).

B. Evidence of impairment in 3 or more of the following central nervous system domains: hard and soft neurologic signs; brain structure; cognition; communication; academic achievement; memory; executive functioning and abstract reasoning; attention deficit/hyperactivity; adaptive behaviour, social skills, social communication.
C. Confirmed maternal alcohol exposure.

The diagnostic criteria for alcohol-related neurodevelopmental disorder, after excluding other diagnoses, are:
A. Evidence of impairment in 3 or more of the following central nervous system domains: hard and soft neurologic signs; brain structure; cognition; communication; academic achievement; memory; executive functioning and abstract reasoning; attention deficit/hyperactivity; adaptive behaviour, social skills, social communication.
B. Confirmed maternal alcohol exposure.

The term alcohol-related birth defects (ARBD) should not be used as an umbrella or diagnostic term, for the spectrum of alcohol effects. ARBD constitutes a list of congenital anomalies, including malforma-tions and dysplasias and should be used with caution ing in regard to possible damages. Discussions are still taking place about how to diagnose the different syndromes of the Foetal Alcohol Spectrum Disorder (FASD). Loeser H. and Streissguth AP. proposed to differentiate between foetal alcohol effects and the foetal alcohol syndrome according to the definitions of Majewski F. (Loeser H. 1995, Streissguth AP. et al. 1990, Majewski F. 1987). We will follow the Canadian Guidelines for Diagnosis of the Foetal Alcohol Spectrum Disorder published by Chudley A.E. et al. 2005. They proposed to separate the Foetal Alcohol Syndrome (FAS, Fig. 9) from the partial FAS and Alcohol Related Neurodevelopmental Disorder.

An early diagnosis is essential to allow access to interventions and resources that may mitigate the development of subsequent "secondary disabilities" (e.g., unemployment, mental health problems, trouble with the law, inappropriate sexual behaviour, disrupted school experience) among affected people. Furthermore, an early diagnosis will also allow appropriate intervention, counselling and treatment for the mother and may prevent the birth of affected children in the future.

3.5 Aetiological aspects of tobacco and alcohol dependence from an epidemiological perspective

Research carried out by our group was able to examine the aetiological connection between smoking and alcohol consumption. Our findings indicate, that severely nicotine dependent adolescents (Heavy Smoking index-HSI ≥ 4 = defined by the two questions of the Fagerstroem Test: After waking up when do you smoke your first cigarette? How many cigarettes do you smoke per day? Heatherton TF et al. 1989) show a significantly increased rate of both alcohol abuse and alcohol dependence. Further, the abuse of illegal drugs also correlates positively with these data, suggesting a strong, possibly common, biological link across all addictive drugs.

In a study, 1,870 18-year old men from a certain catchment area, (4 % of all 18 years old men in Austria), were tested by using questionnaires and biological markers and results showed that the frequency of drug abuse is different depending on region. 962 (51.5 %) of these 1870 men smoke and 145 (7.8 %) smoke with a HSI-index of ≥ 4, with this being characterized as strongly addicted. The size of the hometown and the accessibility of the city of Vienna played a crucial role in determining the frequency of illegal drugs taken. Whether these 18-year olds live in a wine-growing district or an industrial area had no impact on the occurrence of alcohol addictions (Kapusta ND et al. 2006, 2007).

When smoking behaviour was correlated with drinking behaviour, smokers stated significantly more often that they drink alcohol because they desire its psychopharmacological effects. The CAGE Questionnaire consists of four questions and when a question is answered positively, alcohol abuse according to DSM-IV can be hypothesized. When two questions are answered positively, the diagnosis "alcohol addiction" can be made according to DSM-IV and ICD-10 (Kapusta ND et al.2006, 2007, Fig. 11).

When this tool was used with smokers and non-smokers, a significantly higher number of alcohol abus-

Fig. 11 CAGE questionnaire (Mayfield D et al. 1974 and Ewing JA.1984):

CUT DOWN: Have you ever thought to cut down your drinking?

ANNOYED BY CRITICISM: Have you ever been upset because someone criticized your drinking behaviour?

GUILT FEELINGS: Have you ever felt badly or guilty because of your drinking?

EYE OPENER: Have you ever drunk alcohol first thing in the morning (a pick-me-up) to ease your nerves or to get rid of a hangover?

ing and alcohol addicted adolescents were found amongst the smokers. Alcohol addiction is twice as prevalent in smokers who were shown to have 14 times more cannabis in their urine. Non-smokers consume opiates more frequently than smokers, but all other substances correlate with those of the smokers' group.

If the severity of tobacco addiction is being considered, and the question "when do you smoke your first cigarette after waking up in the morning?" is asked, the relationship becomes even more explicit (Fagerstroem KO and Schneider NG. 1989). The severity of biological nicotine addiction significantly correlates with all other addictive drugs. 11.1% of smokers who smoke their first cigarette immediately after waking up fulfil the criteria of an alcohol addiction (CAGE ≥ 2). Also, the consumption of opiates significantly correlates with the severity of a biolo-

Fig. 12 Smoking as a predictor for drug abuse

	Smoker (n = 978) %	Non–smoker (n = 907) %	Chi²	p
Alcohol for taste	78.4	62.0	61.329	<0.001*
Alcohol for effect	36.0	21.8	45.471	<0.001*
CAGE >=1	19.6	10.4	31.409	<0.001*
CAGE >=2	4.2	2.1	6.719	<0.01*
THC	10.0	0.7	69.939	<0.001*
Opiate	2.2	3.1	1.286	0.257
Cocaine	0.7	0	6.510	(0.011*)
Amphetamine	0.5	0	4.645	(0.031*)
Benzodiazepine	0.1	0.2	0.262	0.609
Minimal one Ilicit drug	10.9	3.9	33.810	<0.001*

Kapusta ND et al. (2006) Epidemiology of substance use in a representative sample of 18-year-old males. Alcohol & Alcoholism 41/2: 188-192.

Fig. 13 The first cigarette after rising and urine drug tests

Item	till 5 min. (n=107) %	6–30 min. (n=390) %	31–60 min. (n=183) %	>60 min. (n=282) %	NR (n=907) %	Chi²	p
Alcohol tastes good	77.1	78.1	77.7	80.1	62.0	62.2	<0.001*
Drinking because of the effect	44.9	38.7	30.9	32.1	21.8	56.1	<0.001*
CAGE=1	29.4	23.4	18.5	11.3	10.4	59.5	<0.001*
CAGE=2	11.1	4.5	2.1	2.1	2.1	28.5	<0.001*
THC	16.3	9.3	9.2	5.6	0.7	88.8	<0.001*
Opiates	4.5	2.0	2.7	1.4	3.1	4.5	0.345
Cocaine	3.6	0.3	1.1	-	-	38.8	<0.001*
Amphetamines	2.7	-	0.5	-	-	37.1	<0.001*
at least 1 illegal drug	20.0	10.8	11.4	7.1	3.9	52.7	<0.001*

Kapusta ND et al. (2007) Multiple substance use among yooung males. Pharmacology, Biochemistry and Behavior 86:306-311

gical nicotine addiction, whereas the non-smoking group showed a higher use of opiates than e.g. smokers who smoke their first cigarette after one hour of awakening (3.1 % vs. 1.4 %). These results show that there is a common aetiology of tobacco and alcohol addiction and cannabis abuse, while in regard to opiates there are different aetiological paths to addiction (Figs. 12 and 13).

Although it is well known that alcohol addicts often smoke it is important to know which smoking behaviour is used by which group of alcohol addicts (e.g. Fagerstroem positive vs. Fagerstroem negative). We therefore conducted a study with 100 smoking alcoholics and we were able to show that the smoking behaviour varies depending on the subgroups of alcohol addicts. Lesch types I, III, IV smoked exceedingly more (Fagerstroem-positive), whereas individuals of Lesch type II didn't even meet 50 % of the criteria for a smoking addiction (Fig. 14).

Fig. 14 Nicotine dependence according to alcohol typology (Lesch)

N=100	Type I	Type II	Type III	Type IV	Total
Smoking without dependence	6	18	10	2	36
Nicotine dependence	14	13	20	17	64
Total	20	31	30	19	100

Publication in preparation

3.6 Aetiology of addiction from a psychiatric perspective

Emotions, contentment, but also happiness are important in people's life and Damasio AR. (Damasio AR. 2003) was able to differentiate these from a more purely biological perspective. Damasio contrasts six primary emotions: fear, anger, sadness, disgust, surprise and happiness and distinguishes these from secondary emotions like embarrassment, jealousy, guilt and pride. These are followed by tertiary emotions like contentment, uneasiness, serenity, tenseness and others. These emotions are represented by very complex circuits in the brain and a lack of balance in these circuits can certainly never be explained by an isolated dysfunction. Biological explanation models often merely illuminate singular features (e.g. the serotonergic system). Although these simplifications can be very important for scientific research as far as clinical use is concerned, they are the main reason why medicines (like SSRIs) often have limited effectiveness in the therapy of addiction despite research showing their effectiveness.

The interplay of the basal ganglia, frontal brain, pituitary thyroid axis, adrenal gland and fat metabolism is very important for the well-being of every individual. In 2004, Manzanares explained how alcohol affects each circuit and furthermore showed that each area of addiction development, and therapeutic strategies, have different points of action (Manzanares J. 2005) (Fig. 15).

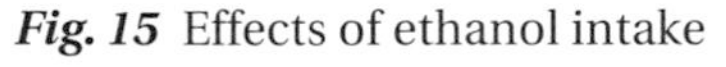

Fig. 15 Effects of ethanol intake

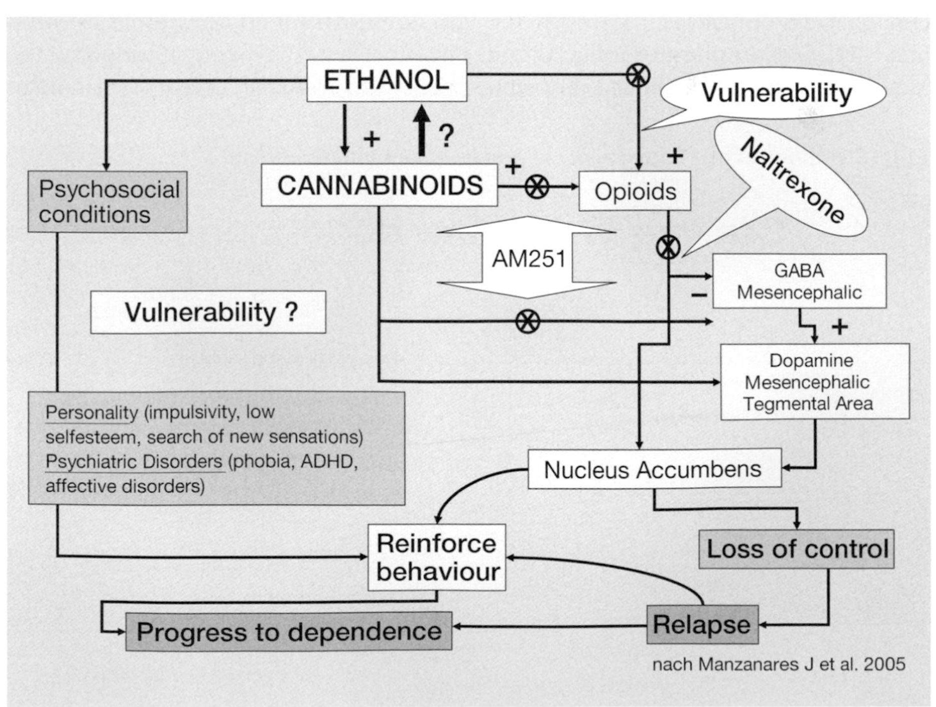

In 2003 Johnson simplified this system for pharmacotherapy and described the interactions between the nucleus accumbens, the ventral tegmental area and the cortex (Johnson BA et al. 2003). The primary emotional state is regulated by activity in the nucleus accumbens. External stimuli are regulated by the frontal basal brain region which generates expectations in regard to the effect of the addictive drug. These can be appraised as either pleasurable, desirable but also as not acceptable. These functions are ascribed to the ventral tegmental area (Fig. 16).

In 1993, based upon our prospective long-term studies of patients, we summarized the developmental process of an addiction in a dynamic model from a clinical perspective (Lesch OM et al. 1993).

At the start of every addiction, the substance's effect is quickly experienced as very enjoyable. However, the very first consumption of tobacco and alcohol is often experienced as negative and use only becomes more frequent after several attempts, typically as a result of peer group pressure. The addictive drug is then taken more frequently when the pharmacological effects of smoking and tobacco ingredients or alcohol begin to have a positive pharmacological effect (key-lock principle). The conditions which lead to the use of addictive drugs are very heterogenic (e.g. fear, difficulties relating to people, tests of courage, depression, desired behaviour in a group and many more), and are therefore portrayed in a broad form as the input of the funnel in Fig. 17.

With increased consumption, the affected individual often shifts between poisoning, withdrawal and its sequelae and a certain percentage actually develop withdrawal symptoms. Alcohol causes a variety of neuropsychological difficulties which can lead to a decline in cognitive functioning such as intelligence, creativity, imagination and the ability to think critically. As a conse-

Fig. 16 Biological mechanisms of craving in alcohol dependence

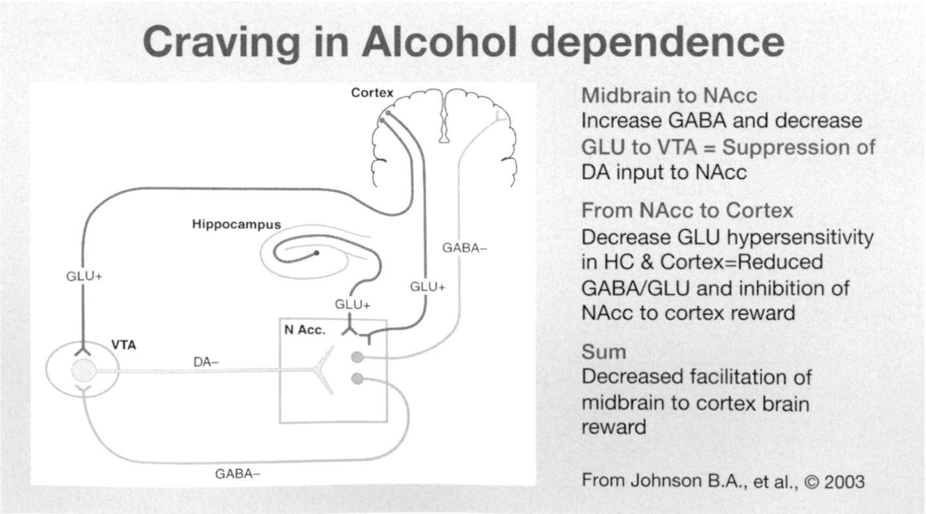

Fig. 17 Funnel model

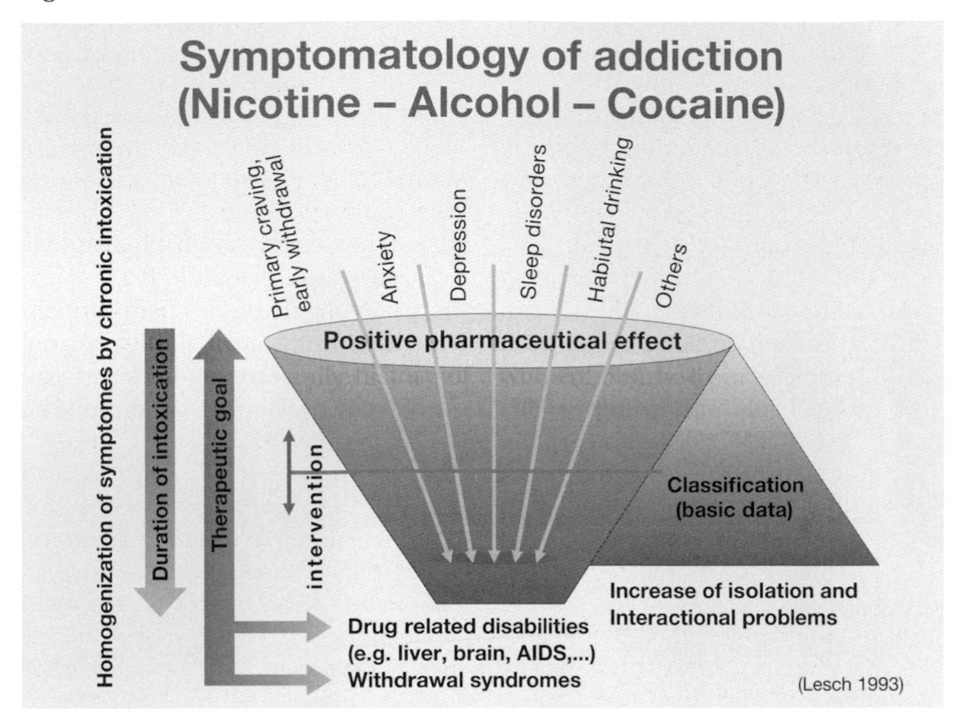

quence, alcohol addicts are often rejected by their social environment, leading to increased isolation. The later a patient is encountered in the developmental process of an addiction, the more dramatic are the symptoms of intoxication, sequelae, withdrawal and social isolation, and the more closely do the clinical pictures of these patients (in regard to their behaviour, reactions and symptoms) resemble each other. The diagnostic criteria of ICD-10 and DSM-IV describe the clinical picture but fail to sufficiently consider the distinct aetiologies and primary personality traits. Only after several weeks of abstinence do the sequelae regress and the personality traits become visible again, thus permitting a psychotherapeutic treatment of the problem. Only after the patient has reached this state, is he able to be compliant with treatment, and long-time therapy goals can then be rationally defined in way that is acceptable to both patient and therapist.

Smoking causes similar changes to those produced by alcohol, although it does not lead to social isolation and causes rather different sequelae (e.g. breathing difficulties). It is these sequelae that often lead the smoker to start therapy. When the patient has both a nicotine and alcohol addiction, he often displays more severe sequelae and more acute withdrawal symptoms.

4

Prevention strategies

4.1 Attitudes towards addictive drugs

4.1.1 Attitudes towards alcohol consumption

For many centuries, many kinds of alcoholic beverages (wine, beer and spirits) have been produced in central Europe. Adolescents grow up in an alcohol permissive milieu and see that adult drinking is socially accepted and even desired behaviour. The advantage of initiating this consumption at a young age is that adolescents often learn how to use alcoholic beverages at an early stage. A primary disadvantage are the increased risks associated with this early consumption and the development of physical and psychological dysfunctions, as well as the learned attitude that alcohol can be used as a basic food.

Almost 50 % of adults think that it is acceptable for adolescents between the age of 16 and 18 to consume alcohol at home or at parties, an attitude which generally complies with regulations of the protection of minors (child welfare). Depending upon the situation, 9-18 % think that alcohol consumption is acceptable even before the age of 16. However 40 % of respondents would not dispense alcohol to their children until the age of at least 18 years. More recently, girls have started drinking at an even earlier age, while boys have slightly reduced and delayed their drinking behaviour (Eisenbach-Stangl I. 1991, 1994).

The consumption of alcohol in Europe is higher than for other continents (Eisenbach-Stangl I. 1991; Hurst W et al. 1997), with central European countries showing a consumption of 14 litres per capita per year..

Around 1900, a large-scale epidemiological study was conducted in Austria in which adolescents of different age groups from different types of school were interviewed about their alcohol consumption. It was found that adolescent alcohol consumption in 1900 was about the same as adolescent alcohol consumption in 1975, as measured by sales data or other studies.

Around 1900, 3.2 % of 14-year old boys had already consumed hard alcohol (40 Vol.-% and over), mostly spirits of low quality. It can be assumed that today slightly over 3 % of 14-year olds have already repeatedly consumed hard alcohol. Reports in the media which denounce adolescent binge drinking as boundary testing, and thereby serve to make drinking a focus of adolescent interest, were already published in middle Europe around 1900 and since then adolescent drinking has at repeated intervals been a focus of news coverage.

Representing a personal-political mandate, the slogan of the social democratic party at the beginning of the 20th century was "A thinking worker doesn't drink and a drinking worker doesn't think". This led to a decline in alcohol consumption up until World War I. However, with increasing prosperity after World War II, the use of alcohol has been growing in Europe and elsewhere. Since the mid 70's, the typical working environment has drastically changed (shorter work breaks, more regulated and controlled working hours and laws which prohibit alcohol use while driving a motor vehicle, while at work etc.). This has lead to a restriction in the consumption of alcoholic beverages. As a consequence, a tendency to consume "lighter, lower calorie alcohol" developed all over Europe. In the 1990's, the percent volume of pure alcohol which is enjoyed in different forms of beer, increased, while wine consumption decreased. The consumption of spirits has halved since World War II (Eisenbach-Stangl I. 1991, 1994) (Fig. 18).

In Austria about 15–36% of the adult population are considered to be vulnerable to alcoholism, and 2.2–4% of the total population are known to have an alcohol addiction. These numbers vary according to a gender specific vulnerability ratio. While Rathner G and Dunkel D assume a 3:1 gender ratio (men to women), other studies suggest a ratio of 14:1 (Lesch OM. et al. 1989; Rathner G. and Dunkel D. 1998). Even if just usual hospital admissions of alcohol-addicted individuals are considered, a ratio of 5:2 (men to women) is observed (Fig. 19).

Fig. 18 Development of alcohol consumption in Austria 1881–1992

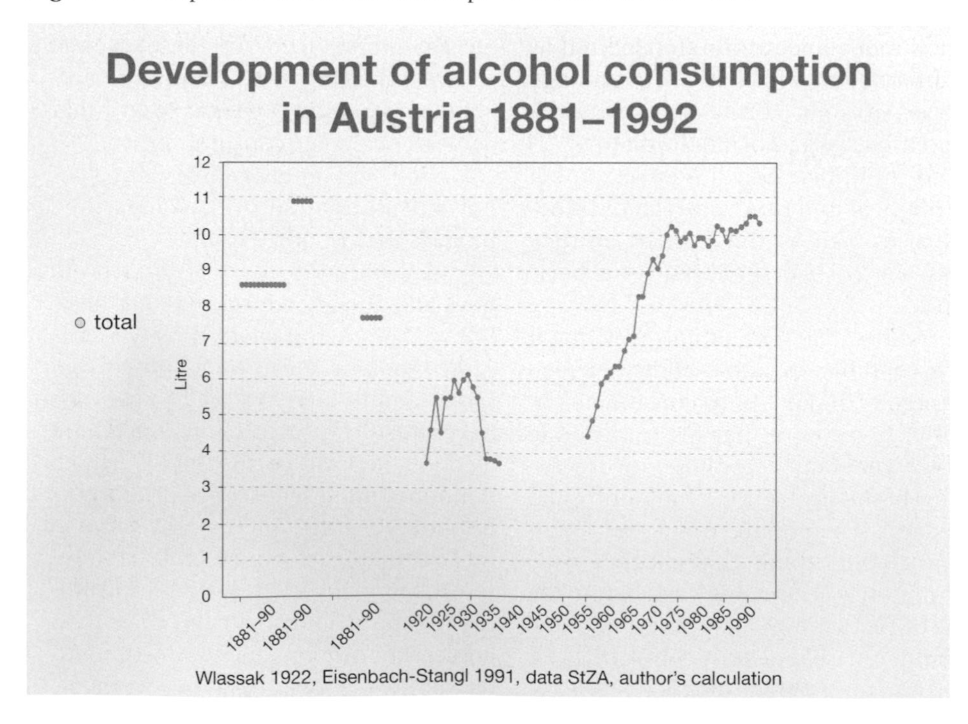

Fig. 19 Alcohol use in Austria according to regions

Pure alcohol/week		Federal states								
		B	W	NÖ	St	K	OÖ	S	T	V
≤245 g	♂	34	56	40	43	59	39	53	57	39
	♀	61	74	68	73	73	73	68	69	75
246 g–420 g	♂	26	7	7	18	13	21	20	9	22
	♀	6	5	1	7	5	10	5	2	–
>420 g	♂	33	17	35	31	22	32	21	17	21
	♀	2	2	2	1	2	2	1	–	1

Uhl A. Springer A. representative sample 1993–94; Lesch OM et al. 1989

A sample survey of 60 to 69 year olds found a per capita alcohol consumption of 25 g alcohol/d, while the 70 to 99 year old age group consumed 26 g alcohol/d (1 unit = 10 g of pure alcohol = ca. 1/8 wine or 1/3 l beer) (Uhl A and Springer A. 1996).

4.1.2 Attitudes towards tobacco consumption

Although it has been known for many years that the ingredients of cigarettes can cause various types of damage to the body, the tobacco industry has blocked all effective methods to reduce smoking. For many years it was claimed that nicotine is not addictive and the tobacco industry produced new "light" cigarettes which were advertised as being "healthier cigarettes". Only in the last fifteen years has this argumentation collapsed, and today it is quite obvious that there is no such thing as a "healthy cigarette". Nicotine is a highly addictive compound and the ingredients of a cigarette are known to produce damage in different areas of the entire body. The European community has finally begun to restrict tobacco advertisements and over the last 10 years, individual countries have started to advise about the damaging effects of cigarettes and to label cigarette boxes with health warnings. Apart from references to the damaging consequences of smoking, such as "Smoking kills" or "Smoking leads to a slow and painful death", the ingredients of cigarettes like tar, nicotine, and carbon monoxide are also listed. Despite this, the smoking behaviour of adolescents has not significantly changed and, today, smoking is still the addiction with the highest mortality rate. (The only one single effective prevention against bronchial carcinoma is a smoke-free life). As it has become more widely known that passive smoking also damages health, smoke-free zones have been set-up in several countries. In Austria this is only being slowly introduced and in some stressful situations (e.g. in hospitals) people still smoke.

Approximately 30% of the population smoke, although smoking behaviour decreases with age. At the age of 18, more than 50% of men smoke and similar kinds of smoking behaviour can be expected in women. Studies of female smokers are needed in almost all areas. 20.3% of 18-year old men who smoke score five or more points on the Fagerstroem scale: this group can be identified as biologically addicted according to the ICD-10 and DSM-IV criteria (Fagerstroem KO. et al. 1989; Heatherton TF. et al. 1089, 1991; Kapusta ND. et al. 2007)

Half of all smokers are displeased with their tobacco consumption ("dissonant smokers"). It is therefore not surprising that by the age of 50, just under 30% of the population still smoke. Yet it can be assumed that education and the awareness of the risks of smoking only seem to reach those individuals who either abstain or abuse only tobacco, while those smokers who meet criteria for a biological addiction are not influenced by prevention programmes. It is this group that develops a withdrawal symptom when the number of cigarettes smoked is reduced and later also shows severe bodily sequelae as a result of their smoking.

4.2 Primary prevention of tobacco and alcohol addiction

By "primary prevention of tobacco and alcohol addiction", we mean measures which attempt to change society by decreasing the demand for an addictive drug. Addictive drugs and smoking are as old as humanity. There has never been a drug-free society and whether this is desirable is still controversially discussed. Yet it is important to change the attitudes of a society in such a way that life without tobacco and alcohol, and all other addictive drugs, is perceived as desirable (catchphrase: happiness is life without drugs). When the reasons why adolescents start the consumption of a drug are investigated, the following motives for starting to smoke and drink include:

- "I just wanted to try it out". Here experimentation is seen as part of natural development.
- Adolescents use tobacco and alcohol to feel "like adults". (The label "Smoking: only for adults" leads to an increase in smoking among adolescents).
- Adolescents want to smoke because they want to be integrated into peer groups. If smoking is a desired behaviour in a particular peer group, it is difficult not to smoke.
- To demonstrate autonomy
- To have fun. Curiosity plays a big role in the initiation of smoking and drinking
- To decrease anxiety in specific situations, e.g. before exams.
- Tobacco is a psychotropic substance which enhances memory in the short-run. This is why adolescents use it for studying. It also has an anti-depressive effect and is used to lift one's spirits (Balfour DJ. and Ridley DL. 2000; Best JA. et al. 1988; Merrill JC et al. 1999; Sutherland I et al. 1998).

For primary prevention efforts to be effective, all socio cultural factors and in-

Fig. 20 Socio cultural model of alcohol and tobacco use and abuse in adolescent and young adults (Johnson BA et al., p. 34, 2003)

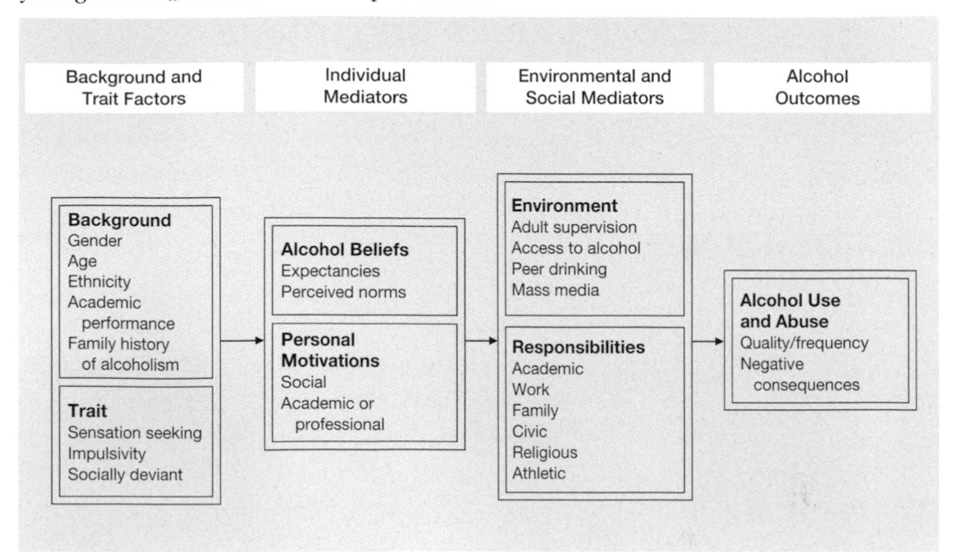

dividual models must be drawn upon. Accordingly, primary prevention uses a plethora of measures and attempts to influence all factors in order to reduce the demand for addictive drugs (Fig. 20).

From a socio-cultural perspective, the individual causes leading to tobacco and alcohol consumption remain in the background. Included in the socio-cultural model are factors, identified in quality of life research, which significantly influence the consumption behaviour of adolescents and adults. Preventative factors which protect against substance abuse include, for example, a high level of satisfaction in adolescents, and a social environment can be created which enables adolescents to feel stable and secure.

Another preventive element is being a member of a group which values living without addictive substances. Research has identified vulnerability factors such as psychological pain, poverty and a drug permissive milieu, which are more likely to push adolescents towards the path of addiction (tobacco, alcohol and other addictive drugs).

As regards alcohol, tobacco and marijuana consumption, 78.9 % describe curiosity as the most important motivating factor, compared to 57.9 % who stated this reason for trying opium and cocaine; on the other hand, 42.1 % stated interpersonal conflicts as being the primary motivation for starting to abuse opium and cocaine, while only 5.3 % of alcohol, tobacco or marijuana abusers indicated poor interpersonal relations as the main reason (Fig. 21.)

Tobacco and alcohol consumption (including abuse) can be influenced by increasing the unit price and taxes, and by other such measures, which make smoking and drinking more expensive. However, individuals who already show a tobacco or alcohol addiction are typically not influenced

Fig. 21 Substance abuse factors which influence alcohol use in society

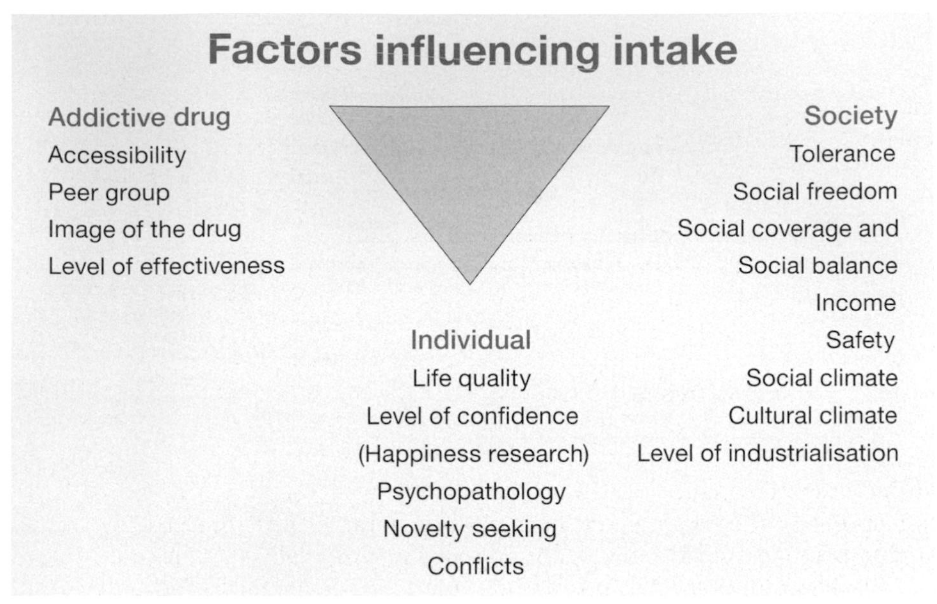

by such measures. The so-called "war against drugs", as has been proclaimed in some countries, is useless without the provision of measures to help affected adolescents, and normally leads to a shift to other addictive substances (drugs, pills etc) or to other behavioural disorders (e. g. eating disorders).

As illustrated in chapter 6.2, 6.3, addiction is clinically very heterogeneous. If we consider a separate aetiology for each subgroup, three entirely different paths to an addiction arise. These different paths obviously need different preventive measures. It is unrealistic to expect that measures can be instituted to entirely prevent these developments. Yet it is possible to imagine that an awareness of these mechanisms could facilitate early detection and support could thus be initiated earlier. Today it is widely agreed that secondary prevention is the ideal way of prevention.

4.3 Secondary prevention: early diagnosis and intervention

In many peer groups, smoking and drinking is a desired behaviour and is used as a ritual to demonstrate group cohesion. This often leads the adolescent member to abuse addictive drugs like tobacco or alcohol in high doses and over a long period of time. Adolescents who show a psychological or biological vulnerability (Rommelspacher H. 2007) often develop an addiction syndrome. This vulnerability sometimes begins in the womb when the mother regularly "poisons" the unborn child by active or passive smoking. Today we know that, especially up until the eighth week of pregnancy, the developing brain can be massively influenced by alcohol and nicotine exposure, similary the reward system and addiction memory (Chantenoud L et al. 1998; Haustein

KO. 2000; Ledermair O. 1988; Salafia C and Shiverick K. 1999).

Within the socialisation process of the adolescent, traumata can lead to an insecure personality which is very dependent on affection from his environment. Insecure adolescents often fear they are not good enough or that they can't meet their own expectations or the expectations of others. They go out of their way to serve their peer group and forget how to say "no", and often this insecurity is mirrored in their choice of partner: they tend to seek powerful partners who reinforce their insecurity. These interactions between an insecure personality and social expectations lead to taxing situations, anxiety and stress, sometimes leading the adolescent to use addictive drugs such as tobacco and alcohol to cope with the taxing situations of every day life.

Some adolescents experience a very strict upbringing based on rigid values. The children love their adult attachment figure very much and this is why they try to accept their values as absolute and to adopt them as their own. As adolescents, they later learn that these values and rules can't always be realised (e.g. the 'internal' command is: "Be a good student!" – but performance at school shows a different picture), and this leads to anxious-depressive reactions and the realization that this uneasiness can be compensated by the pharmacological action of the addictive drug. The beloved adults often demonstrate double standards. Parents always talk about having to be well behaved and not being allowed to consume any drug. However, parents may show a completely different behaviour pattern themselves and serve as a role model by smoking and drinking (smoking and drinking parents, youth coach, teachers etc.). Adolescents learn from role models and often unintentionally adjust to these double standards. Aside from the above-described mechanism of the development of addiction, many other susceptibility factors certainly exist. Early cerebral and psychological damage often leads to early problems and behavioural abnormalities (Brückensymptome = Bridge symptoms) which are so severe that those affected are not able to attend school and finish their diploma or degree, they often show socially deviant behaviour and sometimes even come into conflict with the law. These marginal groups of society, which represent about 10 % of the general population, should be offered help in due time. Furthermore, interventions that are acceptable to those affected should be the primary interventions offered.

4.3.1 Conclusions for secondary prevention

4.3.1.1 Measures concerning the addictive drug

A reduction in the general availability of alcohol and tobacco products typically reduces the abuse rate in the general population. A few examples are: to offer tobacco products only at tobacconists and only at certain times (approximately from 5 am to 11am); no sale of cigarettes at petrol stations, in restaurants or through vending machines; imposing a smoking ban for all public buildings such as hospitals, schools, agencies etc., including restaurants. Further, the public designation of smoking and non-smoking pubs would lead to the consumer being able to chose whether or not he wants to be exposed to tobacco substances. Pubs with an area of less than 50 m^2 and which do not employ staff, should be allowed to call themselves smoking bars (Employee Protection Law).

It would certainly be an improvement if adolescent protection laws regarding both alcohol and tobacco were adhered to, and if alcohol and tobacco were only available in selected shops and at certain times of the day. Thus, availability would be limited. The sale of alcohol in restaurants should be coupled with food consumption during the day and, in principle, only alcoholic drinks with low alcoholic content should be served (an example of this can be found in Sweden). Additionally, prices (including taxes) should be increased, making it difficult for adolescents to regularly drink and smoke. Ten percent of the taxes collected for alcohol and tobacco should be used for the prevention and therapy of addiction.

Regular advertisement campaigns should educate the public about the addictive nature of tobacco and the many toxic substances it contains, emphasizing that tobacco isn't a safe or a pleasurable stimulant. Not only is a large amount of nicotine inhaled by smoking, but so are many other toxic substances which play an important role in the development of an addiction. Once a tobacco addiction has developed, this addiction seems to be a precursor for many other kinds of addictions. Addicted smokers are much more likely to become addicted to other legal and illegal drugs than smokers not biologically addicted (Kapusta ND et al. 2006, 2007). The interrelationship of these addictions should be included in all educational programmes. Of course, alcohol consumed in low amounts as a pleasurable stimulant should not be demonized, but it should be emphasized that alcohol is a drug which, even when consumed in low amounts, reduces cognitive skills and coordination. Alcohol should not be used when working with dangerous machinery, when driving a car or when using public transport (taxi, train, etc.). Like tobacco consumption, the regular consumption of alcohol can damage the whole organism.

Active smoking (and also passive smoking) during pregnancy should be an important topic in prevention. Not only should educational and public service brochures ("0.0 ‰, 0 ppm") be distributed, but pregnant women who smoke should be motivated as early as possible to stop or at least reduce their smoking behaviour (Report of the medical-scientific fonds by the mayor of the federal capital Vienna, 2005) and offered medical intervention (e.g. varenicline), when appropriate.

4.3.1.2 Measures to help adolescents live a drug-free life

All preventive measures should consider the following principles:

"The political credo of society should be based upon the following principles:

In our society no child will be lost. We care for every single child. There are resources available to support a child regardless of age, and every child should be provided with ideal educational opportunities, necessary medical care and social opportunities."

Adolescents who face difficult situations (e.g. family, in school or at work) should be offered help. Here the basic rule is: "Look closely at the problem and don't look away". The earlier the adolescent's seemingly unresolved problem is recognized, and the earlier solutions can be offered and accepted by the adolescent, the less likely it is that the drug will be a problem for the adolescent. Young people are valuable members of society and the adults of this society should be encouraged to support and assist difficult adolescents. In Finland, for example, it is more difficult than in German-speaking countries or the US to "expel or suspend" adolescents from class or school. This responsibility of the part of families, schools and all those involved, leads to good results, as is reflected by the "PISA study".

The peer group can provide a very important protective element and these groups should be provided with the activities they desire, for example active cultural activities (music or theatre groups), sport activities (from athletics to ball games) and especially sufficient time and space to participate in these activities safely whilst still offering some independence and adventure. In terms of prevention, it is known that these low-risk forms of education enable adolescents to live out their curiosity and are important to the development of a healthy and positive personality. Prohibitions and rules that aren't accepted by the group are counterproductive and can lead to the growth of marginal groups and an increase in the number of drug-taking adolescents.

Improvement of the adolescents' social situation is a very crucial prevention factor. The loss of the peer group as a result of academic failure could be another risk factor for the development of drug problems. The clearer the personal development possibilities are, the lower the addictive drug consumption. A feeling of security provided by the family, a circle of friends, and also by one's own occupational situation can protect against substance abuse. The more purposeful the adolescent perceives his function in the family and social situation to be, and the more defined his role, the lower the risk of regular consumption of addictive drugs.

In puberty, adolescents often find it difficult to develop their own identity. Their parents' moral and ethic values are questioned and compared with others. Therefore adolescents need opportunities to experiment, through which they can try to develop their own identity and to set boundaries for themselves. Opportunities to experiment should be supported by society so that the risk of adolescent physical and psychological problems are reduced and kept as low as possible. Furthermore, the influence of adults should be kept to a minimum. Some adolescents can only accept something after having experienced it themselves, and this experience can be painful. If an adolescent group can manage this pain without the influence of adults, a feeling of solidarity can form within the group which can provide protection against the danger of addictive drugs.

Specific preventative strategies should be offered to risk groups and different measures are needed according to the nature of the risk group. An adolescent who is admitted to an inpatient clinic due to severe intoxication, is an emergency case who will certainly need psychological-psychiatric support after he has been medically treated (crisis concept). Families with multiple

Fig. 22 Risk groups

Target groups for the prevention of addiction
- Adolescents after severe intoxications
- Adolescents in emergency hospitalization
- Adolescents of addicted parents
- Adolescents, who were in touch with the police
- Children and adolescents from the streets
- Children and adolescents in corrective training

addicted members require help for the whole family system. Children of these families are highly vulnerable and need intensive support and intervention.

Even if the diagnosis of "addiction" is absent, these target groups need the help of a therapeutic team (social worker, psychologist, physician etc.) that is able to offer support to the adolescent for many years. Furthermore, these teams may need to intensify their efforts when those affected individuals show negative outcomes.

4.4 Tertiary prevention (see chapter 9)

As already stated, almost half of all adolescents are biologically addicted smokers (= Fagerstroem 5 or above). The above-mentioned measures are typically not effective in reducing substance abuse in these groups. Although the adolescents feel uncomfortable about their smoking, they are rarely able to change their smoking behaviour. Here, therapeutic approaches for tobacco addicts, as described in the following chapters, should be applied.

From the medical perspective, alcohol addicts are ill and therefore need therapeutic help. It is not useful to create rules regarding drinking behaviour nor is constructive to tell them to pull themselves together. They need professional therapeutic intervention. It can also be beneficial to provide an environment in which they can talk to other affected individuals so that they become aware that their symptoms can be improved and that there is someone to support them in solving their problems. This help should be sought outside of their usual environment (family, work, school) and the therapists should have psychological and pharmacological knowledge. An addict who feels that an interest is being taken in him that isn't too intrusive can often become allied with a therapeutic network. These alliances over a long period of time are an important therapeutic agent (see chapter 9).

Successfully treated alcohol or tobacco addicts are able to lead abstinent and smoke-free lives. In doing this, they are excellent role models for adolescents by demonstrating how to live a drug-free life.

5

Diagnosis of abuse and addiction

5.1 Problems concerning psychiatric diagnoses

The diagnostic systems typically used in psychiatric hospitals are designed to define homogenous groups of patients whose specific aetiology leads to certain symptoms. From this aetiology, a therapy that is most effective for this disease group should be planned. For a diagnosis of a disease the following should be provided:

By defining a disease, its aetiology is also automatically defined. In addictions, smoking and drinking are often only secondary phenomena. The aetiology of abuse and the causes of addiction have always been seen as two different constructs.

The implementation of the therapy is scientifically supported and defined according to the theoretical aetiology and the clinical conditions at the initiation of the therapy. At least 88 different therapies for addictions are used all over the world: these therapies lead to both positive and negative results (Hester RK and Miller WR. 2003). The therapeutic procedure depends on many factors, but not usually on the consumption behaviour. The diagnosis of addiction merely describes one aspect of the whole problem.

In many cases the natural course of a disease can be predicted on the basis of the diagnosis. However, abuse and addiction have completely different developmental trajectories which depend the least on substance consumption behaviour (see chapter 6.3).

As not all of the preconditions for addiction related disorders have been established, more and more subgroups of different addictions are being identified (see chapter 6). Nevertheless, two international classification systems (ICD-10 and DSM-IV) have been established which have widespread use. The advantage of these systems is that epidemiological studies can compare the incidence and prevalence of addictions in different cultures. Further, in central Europe this schema of diagnosis has been proven to be effective for invoicing insurers and other payment agencies. Therefore it was important that tobacco addiction was included in ICD-10 as a separate disorder. Unfortunately, in meeting the needs of these two goals (epidemiology and the cover of costs) both systems became too general and insufficient to allow development of specific therapies. The therapies which are offered at the moment have very rigid guidelines and primarily comply with the needs of the inpatient and outpatient institutions. Yet, they don't sufficiently address the real needs and capabilities of affected individuals. Results from basic research and pharmacological research can never actually be applied to all addicts (Koob GF and Le Moal M. 2006). For both therapeutic and research reasons, subgroups of addicted individuals were identified from these two classification systems to better meet the requirements of therapy and research.

Different factors are relevant for therapy in the course of the illness. These could be either somatic factors, or factors occurring in the environment or the individual. In Fig. 23 the major elements are shown, constituting the basis for a multidimensional approach.

5.2 Development of the term "addiction"

From a historical perspective, the term "alcoholism" was introduced into the medical literature by Magnus Huss in 1852 (Huss M.1852), but already by the beginning of the 20th century different aetiologies for alcoholism had begun to evolve. Primary or secondary alcoholism, alcoholism caused by a neurotic, psychiatric or psychopathic personality and alcoholism due to physical vulnerabilities were also defined at that time (see Feuerlein W. 1975). In 1952, the

Fig. 23 Factors influencing therapy

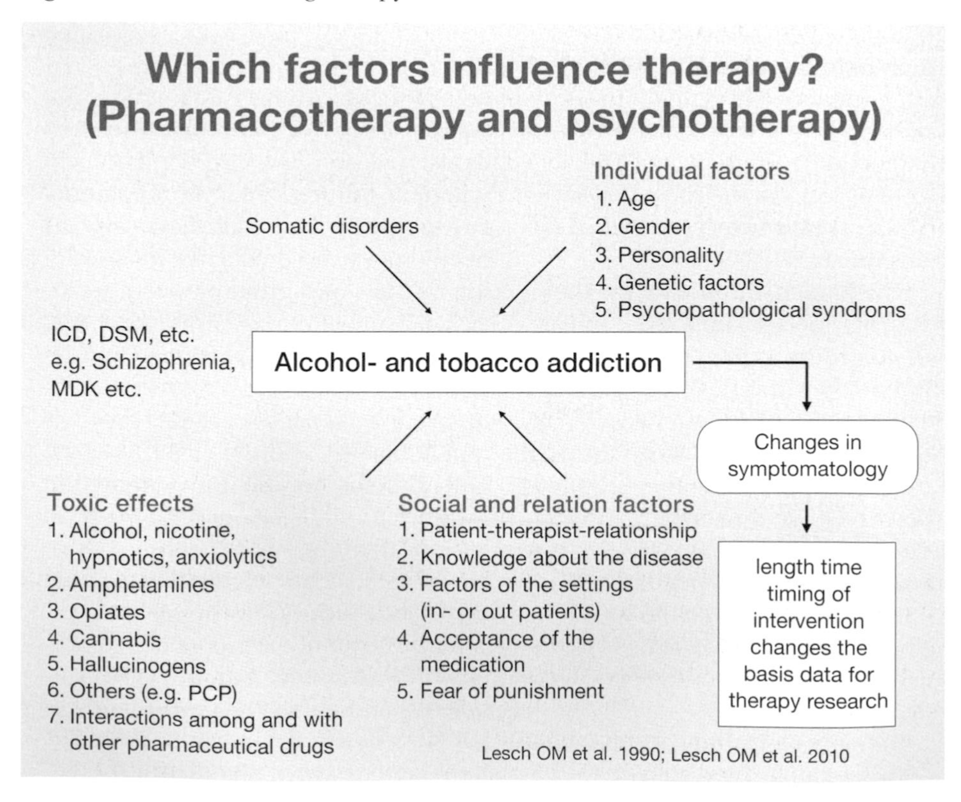

World Health Organisation highlighted the physical, psychological, social and economic consequences of excessive drinking. An expert commission of the WHO suggested in 1977 a distinction between alcohol addiction and alcohol-related sequelae. The symptoms of addiction were defined by three criteria:

- increase in dosage
- withdrawal symptoms (psychological and physical)
- loss of control over use of the drug.

These three criteria are still part of the ICD-10- and DSM-IV diagnostic criteria, although with regards to the development of ICD-11 and DSM-V, there is still considerable discussion about whether an increase in dosage should remain a symptom of addiction. (The problem is that all tobacco and alcohol consumers increase their intake/dosage over time whether or not they have an addiction). About 1977, a distinction between alcohol abuse and alcohol addiction was established and this differentiation is found today in all current classification systems. It is now widely accepted that the term "abuse" depends on socio-cultural factors. Temperance societies, such as those found in Scandinavian countries or the US, define every immoderate use as an abuse (e. g. "one-off drunk driving " or "smoking a cigarette" already meets the criteria for abuse), while alcohol permissive and alcohol producing countries use this term more broadly. The first high-level use, taken over longer periods of time, is defined as abuse. This fact is often mirrored in the definition of an alcohol unit. In Northern Europe, eight grams of alcohol per unit are allowed, whereas Mediterranean countries typically consider twelve grams as a unit. Within the definition of addiction, the consumption of an addictive drug is accepted as an epiphenomenon. This is why the ICD-10 criteria, for example, code the addictive drug only as secondary. Only in a few cases does abuse turn into an addiction. Usually abuse remains a stable behaviour over many years (Widiger TA et al. 1994).

5.3 Substance related diagnoses in the ICD-10

The WHO has developed the ICD classification system on the basic principle that a person can only be called healthy if he/she doesn't suffer from somatic illness, is psychologically healthy and has a stable and supportive social network. To achieve this goal, the WHO is trying to support prevention programmes and the health care systems of many countries. With the introduction of the ICD-10 (Dilling H et al. 1991) hospitals were advised to "follow the general rule to code as many diagnoses as required for the description of the clinical image/condition. If there is more than one diagnosis, a primary diagnosis with the "highest significance for therapy and development" should be made. The ICD-10 captures addicts with all their sequelae (somatic-psychiatric), development and therapeutic settings. Under F1 all psychological and behavioural disorders which are caused by psychotropic substances, are coded. Secondly, the addictive substance is indicated (F10 dysfunctions caused by alcohol, F17 dysfunctions caused by tobacco). The fourth and fifth points describe the clinical image (F10.00-07 or F17.00-07), the acute intoxication with or without complications, the damaging use (F10.1, F17.1) or the addiction syndrome (F10.2, F17.2). These points will be discussed further below; other points to be considered include drinking behaviour, withdrawal symptoms, psychotic dysfunctions, amnesic syndromes and other psychological or behavioural dysfunctions. This more precise specification should allow comparisons between different countries and should lead to therapeutic thinking such as: "Does this group of patients need hospitalization?" "Which clinical profession offers the best therapeutic setting?" etc.

5.3.1 Harmful use (ICD 10 F10.1, F 17.1)

A pattern of psychoactive substance use that is causing damage to health.

The damage may be physical (as in cases of hepatitis from the self-administration of injected psychoactive substances) or mental (e.g. episodes of depressive disorder secondary to the heavy consumption of alcohol).

Psychoactive substance abuse
Diagnostic criteria

A. Clear evidence that the substance use was responsible for (or substantially contributed to) physical or psychological harm, including impaired judgement or dysfunctional behaviour.
B. The nature of the harm should be clearly identifiable (and specified).
C. The pattern of use has persisted for at least one month or has occurred repeatedly within a twelve-month period.
D. The disorder does not meet the criteria for any other mental or behavioural disorder related to the same drug in the same time period (except for acute intoxication ICD 10 F1x.0).

5.3.2 Dependence syndrome (ICD 10 F10.2, F 17.2)

A cluster of behavioural, cognitive, and physiological phenomena that develop after repeated substance use and that typically include a strong desire to take the drug, difficulties in controlling its use, persistent use despite harmful consequences, a higher priority given to drug use than to other activities and obligations, increased tolerance and sometimes a physical withdrawal state.

The dependence syndrome may be present for a specific psychoactive substance (e.g. tobacco, alcohol, or diazepam), for a class of substances (e.g. opioid drugs), or for a wider range of pharmacologically different psychoactive substances.

Diagnostic criteria
Three or more of the following manifestations should have occurred together for at least one month or, if they have persisted for periods of less than one month, then they should have occurred together repeatedly within a twelve month period.

(1) A strong desire or sense of compulsion to take the substance.
(2) Impaired capacity to control substance-taking behaviour in terms of onset, termination or level of use, as evidenced by the substance often being taken in larger amounts or over a longer period than intended, or any unsuccessful effort, or persistent desire, to cut down or control substance use.

(3) A physiological withdrawal state (see F1x.3 and F1x.4) when substance use is reduced or ceased, as evidenced by the characteristic withdrawal syndrome for the substance, or use of the same (or closely related) substance with the intention of relieving or avoiding withdrawal symptoms.
(4) Evidence of tolerance to the effects of the substance, such that there is a need for markedly increased amounts of the substance to achieve intoxication or desired effect, or that there is a markedly diminished effect with continued use of the same amount of the substance.
(5) Preoccupation with substance use, as manifested by important alternative pleasures or interests being given up or reduced because of substance use; or a great deal of time being spent in activities necessary to obtain the substance, take the substance, or recover from its effects.
(6) Persisting with substance use despite clear evidence of harmful consequences (see ICD 10 F1x.1), as evidenced by continued use when the person was actually aware of, or could be expected to have been aware of the nature and extent of harm.

Specfiers
The diagnosis of the dependence syndrome may be further specified by the following five character codes:

- F1x.20 Currently abstinent
- F1x.200 Early remission
- F1x.201 Partial remission
- F1x.202 Full remission
- F1x.21 Currently abstinent but in a protected environment (e.g. in hospital, in a therapeutic community, in prison etc.)
- F1x.22 Currently on a clinically supervised maintenance or replacement regime [controlled dependence]
- Flx.23 Currently abstinent, but receiving treatment with aversive or blocking drugs (e.g. naltrexone or disulfiram)
- Flx.24 Currently using the substance [active dependence]
- F1x.240 Without physical features
- F1x.241 With physical features

The course of the dependence may be further specified, if desired, as follows:

- Flx.25 Continuous use
- F1x.26 Episodic use [dipsomania]

5.3.3 Withdrawal state (ICD 10 F10.3)

A group of symptoms of variable clustering and severity occurring on absolute or relative withdrawal of a psychoactive substance, after persistent use of that substance. The onset and course of the withdrawal state are time-limited and are related to the type of psychoactive substance and dose being used immediately before cessation or reduction of use. The withdrawal state may be complicated by convulsions.

Diagnostic Criteria
G1. Clear evidence of recent cessation or reduction of substance use, after repeated and usually prolonged and/or high-dose use of that substance.
G2. Symptoms and signs compatible with the known features of a with-

drawal state from the particular substance or substances (see below).

G3. Not accounted for by a medical disorder unrelated to substance use, and not better accounted for by another mental or behavioural disorder.

5.4 Substance-related diagnosis in DSM-IV (American Psychiatric Association. 1994)

As the American Psychiatric Association would like to make the classification system more comparable for research and has acknowledged that psychiatric diagnoses (affective disorder, schizophrenia, addiction) are too general, it was decided to include other categories that are additional to axis I (diagnosis of abuse, addiction, withdrawal syndrome) to be able to better describe the examined groups of patients.

Today it is commonly known that the long-term course of every psychiatric disorder is not only determined by an axis-I-diagnosis, but also by personality characteristics, somatic conditions, the degree of social deprivation and the level of social functioning. This multidimensional approach might be commonly known, but in most publications only axis-I-diagnoses are indicated so that the results usually aren't transferrable to groups who have the same disorder, but different psychosocial positions. A 50-year old homeless person with a drinking problem and with severe liver cirrhosis obviously needs different treatment than a 30-year old depressive drinking woman with a dominant partner who starves his wife emotionally. Every diagnostic process should therefore include all five axes and should at least be described next to the axis-I diagnosis so that the reader knows which group is the one concerned.

5.4.1 DSM-IV and the multidimensional diagnostic in five axes

- Axis I
  Clinical Disorders
  Other Conditions That May Be a Focus of Clinical Attention
  Alcohol and or Tobacco dependence, withdrawal states
- Axis II
  Personality Disorders and Mental Retardation e. g. Antisocial Personality Disorder, Cloninger Personality Dimensions
- Axis III
  General Medical Condition
  Deseases of the Respiratory System, Deseases of the Digestive System
- Axis IV
  Psychosocial and Environmental Factors
  Degree of Social Support, Interactions with the Legal System, Occupational Problems, Housing Problems, Oeconomic Problems
- Axis V
  Global Assessment of Functioning

5.4.2 Diagnosis according to DSM-IV axis I

5.4.2.1 Tobacco or alcohol abuse

Friends and family members of the alcoholic are often the first to notice problems and seek professional help. Often, the alcoholic does not realize the severity of the problem or denies it. Some signs cannot go unnoticed, such as loss of a job, family problems, or penalties for driving under the influence of alcohol. Dependence is indicated by symptoms such as withdrawal, injuries from accidents, or blackouts.

The American Psychiatric Association has developed strict criteria for the clinical diagnosis of abuse and dependence.

The *Diagnostic and Statistical Manual-IV (DSM-IV)* defines **abuse** as follows:

Criteria for Alcohol and Tobacco Abuse

- A maladaptive pattern of substance use leading to clinically significant impairment or distress, as manifested by one (or more) of the following, occurring within a 12-month period:
  1. recurrent substance use resulting in a failure to fulfill major role obligations at work, school, home (e.g. repeated absences or poor work performance related to substance use; substance-related absences, suspensions, or expulsions from school; neglect of children or household)
  2. recurrent substance use in situations in which it is physically hazardous (e.g. driving an automobile or operating a machine when impaired by substance use)
  3. recurrent substance-related legal problems (e.g. arrests for substance-related disorderly conduct)
  4. continued substance use despite having persistent or recurrent social or interpersonal problems, caused or exacerbated by the effects of the substance (e.g. arguments with spouse about consequences of intoxication, physical fights)
- B The symptoms have never met the criteria for Substance Dependence for this class of substances.

Most often, abuse is diagnosed in individuals who have recently begun using alcohol. Over time, abuse may progress to dependence. However, some alcohol users abuse alcohol for long periods without developing dependence.

5.4.2.2 Tobacco-alcohol addiction

DSM-IV defines **dependence** as:

Criteria for Substance Dependence

- A maladaptive pattern of substance use, leading to clinically significant impairment or distress, as manifested by three (or more) of the following, occurring at any time in the same 12-month period:
  1. tolerance, as defined by either of the following:
     - a need for markedly increased amounts of the substance to achieve intoxication or desired effect
     - markedly diminished effect with continued use of the same amount of substance
  2. withdrawal, as manifested by either of the following:
     - he characteristic withdrawal syndrome for the substance
     - the same (or a closely related) substance is taken to relieve or avoid withdrawal symptoms

3. the substance is often taken in larger amounts or over a longer period than was intended
4. there is a persistent desire or unsuccessful efforts to cut down or control substance use
5. a great deal of time is spent in activities to obtain the substance, use the substance, or recover from its effects
6. important social, occupational or recreational activities are given up or reduced because of substance use
7. the substance use is continued despite knowledge of having a persistent or recurrent physical or psychological problem that is likely to have been caused or exacerbated by the substance (e.g. continued drinking despite recognition that an ulcer was made worse by alcohol consumption)

5.4.3. Specifiers defining subgroups of dependence

Tolerance and withdrawal may be associated with a higher risk for immediate general medical problems and a higher relapse rate. Specifiers are provided to note their presence or absence:

5.4.3.1 Tolerance and withdrawal

1. With Physiological Dependence. This specifier should be used when Substance Dependence is accompanied by evidence of tolerance (Criterion 1) or withdrawal (Criterion 2).
2. Without Physological Dependence. This specifier should be used when there is no evidence of tolerance (Criterion 1) with withdrawal (Criterion 2). In these individuals, Substance Dependence is characterized by a pattern of compulsive use (at least three items from Criteria 3–7).

5.4.3.2 Course specifiers

Early Full Remission

- Early Partial Remission
- Sustained Full Remission
- Sustained Partial Remission
- On Agonist Therapy
- In a Controlled Environment

Six course specifiers are available for Substance Dependence. The four Remission specifiers can be applied only after none of the criteria for Substance Dependence or Substance Abuse have been present for at least one month. The definition of these four types of Remission is based on the interval of time that has elapsed since the cessation of Dependence (Early versus Sustained Remission) and whether there is a continued presence of one or more of the items included in the criteria sets for Dependence or Abuse (Partial versus Full Remission). A diagnosis of Substance Abuse is preempted by the diagnosis of Substance Dependence if the individual's pattern of substance use has at any point met the criteria for Dependence for that class of substances.

Early Remission: Because the first 12 months following Dependence is a time of particularly high risk for relapse, this period is designated Early Remission. There are two categories:

- Early Full Remission: This specifier is used if, for at least 1 month,

but for less than 12 months, no criteria for Dependence or Abuse have been met.
- Early Partial Remission: This specifier is used if, for at least 1 month, but less than 12 months, one or more criteria for Dependence or Abuse have been met (but the full criteria for Dependence have not been met).

Sustained Remission:
After 12 months of Early Remission have passed without relapse to Dependence, the person enters into Sustained Remission. There are two categories: Sustained Full Remission: this specifier is used, if none of the criteria for Dependence or Abuse have been met at any time during a period of 12 months or longer. Sustained Partial Remission: this specifier is used if full criteria for Dependence have not been met for a period of 12 months or longer; however, one or more criteria for Dependence or Abuse have been met.

5.4.4 Therapeutic approach

The following specifiers apply if the individual is on agonist therapy or in a controlled environment:

- On Agonist Therapy: This specifier is used if the individual is on a prescribed agonist medication, and no criteria for Dependence or Abuse have been met for that class of medication for at least the past month (except tolerance to, or withdrawal from, the agonist). This category also applies to those being treated for dependence using a partial agonist or an agonist/antagonist.
- In a Controlled Environment: This specifier is used if the individual is in an environment where access to alcohol and controlled substances is restricted, and no criteria for Dependence or Abuse have been met for at least the past month. Examples of these environments are closely supervised and substance-free jails, therapeutic communities, or locked hospital units.

5.4.5 Withdrawal symptoms of tobacco and alcohol

After prolonged abuse of alcohol and/or tobacco, reduction or cessation of intake often lead to maladaptive behavioural changes with psychological and cognitive concomitants. Alcohol and tobacco produce different symptoms during withdrawal and it is important to establish that the 'withdrawal' is really substance related before the definition can be applied. During withdrawal, craving is important and, especially in smoking, a main cause of relapse. In alcohol withdrawal, the leading symptoms are tremor, hyperhidrosis and agitation.

Criteria for alcohol/tobacco withdrawal

A. The development of an alcohol/tobacco-specific syndrome due to the cessation of (or reduction in) substance use that has been heavy and prolonged.
B. The alcohol/tobacco-specific syndrome causes clinically significant distress or impairment in social, occupational, or other important areas of functioning.
C. The symptoms are not due to a general medical condition and are

not better accounted for by another mental disorder.

5.5 Commonalities and differences of ICD-10 and DSM-IV

Both diagnostic systems emphasize that compulsive consumption and the lack of motivation to refrain from addictive drugs are a fundamental part of the diagnosis. Thus, motivational work is always the starting point of every therapy. Furthermore, a further criterion of diagnosis is that the craving for an addictive substance is so strong that it cannot be deliberately or sufficiently reduced. Therefore relapses become an essential part of addiction. The ICD-10 describes "craving" as a strong subjective urge to consume a substance and craving is listed as the first criterion of a diagnosis. This phenomenon is a central symptom of an addiction and is of prime importance for smoking and alcohol, but also for other addictive drugs. The DSM-IV does not put "craving" in the centre of the diagnosis. Strong craving, irrespective of addictive substance, e.g. the urge to gamble or the compelling urge to eat etc., is coded as a behavioural disorder in both classification systems. These monomanias are viewed as completely different phenomena. From my experience, phenomena that can be seen in a gambling addiction, for example, are predominant in a similar way in the interpretations of normal perception. Sometimes pathological perceptions can be found and at times even delusions can be seen. Future classification systems should subsume psychological addictions in the category of impulse control disorders. Discussions of expert panels on DSM-V and ICD-11 are already heading in this direction. In regard to eating disorders, and especially anorexic patients, this delusional system has frequently been described. This classification, which is still under discussion from various perspectives, is particularly important in regard to treatment with anti-craving substances. Yet, craving in both, smoking and drinking is a phenomenon whose strength can vary in the course of addiction. It can be heavily reinforced by situations and emotions and therefore three different kinds of craving need to be differentiated: 1.) Craving to enhance mood. 2.) Craving to inhibit aggravating feelings. 3.) Craving which is supported by situations and other stimuli ("key exposure"; Pavlov's principle). During in-patient therapy craving is rarely reported because drinking has never been conditioned in these institutions (cool spots). The in-patient clinical staff therefore often underrates craving and only 6% of addicts leave their in-patient therapy with an anti-craving medication.

5.6 Implication of these classification systems for therapy and research

5.6.1 Alcohol

Above all, as a result of these far too broad systems of classification, there are various therapeutic approaches which are defined primarily by their organisational backgrounds or an ideological perspective. There is no one method or medication which can consistently claim positive effects (e.g. longer abstinence rates), either from a pharmacological or a psychotherapeutic perspective. Research leading to a definition of an addiction-vulnerable personality can now be viewed as completed (McCord W et al. 1960; Lesch OM. 1985). Sociological research, which tries to explain the addiction process by poverty, unemployment, cultural conditions or "broken-home"situations, is discovering more and more that addiction occurs in all social situations and classes. However, the course of addiction seems to be influenced by social factors and personality dimensions. Biologically based genetic research ranging from pharmacological studies on animals to therapy studies of addicts consistently delivers positive results and highlights are published in leading journals which, however, are then either not replicable or are refuted by other research groups (Koob GF and Le Moal M. 2006).

Pharmacotherapy research has clearly shown that the recommended detox medication in the case of alcohol depends on the patient's socio-cultural background, medical care system and, last but not least, the selection criteria which indicate which subgroup of addicts should be treated by which medication, for example, in France with Diazepam and Meprobamat, in Germany with Clometiazol, Tiapride and Carbamazepine, and in Italy with Gammahydroxibutanoic acid and Baclofen. In Austria, it can be clearly seen that Benzodiazepines are used particularly in intensive care units, while Tiapride and Carbamazepine are mostly used in psychiatric hospitals. Meprobamate is also still prescribed although no longer recommended in the literature. Currently it is being taken off the market in Austria (Lesch OM et al. 2010). At the Medical University of Vienna, Department of Psychiatry, withdrawal medications are used according to specific subgroups (see chapter 9.3). Hester RK and Miller WR have compiled therapy methods which are internationally used as relapse prophylaxis. If examples of medication, psychotherapy and sociotherapy are chosen from this book, it should be recognized that there is no method with completely positive data. Today, Disulfiram, Naltrexone and Acamprosate are the primary medications used for relapse prophylaxis.

5.6.1.1 Studies on pharmacotherapy in relapse prevention (according to Hester RK and Miller WR 2003)

Fig. 24 Studies on Disulfiram used for relapse prevention in alcohol addicts

Disulfiram

16 studies of good quality:

- **6 studies – positive results, few relapses** (Fuller RK et al. 1986; Caroll KM et al. 2000; Azrin NH et al. 1982; Chick J et al. 1992; Wilson A et al. 1978 and 1980)
- **6 studies – negative results, increased relapses** (Aliyev NN. 1993; Ling W et al. 1983; Powell BJ et al. 1985; Johnsen J et al. 1987; Dahlgren L and Willander A. 1989; Johnsen and Morland J. 1991)
- **4 studies – no significant changes in the rate of relapses** (Ludwig A et al. 1969; Miller WR et al. 2001; Smith JE et al. 1998; Fuller RK and Roth HP, 1979)

Fig. 25 Studies on Naltrexone and Acamprosate for relapse prevention in alcohol addiction

Naltrexone and Acamprosate

Several studies show that Naltrexone and Acamprosate significantly improve the relapse rates (Volpicelli et al. 1992; O'Malley et al. 1992; Geerlings et al. 1995; Pelc et al. 1997; Sass et al. 1996; Whitworth et al. 1996).

Several studies show no effect of Naltrexone and Acamprosate (Gastpar et al. 2002; Krystal et al. 2001; Chick et al. 2000; Mason et al. 2001).

Conclusion from the existent studies:
Acamprosate prolongs the duration of abstinence, while Naltrexone ameliorates the severity and the duration of the drinking episodes.

5.6.1.2 Studies on relapse prevention using psychotherapy

Controlled studies of individual or group psychotherapy show surprisingly consistent, negative results in regard to relapse prophylaxis. An exception is Client-centred Therapy according to Rogers CR (1951). Confrontational psychotherapeutic methods, like those used for a while in the USA, show continuously negative results. "Motivational in-

Fig. 26 Studies on psychotherapy used for relapse prevention in alcohol addicts

Psychotherapy

6 studies of good quality:

- **4 studies – negative results, increased relapses** (Wells-Parker E et al. 1988; Peniston EG and Kulkosky PJ. 1989; Bowers TG and Al-Redha MR. 1990; Formigoni MLOS and Neumann BRG. 1995)
- **2 studies – no significant changes in relapse rate** (Ludwig A et al. 1969; Oejehagen A et al. 1992).

13 studies of low quality:

- **2 studies – positive results, few relapses** (Rhead JC et al. 1977; Smith TL et al. 1999)
- **3 studies – negative results, increases relapses** (Conrad KJ et al. 1998; Swenson PR et al. 1981; Olson RP et al. 1981)
- **8 studies – no significant changes in relapses** (Potamianos G et al.1986; Kish GB et al. 1980; Sandahl C et al. 1998; Glotzbach LD. 1984; Johnson FG. 1970; Bruun K. 1963; Jacobson NO and Silfverskiold NP. 1973; Zimberg S. 1974)

terviewing", according to Miller WR and Rollnick S., in combination with client-centred therapy, however, has shown the best results (Miller WR and Rollnick S. 2002).

Social learning and behavioural therapeutic learning methods are often used for self-monitoring. Here the data are also equivocal.

Research on sociotherapy also shows varied results, as can be seen, for example, in milieu therapy or participation in AA groups. These results can be explained by the heterogeneity of patients included in these studies. Therefore it is absolutely necessary to identify homogeneous subgroups of patients, for which specific therapy methods should be made available. For more than 100 years, attempts have been made to describe the various dimensions of addiction and the specific therapies which should be used to treat them. Practising therapists often use catchphrases like

Fig. 27 Studies on behavioural therapy for relapse prevention in alcohol addicts

Behavioural therapeutic learning for self-control

22 studies of good quality:

- **7 studies – positive results, less relapses** (Harris KB and Miller WR. 1990; Brown RA. 1980; Alden LE. 1988; Baker TB et al. 1975; Sobell MB and Sobell LC. 1973; Caddy GR and Lovibond SH. 1976; Hester RK and Delaney HD. 1997)
- **2 studies – negative results, increase of relapses** (Connors GJ et al. 1992; Foy DW et al. 1984)
- **13 studies – no significant changes in relapse rate** (Miller WR et al. 1980b; Robertson I et al. 1986; Baldwin S et al. 1991; Alden L. 1980; Vogler RE et al. 1977; Miller WR et al. 1981; Pomerleau O et al. 1978; Sanchez-Craig M et al. 1989; Skutle A and Berg G. 1987; Miller WR. 1978; Sanchez-Craig M. et al. 1984; 1991; Miller WR and Taylor CA. 1980a)

Fig. 28 Studies on relapse prevention in alcohol addicts with "social learning" therapy

Social learning

8 studies of good quality:

- **4 studies – positive results, less relapses** (Azrin NH et al. 1982; Chaney ER et al. 1978; Erikson L et al. 1986; West PT. 1979)
- **1 study – negative results, increase of relapses** (Sannibale C. 1989)
- **3 studies – no significant changes in number of relapses** (Oei TPS and Jackson PR. 1982; Cooney NL et al. 1991; Miller WR et al. 1980b)

"dimensional diagnostic" and "dimension-related therapy" or therapy according to the patient's resources. These therapists define the patient's treatable resources and in treating these, try to improve the course of disease.

Principally, there is no reason why dimensional or resource-based therapy should not be used, especially when one is in the midst of a long-term therapeutic process with a patient. However, one should not forget that there are generally accepted rules for the pratice of psychiatric therapy and for the processes of therapy of addicted individuals that have proven themselves over many years (Berner P et al. 1986; Bleuer M. 1983; Feuerlein W. 1989; Lenz G. and Kuefferle B. 2002; Lesch OM et al. 2010; Moeller HJ. 1993; Rommelspacher H and Schuckit M. 1996; Uexkuell Tv. 1996).

If one choses not to use an "evidence-based" therapy, justification for not having done so in the specific case concerned, should be documented. The large American study Project MATCH included abusers and addicts and no specific therapy method was found that genuinely fits or benefits a groups' profile.

5.6.1.3 Family psychotherapy

As every therapist who is trained in systemic therapy knows, drinking behaviour and how one handles alcohol is only understood as part of the person's systemic relationships and systemic equilibrium. In systemic therapy, diagnosis is of little or no significance.

The medication that is used to manage withdrawal, relapse prophylaxis and for treatment of a relapse can show considerable differences across patients. In order to appropriately assess these effects it is very important to

Fig. 29 Studies on the relapse prevention in alcohol addicts who take part in AA groups and milieu therapy

AA-Groups

3 studies of good quality:

- **2 studies – negative results, increase of relapses** (Ditman KS et al. 1967; Brandsma JM et al. 1980)
- **1 study – no significant changes in the number of relapses** (Walsh DC et al. 1991)

Milieu therapy

6 studies of good quality:

- **2 studies – negative results, increase of relapses** (Chapman PLH and Huygens I. 1988; Longabaugh R et al. 1983)
- **4 studies – no significant changes in the number of relapses** (McLachlan JFC and Stein RL. 1982; Pittman DJ and Tate RL. 1972; Rychtarik RG et al. 2000; Edwards G and Guthrie S. 1967).

clearly define patient groups with different types of biological dysfunctions which can be favourably treated by medication.

5.6.2 Tobacco

A variety of clinical studies from both the medical and psychological fields also support the heterogeneity of Tobacco-addiction. It has been repeatedly confirmed that clear medical advice for subgroups of addicts – 20–30 % are indicated in the literature – significantly reduces the number of cigarettes smoked per day and may even completely stop smoking (Fiore MC et al. 2000; US Department of Health and Human Services; World Health Organization 2003; Henningfield JE et al. 2005).

Pharmacological therapy, especially nicotine supplements and antidepressants like Bupropion, Nortryptiline and Doxepin, is used, as the effectiveness of these agents is generally accepted. The fact that nicotine supplements are only effective in Fagerstroem positive smokers and antidepressants primarily in tobacco addicts with low Fagerstroem scores, once more demonstrates the heterogeneity of addiction, including nicotine (Benowitz NL et al. 1988; Shiffman S et al. 1996; Henningfield JE et al. 2005; Sweeney CT. et al. 2001; Tonnesen P. et al. 1999; Le Foll B. et al. 2005; J. Clin Psychiatry Monograph 2003; National Institute for Clinical Excellence 2004; Lerman C et al. 2004; Fiore MC. et al. 2000; Scharf D and Shiffman S. 2004; Shiffman S. et al. 2000; Jorenby DE et al. 2004; Ferry LH. 1999; Prochazka AV et al. 1998; Hall SM et al. 1998; Edwards NB. et al. 1988; Murphy JK et al. 1990).

In recent clinical trials, two new classes of medications seem to provide interesting results. Varenicline is effective for those patients in which the vulnerability of the nicotine receptor is the essential pathological factor.

Varenicline is a partial nicotine receptor agonist (Alpha4Beta2). This selectivity leads us to expect that its effectiveness as a nicotine substitute is considerably greater for some smokers. However, smokers in whom other subunits of the receptor play a role might profit less. Clinical studies showed a duplication of abstinence rates and therefore 1 mg Varenicline twice daily can be described for nicotine withdrawal and nicotine craving (Fagerstroem score 5 or more) (Tonstad S. et al. 2006; Zierler-Brown SL and Kyle JA. 2007; Oncken C. et al. 2006; Williams KE. et al. 2007; Coe JW et al. 2005; Gonzales DH. et al. 2006; Cochrane Review Cahill K et al. 2007). In a study comparing Varenicline with Bupropion 150 mg and placebo, the former clearly showed better results. This effect could also be demonstrated 53 weeks later. In a review (Cahill K et al.) of Varenicline, the data for daily practice were summarized as follows:

1. Varenicline improves smoking behaviour three times better than placebo, also in the long run.
2. In smokers, Varenicline is superior to Bupropion. Studies that combine Varenicline and other therapeutic methods are still lacking and most research groups agree that the administration of Varenicline for smoking withdrawal needs further examination.

Other subgroups of tobacco addicts could have vulnerabilities in the CB1-

receptor system and there are data about CB1-antagonists (Rimonabant) which support an amelioration of impulse control in eating, alcohol and smoking. A clinical definition of this subgroup is however still lacking. Studies included occasional smokers as well as smokers with a Fagerstroem-score of five or more and results show a twice as high abstinence rate with simultaneous weight loss, not only in comparison to placebo but also to Bupropion (Despres JP et al. 2005; Pi-Sunyer FX et al. 2006; Cohen C et al. 2002; Anthenelli R. 2004; Klesges RC et al. 1997; Klesges RC et al. 1989; Soyka M. et al. 2007). Based upon our own research, we found that antidepressants are especially effective in the subgroup using tobacco as an antidepressant. Women clearly smoke more frequently because of a chronic depressive mood and for weight control. Our data showed that these subgroups of tobacco addicts respond to 20 mg of Rimonabant daily (Lesch OM et al. 2004; Lesch OM. 2007). The warnings in regard to depressive reactions of Rimonabant need further study. The impact of the absence of tobacco, with its antidepressant effects, should be viewed separately. (see chapter 9.6.8.1.8).

The utilisation of psychotherapy for tobacco addicts is only well studied in relation to behavioural therapeutic approaches. Behavioural therapy self-control techniques paired with strategies for relapse prevention have shown average long-term success rates of 25–30 % abstinence (Hanewinkel, Burow, Ferstl. 1996; Hughes JR. 2000; Prochaska J and DiClemente C. 1992; Schoberberger R. 2006, 2002; Batra A. 2005; Kienast T et al. 2007). Again, these results support the heterogeneity of tobacco addiction and there are data to suggest that tobacco addicts can be grouped into four clusters or subgroups as well, although the craving mechanisms for tobacco vs. alcohol should be viewed differently (see chapter 9.2; European Smoker Classification System – Appendix 2; Lesch OM. 2007).

Over the last 100 years, these craving mechanisms have been extensively investigated, leading to different definitions of types of alcohol and tobacco addicts. These different types of addiction obviously have a different aetiological course and development and therefore need very different therapies. These more specific classifications of homogeneous types of addicts have a stronger validity than just the diagnosis "addiction". Those classifications help guide the initial treatment plan for the addicts and are helpful for medical intervention, for motivating the patient and also for classification into a psychotherapeutic school of thought. Most addicts do not want intensive psychotherapy and often stay with the general practitioner or with social agencies. In relation to the psychotherapeutic process, patient characteristics, his ability to cope with stress and other resources of the patients are clearly more important than the psychiatric diagnosis.

6

Types, dimensions and aetiology

6.1 Alcohol addiction

6.1.1 Development of typology research

As already emphasized in the last chapter, it has long been known that alcohol dependents are not a homogenous group. Studies that have used the DMS-IV in order to categorize alcohol dependents into groups were able to show that the majority of patients either have a second axis-I or an axis-II diagnosis or both an axis-I and an axis-II diagnosis.

A research group lead by Driessen M. described the high co-morbidity on axis-I and axis-II in several studies. More than 50% of the patients show psychiatric co-morbidity with 24% having an additional diagnosis on axis I. In addition, 17.2% have a further axis-I dysfunction as well as another axis-II-dysfunction and 16.4% have, next to the diagnosis of alcohol dependence, an axis-II diagnosis (Zimmermann P et al. 2003; Driessen M et al. 2001).

Due to this heterogeneity, attempts have been made to categorize subgroups of alcohol dependents, in such a way that factors such as drinking history, consumption of other drugs, biographical information and other psychiatric disorders, sequelae or personality disorders are taken into consideration. These factors were usually recorded only once during in-patient admission and lead to very different typologies according to the researcher's point of view and the criteria for selected patients. The number of subgroups of the alcohol dependent typology's ranged from two to ten, but nowadays there is consensus that a four-cluster solution should be preferred. Four groups seem to be most suitable for basis research and therapy (Hesselbrock VM and Hesselbrock MN. 2006).

Typology according to Jellinek

The drinking behaviour-based typology according to Jellinek (Jellinek EM. 1960), which has established itself internationally due to its simplicity, was neither able to support basis research, nor provide information for therapy. Yet this typology was very important for the development of diagnostic methods and especially for the WHO in defining dependence and abuse. Yet this typology is not mentioned by any recognised journal nor is it documented in any therapy study.

Typology according to Foucault

The French school, which has clearly always taken considerably more account of the aetiology and course of mental disorders than the German speaking psychiatric schools, developed by Foucault M. 1980 and Malka R et al. 1983, a typology which pays special attention to aetiology and sequelae. The type "alcoolite" shows gender differences (about 60 % of male and 5 % of female alcohol dependents). The type "alcoolose" is marked by psychological disorders, often displays an episodic intoxicating drinking behaviour and can be found in type III according to Lesch. Independent of drinking behaviour the type "somaalcoolose" often shows somatic symptoms, like severe polyneuropathy or real epilepsies, and it is very similar to Lesch's type IV.

Multivariate and multidimensional typologies (like e. g. Bleuler M. 1983; Rounsaville BJ. et al. 1987; More LC and Blashfield RK. 1981; Skinner HA. 1982; Tarter REH. et al. 1977) have led to research tools which are suitable for defining different groups of alcohol dependents, but further studies in regard to basis research and therapy of these subgroups are still needed.

6.1.2 Important typologies for research and practice

6.1.2.1 Two-cluster-solutions

6.1.2.1.1 Schuckit's typology

In 1985, Schuckit differentiated between primary and secondary alcoholics. Primary alcoholics don't show any mental disorders before the onset of alcohol abuse, whereas secondary alcoholics show psychological disorders before the onset of alcohol addiction. Secondary alcoholics tried to "treat" these disorders by using alcohol as a form of self-therapy. In regard to this process, Schuckit MA showed that the regression of psychical symptoms like those in anxiety or depression occurs in many patients even without a specific therapy within 14 to 21 days only ofabsolute abstinence (Schuckit MA. 1985).

6.1.2.1.2 Cloninger's typology

As a result of genetic studies, in 1981 Bohman MS. et al. and Cloninger CR. et al. differentiated between two types of alcoholics (Knorring et al. 1985).

Type I according to Cloninger is characterized by varying alcohol abuse (sometimes occasional, sometimes heavy). Their fathers don't show any delinquent behaviour and they belong to the upper classes. The biological mother is often alcohol dependent. Type I dependents according to Cloninger have lesser alcohol-related social problems with less frequent in-patient admittances, and the onset of alcohol dependence occurs after the age of 25. The dependents are easily influenced by their environment ("high reward dependence"), very careful and often react with avoidance behaviour ("high harm avoidance"). They are very reluctant to put themselves in risk situations ("low novelty situations") (Kiefer F et al. 2007).

Cloninger type II patients often have more alcoholics in their family next to their alcohol dependent mother. Type II alcohol dependents according to Cloninger grow up in very difficult social conditions and aggression and violence are frequent factors in these families. The patients can also turn aggressive for minor reasons or no reason at all. They often take other drugs and the addiction process starts before the age of 25. According to Cloninger's personality dimensions they can be characterized by a high readiness to enter risk situations ("high novelty seeking"), a love of unstable life situations ("low harm avoidance") and act like they are very independent from their environment ("low reward dependence"). These types are biologically validated (type II shows a high MAO-activity) and the classification has been used by researchers in therapy studies which showed that Acamprosate and Topiramate show different effects in Cloninger's types (Kiefer F. et al. 2005 and Johnson B. et al. 2004). Cloninger types are continuously used for genetic studies. TypeII patients according to Cloninger show higher heritability than type I patients. Furthermore, type II patients are more frequently admitted into in-patient clinics and suffer from severe mental problems (Van den Bree MBM. et al. 1998; Gilligan SB. et al. 1987).

Cloninger's typology has also been included in several pharmaceutical relapse studies, in which type II clearly shows better results in regard to anti-craving substances. Naltrexone reduces relapses in type II (Kiefer F et al. 2007). Ondansetrone also showed better results in type II (Johnson BA et al. 2000). This data shows that the biological mechanisms of craving are heterogenic in type II and this is in line with Lesch's typology, as type IV shows an early onset of addiction and is defined by severe psychiatric and neurological complications.

6.1.2.1.3 Typology according to Babor

In 1992 Babor TF examined 321 female and male alcohol dependents during their in-patient admission. 17 categories were used for a multi-dimensional classification and he recorded premorbid risk factors, abuse of alcohol, the use of other addictive substances, chronifications in the process and alcohol-related sequelae (Babor TF et al. 1992).

Similar to Cloninger's type, Type A according to Babor shows symptoms such as a late onset of dependence, few problems during childhood and less psychopathological symptoms.

Type B according to Babor has a high prevalence of infantile behaviour disorders and multiple alcoholic members in the family; early manifestation of alcohol addiction symptoms in the individual's life and acute life stress factors can be observed. This group of dependents require lengthier treatment and individuals have often been in in-patient care. The symptomatic is very

Fig. 30 Cloninger Type I and II

Type I	Type II
Onset of alcohol dependence after the age of 25 Men and women Mild alcohol-related sequelae Few problems with aggression and the law Avoidance behaviour in regards to social difficulties Doesn't like surprises	Onset of alcohol dependence before the age 25 Only men Problems with the police and aggressions No avoidance behaviour, but acting out their aggressions High "novelty-seeking" potential

similar to Cloninger's type II. Other authors (e.g. Brown J et al. 1994; Del Boca FK. 1994 Del Boca FK and Hesselbrock MN. 1996) were able to verify these syndromes according to Babor A and Babor B, in their patients.

Babor's typology has also been included in therapy studies in which SSRIs lead to an improvement of the process, especially in type B (Kranzler HR et al. 1996). Only recently, Johnson showed that Ondansetrone significantly reduces the relapse rate especially in "early onset" dependents and in Babor type B (Roache JD et al. 2008).

Since 1992, primarily the team around Schuckit MA has continued to research Babor's typology (e.g. Schuckit MA et al. 1995), whereas other researchers were not able to match some cases with the typologies according to Babor and Cloninger, so that the two-cluster solution was described as not satisfactory by some authors (Hesselbrock VM and Hesselbrock MN.2006).

6.1.2.2 The four-cluster solutions

6.1.2.2.1 Del Bocca and Hesselbrock's typology

Several studies have found that two group solutions seldom fully capture the clinical entity or adequately classify general population samples. The variability in the number of subtypes could be a consequence of the data reduction technique used (e.g., cluster analysis, factor analysis), since most are not governed by prescribed rules. Further, the final solution could also be influenced by a variety of factors including sample characteristics and sample size, availability of clinical information and the theory underlying the original analysis. Depending upon the variables of interest and the number of subjects examined, more recent studies typically identify 3–5 subtypes.

The indeterminate nature of cluster-derived typologies (and a limit of the statistical procedure) is best exemplified by a re-analysis of the Babor et al. data by Del Boca and Hesselbrock (1996). Their results showed four clusters as functional solutions that distinguished alcohol dependent persons along gender and several clinically important dimensions.

Cluster Low Risk/Low Severity (LR/LS)
The largest subtype, containing approximately one third of the cases (39 % of female and 29 % of male) was characterized as relatively Low Risk and Low Severity, while 22 % of female and 22 % of male were classified as High Risk and High Severity. The Low Risk/Low Severity (LR/LS) groups were characterized as having a mild form of alcohol dependence, with a late onset of alcoholism, low alcohol involvement, with no alcoholic family members or co-morbid psychopathology

Cluster High Risk/High Severity (HR/HS)
In contrast, the High Risk/High Severity (HR/HS) group was characterized as having a severe form of alcohol dependence, an early onset of alcohol use and dependence, a positive family history of alcoholism, high alcohol involvement, behaviour problems, poly drug use, depression and antisocial personality disorder. There were no gender differences in terms of the proportions or characteristics of subjects among both mild and severe forms of alcohol dependence.

Two other identified clusters can be characterized as moderate forms of alcohol dependence and were labelled as Internalizing and Externalizing groups. Gender specific differences were found for both groups.

Cluster Internalizing type
The Internalizing type included a higher proportion of women (32 %) than men (11 %). This group was characterized as depressed, anxious, and having severe alcohol dependence. They also reported medical and/or physical problems resulting from chronic alcohol use, but a moderate family history of alcoholism risk.

Cluster Externalizing type
The Externalizing subtype was predominantly male (38 % of men and 7 % of women) and was characterized as having a moderate alcoholism family history risk, high levels of alcohol use, social consequences and antisocial personality, but no depression or anxiety disorders.

While many studies of alcoholic typologies do not have long term follow-up or treatment outcome data, subjects in the Del Boca and Hesselbrock's study completed one and three year follow-up interviews. In addition, 25-year mortality data have also been obtained. At the one year follow up, the majority of men in the Externalizing, High Risk/High Severity and Internalizing clusters relapsed to regular drinking and/or sought treatment of alcohol problems (86 %, 74 %, and 72 % respectively) while a little over half (56 %) of men in the Low Risk/Low Severity group reported regular drinking and/or seeking treatment. Among women, five of six who were classified as Externalizers relapsed to regular drinking or received treatment. The remaining subtypes of women fared better; the rates of relapse to regular drinking or treatment ranged from 52 % to 57 % of women in the other three clusters.

At the three-year post-discharge follow-up, a similar trend continued to be found. Both the High Risk/High Severity group and the External group continued to report high rates of relapse to drinking for both the men and women, while the men, regardless of their cluster assignment, tended to report higher rates of relapse than the women. Nearly 4 out of 5 men in the HR/HS group and the Externalizing group continued to relapse to regular drinking or receiving treatment, as compared to approximately half of the men in the LR/LS and the Internalizing groups. There were no differences in the rates of relapse among women by cluster subgroups. Regardless of their cluster assignment, approximately half of the women were either abstinent or engaged only in occasional drinking at the three-year follow-up. However, the number of women in each cluster was small and these findings should be interpreted with caution.

A 25-year post-treatment follow-up of this sample was made through a search of the Social Security Death Index records, death certificates and autopsy results. An overall crude death rate as of December 2005 was 45.7 % for men and 41.7 % for women. The crude death rate was highest among the "Low Risk/Low Severity"(53.0 %) and "Internalizing"(55.6 %) clusters for men and Low Risk/Low Severity cluster for women. Both men and women in the High Risk/High Severity cluster had the lowest crude death rates (29.4 and 21.1 % respectively). These crude death rates are reflective of the discrepancy in the different clusters' ages at the time of their admission to the treatment centre (baseline). The average age of the HR/HS group was youngest at admission, 27.7 years old, followed by the Externalizing and Internalizing groups (40.5 yrs and 40.0 yrs respectively), with LR/LS group being the oldest (44.7 years). Consequently, the age of death for the HR/HS group was youngest, 49.5 yrs for men and 47.8 yrs for women, followed by the Externalizing group (58.6 yrs for men and 53.8 yrs for women). The LR/LS group had the oldest age of death (62.8 for men and 60.2 for women). The available death certificates were reviewed by two physicians and classified into three categories: definitely related to alcohol, definitely not related to alcohol, cannot be determined. The two reviewers were mostly in agreement, but in a few cases, a third person was asked to review the certificates and discuss his reviews with the other two to determine the appropriate category. Among those subjects whose deaths could be determined, 6 of 7 HR/HS men's deaths were alcohol related. Approximately half of the Externalizing and LR/LS men's deaths were related to alcohol, while less than half of the Internalizing group deaths were related to the use of alcohol. There were no statistically significant differences in alcohol-related deaths by cluster among women. Approximately 50 % of all deaths were related to alcohol among all clusters, but the number of women whose cause of death could be determined was too small for meaningful analysis (the number ranged 0 to 6).

We were able to determine the manner of death for 117 subjects. Most subjects died of natural causes (86 % for men and 80 % for women). The suicide rate was higher among women than men (17 % vs 8 %), while accidental death was slightly higher among men than women (6 % vs. 3 %). Among the 7 men who committed suicide, three men each were from the Externalizer and Internalizer groups, while one man was from LR/LS subgroup. Among the 5 women who committed suicide, three were from the Internalizer group and two from the LR/LS groups.

In order to adjust for the variation in age among the four cluster groups, a standard mortality ratio (SMR) was calculated for each cluster by gender using the State of Connecticut mortality table for1980 to 2005. Overall, the SMR was quite high, with the rate for women being much higher than that of men (5.41 (CF 3.77–7.52) for women vs 2.82 (CF 2.30–3.43) for men). The SMR was highest among High Risk/High Severity group men and women (4.72 for men and 6.60 for women). The SMR was also high among men in the Externalizing group (3.18 (2.27–4.33)), while the SMR for both Low Risk/Low Severity and the Internalizing clusters were similar and the lowest (2.42 and 2.09). Unlike the men, the SMR was also high among Low Risk/Low Severity and Internalizing cluster women. However, the results for women could be biased since the number of women in each cluster was very small.

As expected, the grouping of alcohol dependent persons into more homogeneous clusters provided important information regarding the long-term course of alcohol dependence among treated persons. The High Risk, High Severity group was particularly associated with early onset alcohol dependence, severe multiple addictions, psychiatric co-morbidity at baseline, one-year and three-year follow-ups, and impacted on long term survival.

These findings again demonstrate the potential clinical importance of grouping patients into homogeneous clusters since different clusters/typologies do present with different clinical symptom profiles and have different short and long-term prognoses,and such different types of alcoholics also require different treatment plans.

6.1.2.2.2 Windle and Scheidt's typology
These authors also identified four clusters of addiction by using a similar method of data collection as the one used by Babor. They defined a mild progression with multiple addictive drugs and compared this to an alcohol addiction with a depressive symptomatic and a chronic progression with an antisocial personality disorder.

Cluster 1
The mild progression showed less infantile behavioural disorders and a later onset of alcohol addiction with this group drinking less than the other group. Additionally withdrawal syndromes occurred.

Cluster 2
In cluster 2 the highest concomitant use of other addictive drugs, especially Benzodiazepines was found.

Cluster 3
In cluster 3 the most acute manifestation of affective and anxiety disorders was found.

Cluster 4
In cluster 4 the highest level of alcohol abuse in regard to both amount and duration was found.

These clusters showed significant gender differences. In Cluster 4 significantly more men have been defined, whereas more women were defined in clusters 1–3. These clusters are in line with the clusters described by Zucker RA. and Gomberg E, Schuckit MA, Del Boca FK and Hesselbrock MN, Hesselbrock VM and Lesch OM. (Hesselbrock VM. and Hesselbrock MN 2006).

6.1.2.2.3 Foroud's typology
In 1998, Foroud T defined alcohol dependents according to the disease's severity and also described four clusters: patients with almost no alcohol-related sequelae, patients with a minor problematic, a group with medium severity and a group with serious dysfunctions in psycho-socio-biological areas. This classification was also used for genetic studies, however no replicated data is available yet (Foroud T et al. 1998).

6.1.3 Assessment of severity in different dimensions

Besides the establishment of definitions and typologies, attempts have been made for several years to describe the severity of addictive diseases according to several dimensions. The research tools which are required for this, also assess the intensity of the dimensional therapeutic intervention. In particular McLellan AT.'s Addiction Severity Index (ASI) has established itself internationally and in Austria the multidimensional diagnostic by Scholz H is an approved method (McLellan AT et al. 1980; Scholz H. 1996).

6.1.3.1 Addiction Severity Index (ASI)

The ASI divides severity into seven dimensions and defines whether therapy is needed for these specific areas. This

Fig. 31 Addiction severity index (ASI)

Problems	0	1	2	3	4	5	6	7	8	9
physical										
work/expenses										
alcohol										
drugs										
legal										
family/social										
psychological										

0–1	No real problem, no treatment needed
2–3	Minimal problem, possibly no treatment required
4–5	Medium problem, treatment recommended
6–7	High problem, treatment required
8–9	Extreme problem, treatment absolutely required

instrument was developed in the United States and has been adopted in most European countries.

In 2003, Van den Brink stated that a consensus conference of the ECNP in Nizza suggested that all therapy studies on addictive diseases and of course alcohol addiction should use the ASI to ensure that the studies' results from different countries are more comparable. A German language validated version has already been published (Gsellhofer E-M et al. 1993, 1999; van den Brink W et al. 2006).

6.1.3.2 Syndrome diagnosis according to Scholz

In Austria, five dimensions to capture addictive diseases have been proposed by Scholz H.

These strategies are summarized in the book "Syndrome related therapy of alcoholism" by Scholz H (1996). The assessment according to Scholz has also been compared with Lesch's typology. As the types according to Lesch show different profiles, this typology can also be assigned to the method according to Scholz (see chapter 6.3; Lesch OM and Walter H. 2006).

Most of these typologies showed, that they are able to define more homogenous groups of patients than it is

Fig. 32 Diagnosis of syndromes according to Scholz

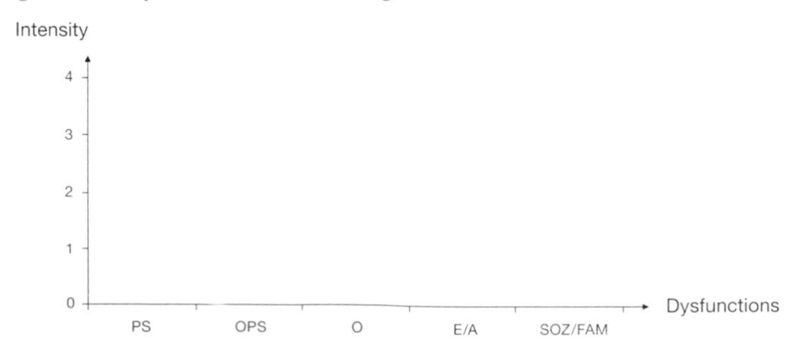

PS:	Actual psychopathological syndrome and basic disturbances
OPS:	Cognitive impairment
O:	Other organ diseases
E/A:	Lack of insight, defensive attitude, lack of motivation
FAM/SOZ:	Family-/social problems

possible to achieve through the diagnosis of addiction according to DSM-IV and ICD-10. Yet, many of these typologies were only described cross-sectionally and psychological, biological and therapeutic validations that record the stability of these types over time are lacking. All these typologies agree about the existence of an acute chronic progression type, a mild progression without serious sequelae, a cluster in which alcohol is used as an anti-depressant and anxiolytic. Furthermore, they agree that the development of an anti-social personality, together with the complicating factors of an alcohol addiction, has its' own pattern of progression.

In their article on subgroups of alcoholics, Hesselbrock VM. and Hesselbrock MN. call for an examination of these clusters in regard to their genetic vulnerability, biological aetiology and in terms of their stability and treatability. As a result, such examinations could lead to detections of the clusters' aetiologies and psychological and pharmacological therapies could then be examined in long-term settings (Lesch OM and Walter H.1996; Kadden RM et al. 2001; Basu D et al. 2004; Kranzler HR et al. 1996).

6.2 Tobacco addiction

6.2.1 Smoking typology according to Schoberberger and Kunze

From a psychiatric perspective, research on tobacco dependence is in its early stages and, so far, specialists in internal medicine, especially pulmonary physicians, have dealt with tobacco research. Social medicine has described subgroups of alcohol addicts according to the Jellinek scheme in regard to their smoking behavior (Schoberberger R and Kunze M. 1999).

Fig. 33 Types of smokers according to Schoberberger R and Kunze M

What kind of smoker are you?

Do you smoke regularly throughout the day, e.g. every half or every hour?

You don't have any desire to smoke throughout the day, but only in certain situations, in which you smoke several cigarettes?

Your smoking is regularly throughout the day and in certain situations you smoke more top?

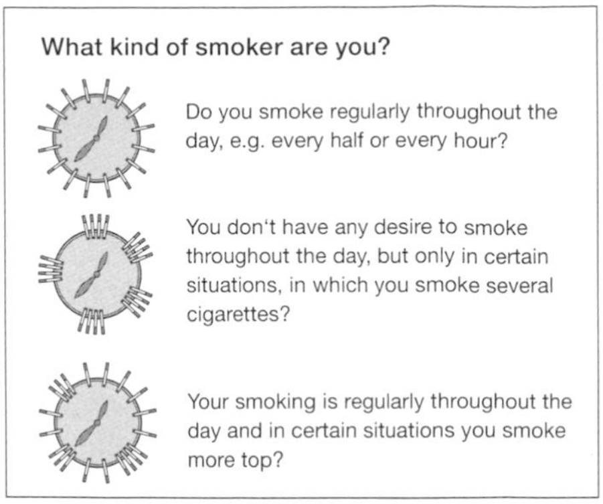

"Level-smokers"

This term describes smokers who smoke evenly throughout the day on a regular basis.

"Peak smokers"

Peak smokers usually smoke few or no cigarettes, but when they get into a stressful situation they smoke a lot within a short time.

Most patients belong to mixed types between these two groups.

About 60 % of smokers are unhappy with their smoking habits (dissonant smokers) and would like to stop or at least reduce their smoking (Schoberberger R and Kunze M. 1999).

6.2.2 Smoking Typology according to Fagerstroem

In 1989, Fagerstroem KO and Schneider NG and later Heatherton TF et al. (1991) developed the Fagerstroem test to measure the severity of biological tobacco addiction. This test enables a classification according to the severity of the nicotine addiction:

Score 0-2: very low (or no) nicotine addiction
Score 3-4: low nicotine addiction
Score 5-10: medium to high nicotine addiction

The Fagerstroem score measures the severity of the biological tobacco addiction and Fig. 35 shows that the Fagerstroem score correlates with carbon monoxide levels and that scores of five or more correlate very strongly with tobacco sequelae and with the severity of withdrawal symptoms.

Two questions of the Fagerstroem Test (question 1 and 4) have turned out to be the most significant and these two questions are being used to define biological tobacco addiction. They are referred to as the Heavy Smoking Index (HSI) (Kapusta ND. et al. 2006; Heatherton TF. et al. 1989, 1991). A HSI-score of 1–3 suggests a low nicotine addiction and a score of four or more is associated with a strong nicotine addiction (Diaz FJ et al. 2005). If these instruments (Fagerstroem Test or HSI) are used to measure smoking behaviour, no correlation between motivation to change the smoking behaviour and smoke-free intervals could be found. The Fagerstroem score also can't predict the nature of tobacco craving. However, this test offers sufficient information about the severity of withdrawal syndromes and about the kind of pharmaceutical therapy needed (Nicotine supplements or Varenicline) in order to determine the dose of nicotine supplement therapy (Henningfield JE et al. 2005; Le Foll B

Fig. 34 Fagerstroem Test

How soon after you wake up do you smoke your first cigarette?

- within 3 minutes (3)
- 6–30 minutes (2)
- 31–60 minutes (1)
- after 60 minutes (0)

Do you find it difficult to refrain from smoking in places where it is forbidden?

- yes (1)
- no (0)

Which cigarette would you hate most to give up?

- the first in the morning (1)
- any other (0)

How many cigarettes per day do you smoke?

- 10 or less (0)
- 11–20 (1)
- 21–30 (2)
- 31 or more (3)

Do you smoke more frequently during the first hours after awakening than during the rest of the day?

- yes (1)
- no (0)

Do you smoke even if you are so ill that you are in bed most of the day?

- yes (1)
- no (0)

Fig. 35 The validity of the Fagerstroem-Test in regard to different dependence dimensions in tobacco dependents according to ICD-10 (Lesch OM et al. 2004)

A Fagerstroem score of ≥ 5 correlates with
1. Severity of dependency (ICD-10)
2. Duration of dependency
3. Level smoking
4. Number of cigarettes
5. Duration and severity of nicotine withdrawal syndrome

n=330

et al. 2005; National Institute for Clinical Excellence 2004).

6.2.3 European smoking classification system

Since 1973 researchers have tried to correlate personality factors with smoking behaviour. Using this procedure, Patton D. et al. developed a typology which includes different personality traits. Unfortunately no longitudinal and no therapy studies in regard to these subgroups have been performed (Eysenck J. 1973; Patton D et al. 1997). Pomerleau together with Fagerstroem described the heterogeneity of tobacco dependence and suggested that three different mechanisms should be differentiated in regard to nicotine craving (Pomerleau CS et al. 2000):

- Smoking to ameliorate negative mood, like depression or anxiety
- Smoking to enhance positive mood
- Smoking as a habit as a result of heavy smoking in the social environment

He also suggests that these three mechanisms are reflected by different biological dysfunctions which should be considered for pharmacotherapy and motivational strategies.

Our research group was able to show that four different dimensions (Fig. 36) of craving need to be differentiated, which are unequally distributed between genders. (Figs. 36 and 37)

It is very likely that these different mechanisms of craving have different biological causes. Within relapse prevention medication has only been examined in regard to all tobacco dependents. Only the Fagerstroem score has been considered in these studies. The various distinct types of craving, such as those described by Pomerleau CS, Fagerstroem KO and the research group around Lesch OM., should be considered in future relapse studies. Gender differences in regard to coping with stress and tobacco craving should be incorporated into such studies. Women smoke mainly to ameliorate a negative mood, while men mostly try to enhance a positive mood state (Lesch OM et al. 2006).

Motivation strategies and diverse relapse prophylaxes are unfortunately still not sufficiently researched. Shiffman has investigated the differences in motivation and differentiated motivation in regard to different types of smoking behaviours (Shiffman S. 1996).

Fig. 36 Factor analysis of craving in tobacco dependents, n=330 (Lesch OM. et al. 2004, 2006, 2007)

Factor analysis: craving for cigarette smoking
- relaxation
- coping
- stress
- depression

Lesch OM et al. 2004

Fig. 37 Tobacco craving according to gender, n = 330 (Lesch OM et al. 2004, 2006, 2007)

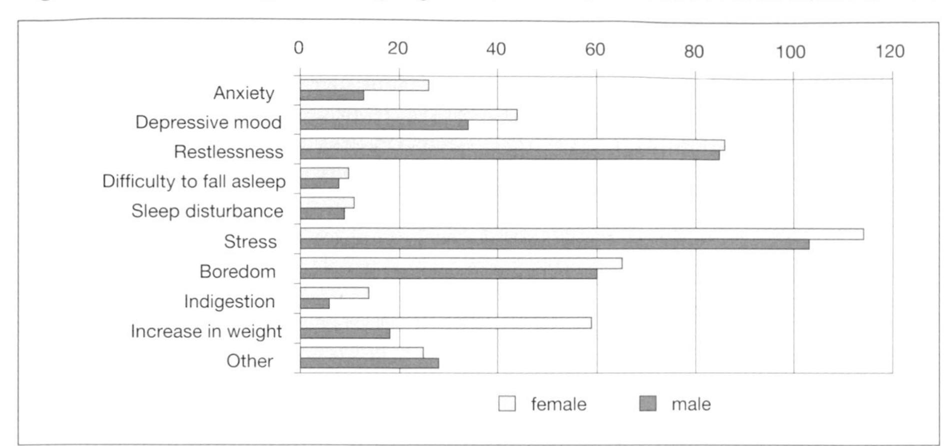

Behavioural therapeutic studies and hypnotherapeutic studies in regard to these subgroups are also seperately needed (Lesch OM. 2007).

6.3 Alcohol addiction – Lesch's typology

6.3.1 Framework for the definition of Lesch's typology

In 1972, a research group was formed at the university hospital for psychiatry in Vienna under the direction of Peter Berner which has devoted itself to the topic of alcohol addiction and which is still active today. At that time, the direction of research at the psychiatric hospital in Vienna was shaped by research on psychopathology and the definition of syndromes which describe psychopathological stages. It was attempted to evaluate these syndromes in therapy studies (e.g. delusional disorders or concurrent disorders) which led to the hypothesis that these syndromes are more suitable for providing information about the choice of therapy and for basis research than the description provided by conventional classification systems. As our clinic always puts equal emphasis on both the French school of thought (Pichot, Alliere) and the German-speaking school of thought (Schneider, Bleuler, Kraepelin), progression research according to the French paradigms and cross-sectional research with instruments according to paradigms from German-speaking countries have always been equally important (Berner P. 1986).

In cooperation with the University Hospital for Psychiatry in Vienna and the Anton-Proksch-Institute, an ambulant care unit for mentally ill was founded in Burgenland, a province of Austria. In 1972, Peter Berner, Head of the University Hospital for Psychiatry and Rudolf Mader, Director of the Anton-Proksch-institute, commissioned me to setup the very patchy outpatient care of this province and also to assume leadership of the team for outpatient care (Lesch OM et al. 1980, 1983, 1984; Lesch OM. 1985; Spielhofer H and Lesch OM. 1980). This activity has led to the Psychosocial Service (PSD) Burgenland which today supplies the entire province. Already in 1973, for scientific purposes, we defined a "catchment area" which encompassed around 160.000 inhabitants (see Fig. 38). The established care system enabled us to prospectively examine the long-term progression of diverse disorders such as paraphrenic psychoses, depressive disorders and alcohol addiction (Lesch OM et al. 1985).

Alcohol dependents were of course also cared for in this setting and these were cross-sectionally assessed so that they could be included in prospective therapy studies and basis research (Lesch OM et al. 1983). The opportunites which were offered here for long-term support and long-term scientific observation, led to Lesch's typology.

6.3.2 Alcohol addiction from a longitudinal perspective 1976–1982–1995

The observable trend in psychiatry to describe medical conditions by using brief psycho-pathogenetic or even solely cross-sectional methods, and then to merely assign these syndromes to common diagnosis systems (ICD-10, DSM-IV), often leads to a diagnosis that is hardly relevant for the patient's long-term progression.

As a result of this fact, very different long-term progressions have been described for all major psychiatric disorders. For instance, Kraeplin and Bleuer observed different progressions in schizophrenic disorders (remission, course of the disease process, progress in episodes, episodic progress). In their prospective longitudinal study, Angst and Perris investigated the progression of affective disorders. Their division of progression into unipolar and bipolar 1 or 2 was not only important for therapy, but also for the co-morbidity of alcohol addiction. Both researchers were able to show that mainly bipolar progressions are linked to alcohol addiction, while this was not the case for unipolar progressions (Bleuler M. 1972; Angst J. 1973; Angst et al. 2006; Berner P. 1986).

6.3.3 The "Burgenland Modell"

Since 1953, the diagnosis "addiction" is accepted, like any other diagnosis, as a diagnosis of disease by national insurance institutions in Austria. Since then, the costs of outpatient as well as in-patient treatment have been funded by public health insurance. If patients are not insured, the local province pays for the costs. The fact that every alcohol dependent has the right to publicly funded therapy has led to the concept of long-term support for alcohol dependents. In the province of Burgenland, nine counselling centres (with social workers, psychologists and doctors) support alcohol dependents either on an outpatient or, if required, on a short-term in-patient basis. This concept is only possible because of the close collaboration between field doctors and medical specialists in psychiatry and neurology. When an alcohol dependent was admitted as an in-patient to one of the following hospitals: University Hospital for Psychiatry in Vienna, University Hospital for Psychiatry in Graz, Psychiatric Hospital Mauer-Oeling, Psychiatric Hospital Graz Sigmund Freud or Anton-Proksch-Institute Vienna, this patient was visited by the staff of the counselling centres responsible. During these visits, the attending therapists were informed about the patient's family situation (home visits were made previously) and patients were encouraged to continue therapy in the counselling centre or in another care institution. If patients were unable to adjust to this setting, they were visited at home during the forthcoming weeks and in some cases it was possible to develop a therapy plan with these patients. The low migration rate during this time and this particular support concept enabled secondary research to be carried out with very low drop-out rates, which ultimately led to the formation of subgroups as summarized by Lesch's typology (Lesch OM. 1985). Longitudinal studies of alcohol addicts showed that smoking behaviour massively affects health even if the patient is totally abstinent. Despite total abstinence, high mortality rates can be ascribed particularly to smoking (Lesch OM and Walter H. 1984). Due to these facts, we started in 2002 to examine smoking behaviour in more detail. For this project, we used findings from alcohol research about typology and research tools (methods of data collection) and from this developed a smoker typology (see Appendix 2; Lesch OM et al. 2004).

Fig. 38 Longitudinal course of alcohol dependent patients, according to DSM-III and ICD-9
Study design (n = 444)

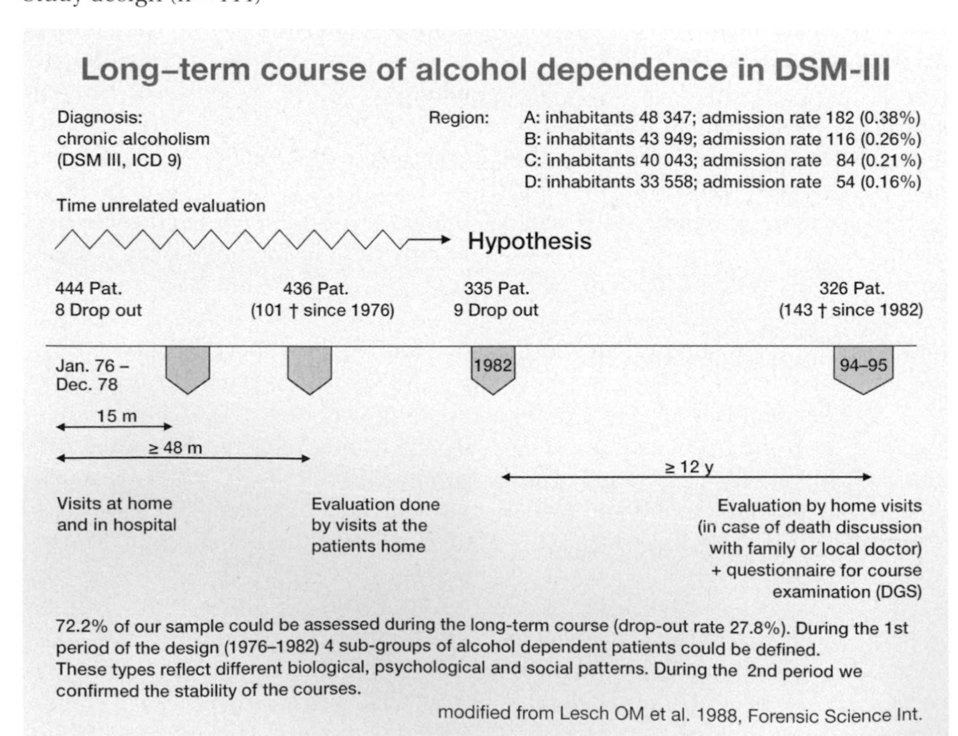

6.3.4 Methodology of the longitudinal study on alcohol dependent patients (according to DSM-III and ICD-9), used for the development of Lesch's typology

From January to December 1978, all patients treated as in-patients and living in the four northern districts of Burgenland were included in the study. A total of 444 patients were recruited of which 8 died within the first 24 hours after admission, therefore only 436 patients could be included in the study. These patients were visited during clinic admission which was followed by an assessment. Patients were assessed by a social worker in the form of a personal interview which took place six times a year over a minimum of four years. The assessment in the hospital was backed up by house calls to the family. After those four years, I could either visit patients at home or in the institutions. I used a multidimensional questionaire with 136 items and this observation stage lasted two years. When patients died (n = 101), family members were asked to document the course of the disease until death. The progress previously defined by the literature was then correlated with the information (biography, diseases) which had been documented at admission. From 1985, the different progressions were published with the data and therapy recorded at admission. Twelve years later (1994/95), the alcoholics who were still alive (335 patients) and/or their family members were examined in a personal interview by two independent psychiatrists, in order to document the stability of progression. Also in an independent evaluation after twelve years, both patients and family members of deceased patients (= 143) were interviewed (Lesch OM et al. 1985, 1988).

The four northern districts of Burgenland were chosen because of their very diverse socio-cultural backgrounds, e.g. region A: rich winegrowers, region C: no wine production and many inhabitants of this region drive to Vienna for work (high commuter rate), region D: rural structures with significantly lower income than region A and no alcohol production. The significantly different admission rates with an ad-

Fig. 39 Long-term progression of alcohol dependent patients according to DSM-III (n = 335)

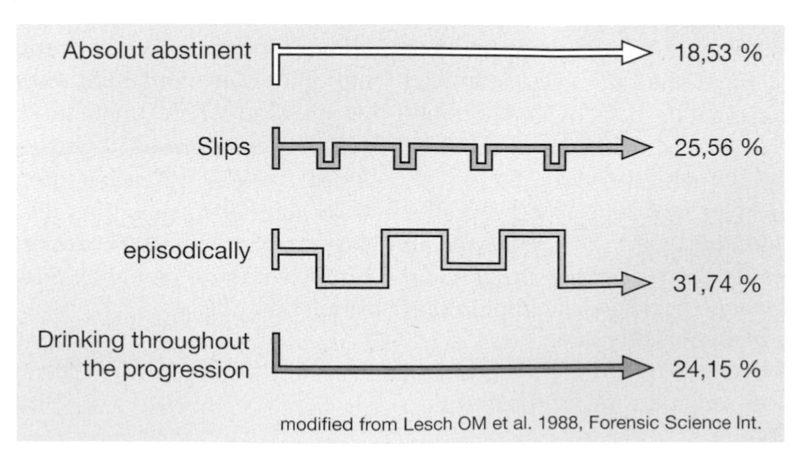

Fig. 40 Location and type of admission and progression (Lesch OM et al. Forensic Science 1988)

Psychiatric hospital :	338 alcohol dependents 307 patients voluntarily 31 patients compulsory
Specilized alcohol unit:	87 patients – all voluntarily
	11 patients both compulsory in the psychiatric hospital and voluntarily in the specialized alcohol unit

There was no correlation between location and type of admission and progression.
Aftercare had a significant influence on the illness course.

Lesch OM et al. 1988, Forensic Science Int.

diction diagnosis (region A has more than twice as many in-patient alcohol admissions than region D) had no effect on the longitudinal progression. After a minimum of four and a maximum of seven years, the progressions were related to drinking behaviour which has led to the definition of four types of progressions.

As illustrated in Fig. 39, we were able to show that 18.5 % of patients were totally abstinent during the entire observation period and also did not report any acute social-psychiatric problems. 25.6 % reported short drinking episodes but no loss of control during the observation period, whereas these short relapses had no negative impact on their mental, social or somatic well-being. 31.7 % showed an alternating progression which could often be observed at regular intervals. Even after in-patient treatment, 24.2 % showed no change in their drinking progression and an acute psychosocial impairment with a high mortality rate.

There was no correlation between location and type of admission and progression.

Aftercare had a significant influence on the illness course (Lesch OM et al. Forensic Science 1988).

No correlation was found between the location of admission (psychiatric hospital vs. specialised addiction clinic) and the further course of the illness.

Furthermore, there was no correlation between voluntarily admitted patients and patients that were admitted involuntarily and longitudinal course (Lesch OM.1985; Lesch OM et al. 1988).

The frequency and regularity of the continuing outpatient therapy had a significant influence on the longitudinal course. The patients who regularly kept appointments more often showed good progression, whereas patients that didn't seek help at counselling centres showed more frequent relapsing progressions with acute sequelae. This data clearly suggests that long-term support is more important than the nature and place of admission (Fig. 41).

Fig. 41 Utilisation of aftercare and illness course

	Regularly	Occasionally or irregularly	None	**Total**
Optimal	44 ↑	10	12	66
Good	50 ↑	29	12	91
Fluctuating	47	43	22	112
Poor	16	38 ↑	32 ↑	86
Total	157	120	78	355

One patient has dropped out, p < 0,0001 Lesch OM. 1983

6.3.5 Stability in the longitudinal course

Twelve years later, this patient group was again examined during home visits by two independent psychiatrists. As 143 patients died during the second observation phase, the recording of the course up until the patient's death via interviews with family members and therapists was extremely important.

Figure 42 A and B illustrates the high stability in the progression of subgroups I, III, and IV.

When the progression of both living and deceased patients during the entire observation phase is included, it becomes apparent that patients whose disease course could be assigned to type II (slips without loss of control) could be reassigned to other groups

Fig. 42A Stability of progressions

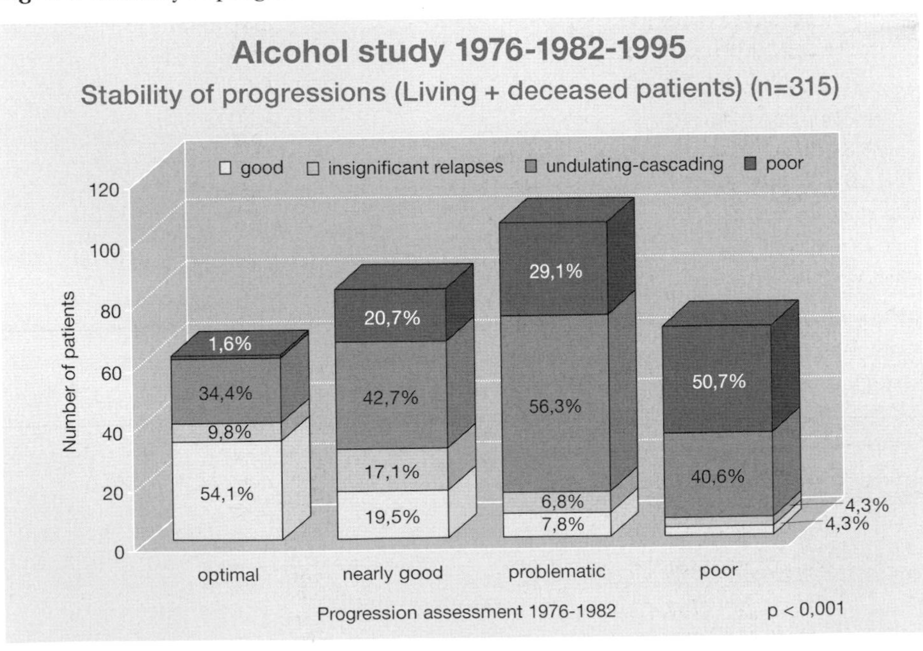

Fig. 42B Stability of illness course

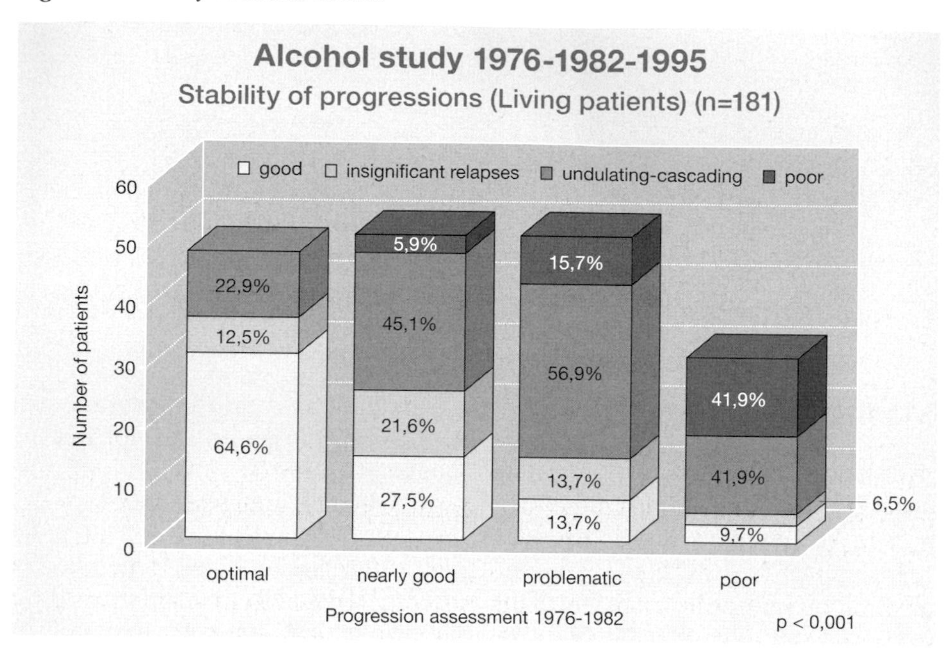

Fig. 43 Long-term course and mortality rates

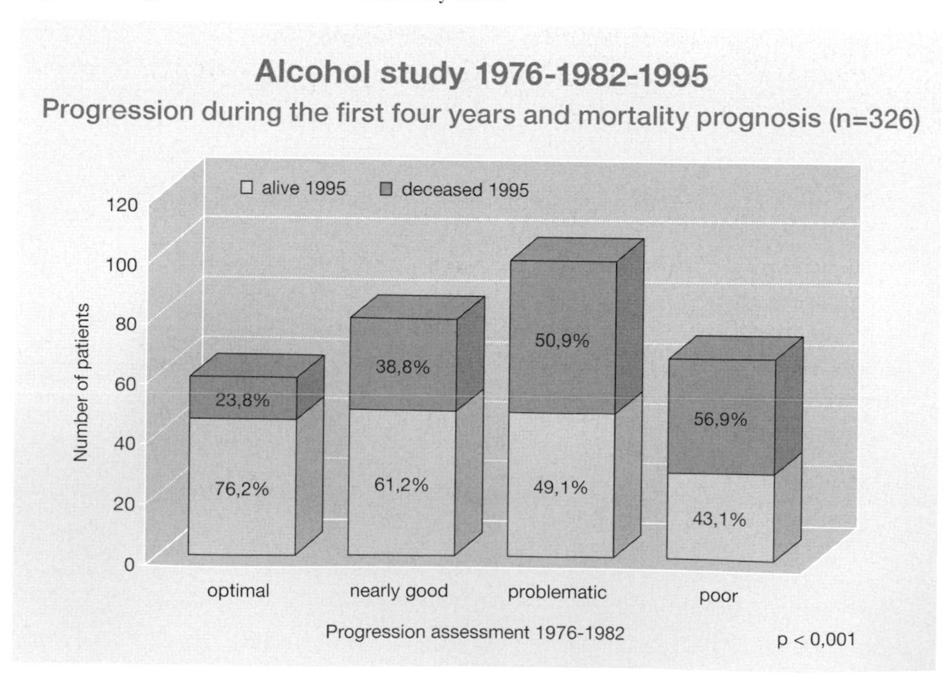

over the following twelve years. Chronic intoxications lead to symptoms, which result in type I, III or IV classifications. In later stages of the progression, cranio-cerebral injury, caused by high intoxication or a withdrawal episode, can simulate type IV progressions. The social deprivation of type IV alcohol addicts can lead to suicide attempts during abstinence and thus need a type III classification etc. The longer the patients are damaged by the addiction, the more their biological sequelae and withdrawal symptoms ressemble each other. If one disregards the deceased patients, and tests only the patients who were still alive at the end of the longitudinal study, the results are much more positive. Only 21,6 % of the type II patients ended up in the group with good progression and insignificant relapses. 27,5 % were entirely abstinent, 45,1 % changed to an episodic progression and only 5,9 % shifted to a very negative drinking progression. Those patients that were classified into the other three groups (type I, III and IV) during the first phase of observation largely remained in their groups, though many patients from groups III and IV died.

The severity of the disease alcohol addiction is demonstrated by this high mortality rate. The fact that 8 out of 436 patients died during the first 24 hours of admission; a further 101 (22.7 %) patients died during the first four years and in the following twelve years another 143 patients (32.2 %) died. When this mortality rate is compared to a non-alcohol dependent control group from the same borough with the help of the borough's practitioners, it shows that the lives of alcohol dependents are on

Fig. 44 Life expectancy of alcohol dependents (Lesch OM et al. 1986)

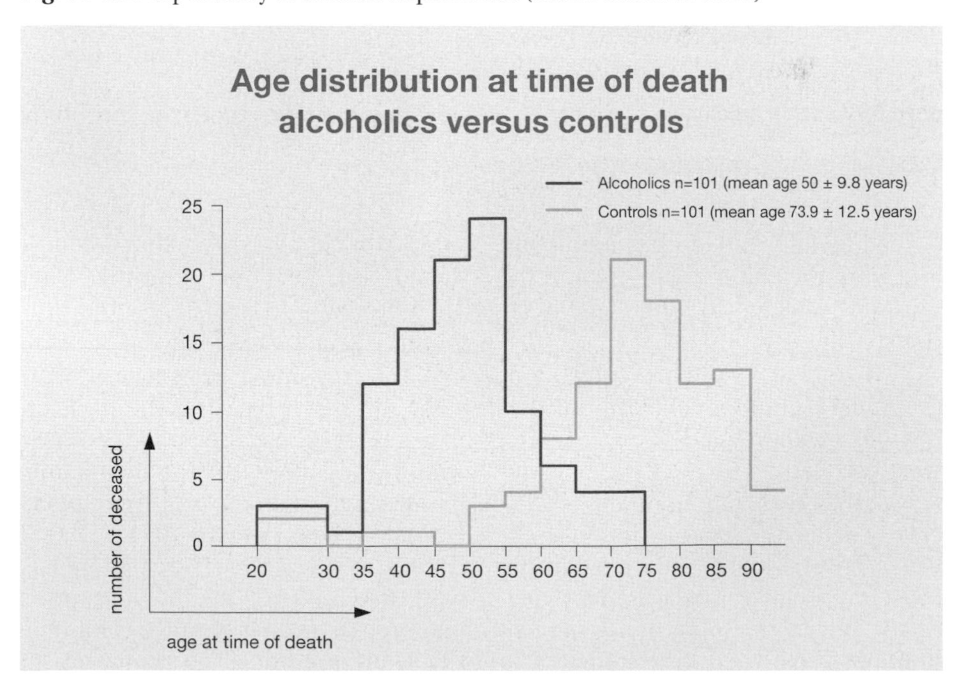

average 23. 9 years shorter than the lifespan of the control group of the same region (Lesch OM and Walter H. 1984).

This high mortality rate also shows that chronic intoxication causes acute somatic damages, although the smoking behaviour of alcohol dependents should not be underestimated (see chapter 7.3). Furthermore this high mortality rate shows the severity of these somatic damages.This is why it is so important to start with therapy as early as possible. There are still therapeutic drop-in centres that hypothesize that in order to be "genuinely" motivated, patients must first hit rock bottom. This thesis must clearly be rejected. The refusal of therapy only because the patient states that he/she doesn't have the motivation for a lifelong abstinence is absolutely to be rejected in view of the high mortality rate of alcohol dependents ("Look at the problem instead of looking away", "Rapid and sufficient help instead of permanent plans").

6.3.6 The four long-term illness courses used for Lesch's typology

These four types of disease courses were correlated with symptoms that were recorded before and during admission and were then later organized and the findings weighted to form "Lesch's typology" in a decision tree.

A total of 136 items (social, biographical, somatic, consumption behaviour, withdrawal symptoms etc.) were correlated with progression and it was shown that only some items were clearly related to disease progression. When several items were related, the most important item was used for diagnostic purposes. Some items were so dominant that they were sufficient to be put into a progression group. For example, it was shown that an acute Enuresis nocturna (more than half a year, socially impairing for the patient e.g. spending the night at a friend's house is impossible) only occurred in irregular and negative progressions. Patients had an episodic progression when a coexistence of Enuresis nocturna and pre-existing psychiatric conditions (comorbidity of an affective disease before, or independent of, drinking behaviour) or a suicide attempt, independent of alcohol and withdrawal, was found. Patients with no additional co-morbidity always showed a negative progression. Patients with Enuresis nocturna mostly showed other acute dysfunctions before the age of 14 such as epileptic convulsions in childhood. Because of this, it was important that these symptoms were weighted in the decision tree because symptoms like acute withdrawal symptoms were less significant for the longitudinal progression than a suicide attempt during abstinence or epilepsy in childhood, for example. The decision tree that was developed in this study was published in 1990 (Lesch OM et al. 1990).

Herbert Poltnig subsequently developed a computer algorithm that produced classifications by group. Data are entered into the computer programme which is based on the decision tree. The programme automatically classifies the Lesch types. In the decision tree the diagnostic procedure starts with the symptoms of type IV and only if none of these items is present, is the patient assigned to type III, I or II, according to symptoms. If the patient has type III symptoms, he/she is grouped into type III, even if symptoms for type I or II are present. If no symptoms of

Fig. 45 Decision tree for Lesch's typology

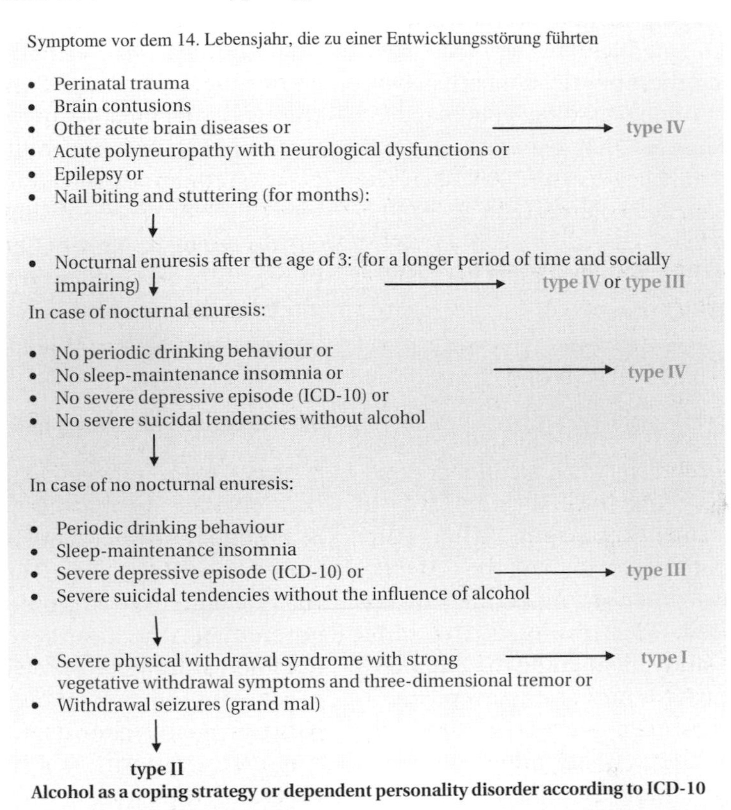

type IV and III are present, severe withdrawal symptoms and/or withdrawal seizures then determine whether the patient is assigned to type I or type II. Type II is a miscellaneousgroup with no symptoms of type I, III or IV, although the diagnosis "alcohol dependence" according to DSM-IV or ICD-10 does exist for this group (type II).

Symptome vor dem 14. Lebensjahr, die zu einer Entwicklungsstörung führten
Perinatal trauma
Brain contusions
Other acute brain diseases or
Acute polyneuropathy with neurological dysfunctions or
Epilepsy or
Nail biting and stuttering (for months):
type IV
Nocturnal enuresis after the age of 3: (for a longer period of time and socially impairing)
type IV or type III
In case of nocturnal enuresis:
No periodic drinking behaviour or
No sleep-maintenance insomnia or
No severe depressive episode (ICD-10) or
No severe suicidal tendencies without alcohol
type IV
In case of no nocturnal enuresis:
Periodic drinking behaviour
Sleep-maintenance insomnia
Severe depressive episode (ICD-10) or
Severe suicidal tendencies without the influence of alcohol
type III
Severe physical withdrawal syndrome with strong vegetative withdrawal symptoms and three-dimensional tremor or
Withdrawal seizures (grand mal)
type I
type II
Alcohol as a coping strategy or dependent personality disorder according to ICD-10
Lesch et al. 1990

As international therapy centres and research groups were keen to make use of this classification system from as early as 1990 onwards, this tool (www.lat-online.at) has been translated into several languages (Bulgarian, Czech, Danish, English, French, Greek, Italian, Norwegian, Portuguese, Russian). Various research groups have validated these subgroups, which were tested in regard to their prognostic significance and therapeutic procedure.

Today, data on typology exists in regard to various kinds of withdrawal symptoms, underlying personality characteristics, different craving and relapse mechanisms, prognosis and mortality as well as different kinds of sequelae. Basis research offers data on alcohol metabolism, condensation products, genetic vulnerabilities, neurophysiological mechanisms like dynamic pupillometry, imaging diagnostics and therapy research (medication, hypnosis therapy, sociotherapeutic concepts; overview on biological data: Hillemacher T and Bleich S. 2008; overview on treatment data: Leggio et al. 2009, Zago-Gomez, et al. 2009, Pombo S et al. 2009).

6.3.7 Results of studies using the Lesch typology

6.3.7.1 Studies on prognosis

In the realm of a prospective appraisal of the prognosis of 84 alcohol dependents according to DSM-IV and ICD-10 in a normal therapeutic setting (after an in-patient admission), the CAD (cumulative duration of abstinence) was measured. The results of the nine-month study highlighted the typology's usefulness for prognosis. Several therapy studies using placebo groups show that the prognosis clearly depends on typology (Walter et al. 2001; Lesch et al. 1996, 2001; Kiefer et al. 2005). After three months, type II patients show the best abstinence rates, type I patients are either abstinent or suffer from an acute relapse (loss of control), while type IV-patients only rarely change their drinking behaviour even after therapy. Therefore in regard to forming a psychiatric opinion, Lesch's typology is recommended as a parameter for a successful prognosis and its therapeutic recommendations (Platz W. 2007). Gender differences have been found in the progression of alcohol dependents. As there are significantly more women belonging to the type III group of patients, and more men in the type IV group, these differences should be taken into account in therapy.

New therapy methods improve the long-term course of alcohol dependent patients. Furthermore, it was shown that 50 % of type IV patients who received specific therapy over a year were able to permanently stay abstinent (graduate dissertation Tiefengraber D. 2008). These results were also supported by W. Platz in Berlin, who reports a 42 % abstinence rate in group IV after having received specific therapy over two years (Platz W. 2007).

6.3.7.2 Studies on biology and genetics

A study with intoxicated alcohol dependents showed that elimination rates of ethanol and methanol significantly correlate with typology (Leitner A et al. 1994). Condensation products like the norharmanes significantly correlate with typology, although this might be linked to smoking behaviour because type I patients nearly almost always smoke (Fagerstroem-positive) (Leitner A et al. 1994). Another study, in which alcohol dependents with or without polyneuropathy were examined, showed that patients with acute polyneuropathy (type IV-patients) eliminated ethanol and methanol at a significantly slower rate than patients with no polyneuropathy (type I, II or III patients). These results suggest that ethanol and methanol are linked to peripheral nerve damages, while central symptoms (withdrawal symptoms or withdrawal attacks) are mainly linked to aldehydes that are centrally active. For many years alcohol addiction has been associated with increased homocysteine levels (Hultberg B et al. 1993; Bleich S et al. 2004). Homocysteine is intensively discussed in regard to damages to the cardiovascular system (Stanger O et al.

2001) although the mechanisms are not entirely clear (De Bree A et al. 2002). In 2004 Bleich was able to show that the homocysteine level is only heightened in intoxicated type I patients with or without epileptic withdrawal convulsions. These high levels rapidly decrease during abstinence or can be reduced with folic acid therapy if drinking behaviour is continued (Bleich et al. 2004). An unpublished study found that especially type I dependents are admitted to cardiologic units. Kiefer F was able to support the notion that only type I patients benefit from Acamprosate. This suggests that homocysteine could be a biological indicator for a successful response to Acamprosate as a relapse prophylaxis in alcohol-related heart diseases (Kiefer F et al. 2005).

Genetic studies from various centres show significant differences between the types (Samochowiec J et al. 2007; Saffroy R et al. 2004; Boensch D et al. 2006).

Neuroendocrinological studies showed that the HPA-axis is linked to drinking behaviour, withdrawal, and craving during abstinence (Hillemacher T et al. 2007; Kiefer F et al. 2001a/2001b, 2005). CRH-and ACTH-changes are associated with craving. Prolactin, which is closely related to dopaminergic functions, is also highly significant in regard to craving. Hillemacher was able to show that especially in the case of type II alcohol dependents, intensity of craving and changes in prolactin levels go hand in hand (Hillemacher T et al. 2006). Another important aspect is the relationship between leptin and ghrelin and the regulation of the intensity of hunger and appetite. Inconsistent findings exist in the literature (Kiefer F et al. 2001a,b; Nicolas JM et al. 2001; Wurst F et al. 2003; Kim DJ et al. 2005; Kraus T et al. 2005; Addolorato G et al. 2006). Hillemacher has pointed to a positive correlation between leptin and Lesch's type I-and type II alcohol dependents, whereas ghrelin only significantly correlated with Lesch's type I (Hillemacher T et al. 2007).

In 1988 Gruenberger J et al. showed that the four types of alcohol dependent patients are significantly different in the assessment with dynamic pupillometry, indicating differences in acetylcholinergic activities (Gruenberger J et al. 1988, 2007). The spontaneous fluctuation of the pupil's diameter, maximal pupil contraction and the absolute change were measured in 117 female and male typologically classified alcohol dependents by means of Josef Gruenberger's dynamic pupillometry. These participants were then compared to 107 control participants (no psychiatric diagnosis and alcohol abuse). Lesch's type I patients differed from both the other types and the control group. In type II and type III, significantly fewer spontaneous fluctuations could be observed in comparison to the control group. All types significantly differed from the control group with regards to an absolute change, whereas type I was characterized by the highest absolute change. During the last two years, these differences were examined in 300 alcoholics and the first results were largely confirmed (presentation ESBRA 2007, publication in preparation, Friedrich F, et al. 2010 in preparation).

6.3.7.3. Relapse prevention studies, anti-craving substances

In 2006 Hillemacher et al. examined alcohol dependents that were classified

Fig. 46 Craving with regards to Lesch's typology (Hillemacher T et al. 2006)

	Mean Values				
	Lesch Type 1 (N = 37)	Lesch Type 2 (N = 94)	Lesch Type 3 (N = 38)	Lesch Type 4 (N = 23)	Population (N = 192)
OCDS Total[a]	17,4 ± 7,3	21,0 ± 7,2	19,0 ± 7,9	24,3 ± 6,9	20,3 ± 7,6
OCDS Activity	6,8 ± 3,7	8,8 ± 4,8	7,7 ± 5,0	9,8 ± 5,3	8,3 ± 4,9
OCDS Compulsive thoughts[a]	10,5 ± 3,7	12,1 ± 3,5	11,3 ± 3,6	14,5 ± 3,2	12,0 ± 3,7
Age (years)	43,3 ± 8,8	43,9 ± 9,0	44,8 ± 8,2	41,4 ± 9,3	43,7 ± 8,8
Onset of disease (years)	25,8 ± 10,6	26,2 ± 9,2	24,9 ± 9,5	22,4 ± 8,1	25,4 ± 9,4
Number of previous detoxification[a]	9,0 ± 10,4	8,2 ± 10,1	14,7 ± 29,1	18,8 ± 17,1	10,9 ± 16,8
Daily intake in g	217,9 ± 123,3	263,3 ± 219,0	233,9 ± 190,0	230,1 ± 108,6	244,8 ± 186,9
[a] significant differences between the types according to Lesch examined by the Kruskal-Wallis-Test for independent samples (OCDS total score Chi-square p < 0,05)					

according to Lesch's typology in regard to different craving mechanisms. By using Anton's OCDS (Anton RF et al. 1995), they were able to show that type IV had the highest craving-scores. Furthermore type II had higher craving scores than type I and III. Type IV had the highest number of acute withdrawal symptoms and correlated with the most severe craving symptoms. A significant relationship between craving and the number of earlier detoxifications could only be found in type I, Fig. 46, (Hillemacher T et al. 2006).

There are different opinions about the craving mechanisms of Lesch's types.

Fig. 47 Craving according to Lesch's typology and scientific hypotheses of craving (Walter et al, 2006)

Type I – The effect of alcohol on withdrawal symptoms (Neuroadaptation)

Type II – Alcohol as an anxiolytic (social learning and cognitive models)

Type III – Alcohol as an antidepressant

Type IV – Alcohol as an impulse control disorder and/or a compulsion with previous cerebral damage, alcohol to cope with social situations (socio-cultural-organic model)

Walter H et al. 2006

Individual subgroups use alcohol as a sedative, anti-depressant or as medication against withdrawal symptoms. These different effects and their possible biological aetiologies have been summarized in 1997. From this, the following considerations for research in regard to animal models and clinical therapy research can be suggested, Fig. 47, (Lesch OM et al. 1997):

These considerations suggest that different etiological vulnerabilities need different pharmacological and psychotherapeutic therapies. Relapse prevention studies with disulfiram, acamprosate, naltrexone, flupentixol, baclofene and neramexane clearly showed that the relapse rate can be both positively and negatively influenced by each individual medication. Acamprosate and naltrexone are internationally used as anti-craving substances. Animal studies clearly show that acamprosate improves abstinence, while naltrexone reduces the amount of alcohol consumed and the duration of periods of drinking. Therefore it can be suggested that abstinent progressions, namely type I and II, can be influenced by acamprosate, while naltrexone has a better effect for sporadic or permanent drinking progressions. Based upon this, David Sinclair administers naltrexone as a so called "extinction method" in alcohol dependents (Sinclair JD. 2001). In a placebo-controlled acamprosate study, in which alcohol dependents received acamprosate over a 1 year period, our research group was able to demonstrate that acamprosate only significantly improves abstinence in type I and type II (Lesch et al. 1996). In a three-monthly acamprosate-naltrexone-placebo study in 2005, Kiefer F et al. showed that acamprosate is only effective in type I, because after three months the abstinence rate in type II patients is still satisfactory and no medication is

Fig. 48 Acamprosate as a relapse prophylaxis in alcohol dependents and Lesch's typology

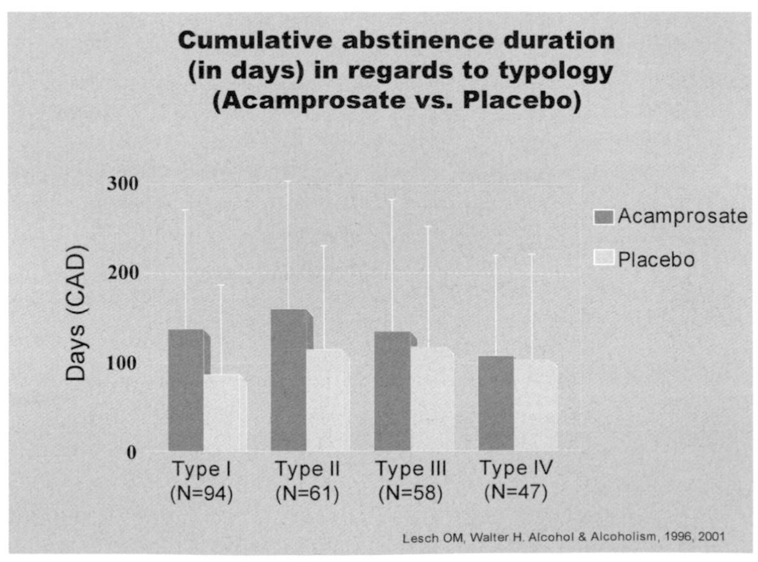

Fig. 49 Acamprosate and naltrexone as relapse prophylaxis in alcohol dependents according to Lesch's typology

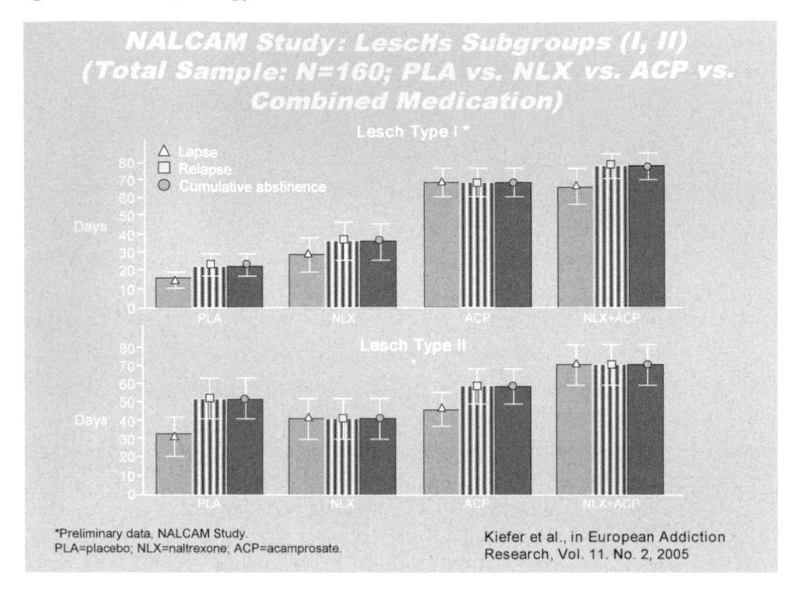

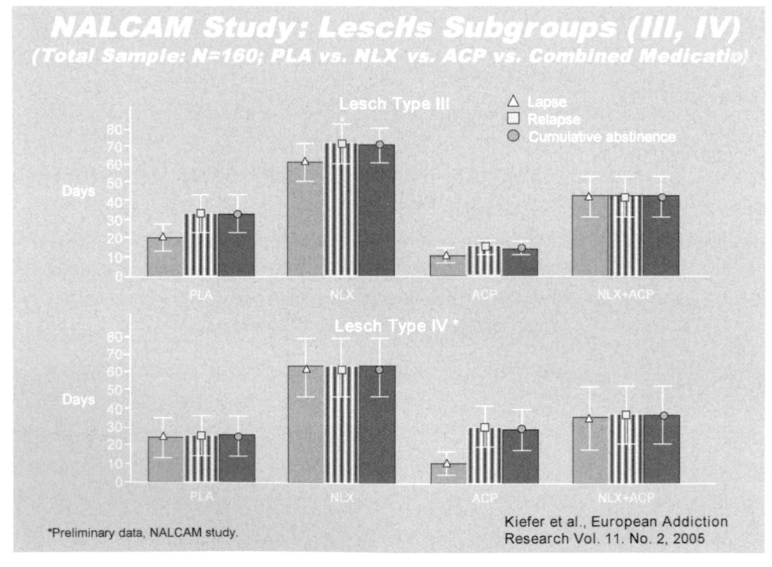

effective. Type III and IV can be significantly improved by naltrexone, which suggests that a combination of naltrexon and acamprosate significantly worsens the results in type III and IV. A flupentixol study (D2-antagonist) was carried out under the direction of Wiesbeck G and it was shown that particularly type I-and type III patients had a higher relapse rate with flupentixol than

Fig. 50 Flupentixol as relapse prophylaxis in alcohol dependents according to Lesch's typology

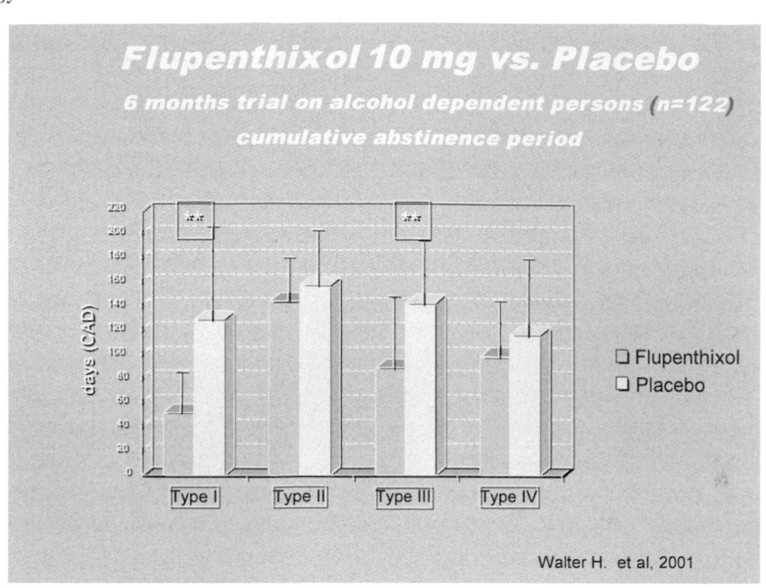

with placebo (Wiesbeck G et al. 2001; Walter H et al. 2001).

Neramexane (NMDA-antagonist) worsened the progression in type III, while it didn't have an impact on type I, II and IV (unpublished data).

CB1-antagonists or SSRIs like Ritansarin showed no changes in drinking behaviour and also no differences in regard to typology (unpublished studies, Soyka M. et al. 2008).

In conclusion, there are data on relapse prophylaxis in regard to typology for various medications and this is why our recommendations for relapse prophylaxis medication are always made in accord with typologies. As the symptomatic of withdrawal symptoms differ with types, withdrawal symptoms should also be treated differently.

From the psychotherapeutic field, only studies on hypnosis therapy are available in regard to typology. It was demonstrated that hypnotherapeutic groups are best suited for Lesch's type II-and type III patients (Hertling I et al. 2002).

Summerizing our results and including our experience of 20 years practical work with withdrawal and relapse prevention treatment we recommend the following medication (Fig. 51, Lesch et al. 2010)

6.3.7.4. Other results regarding Lesch's typology

Sequelae are also expected to differ among types, which explains why the frequency of types admitted into different therapeutic settings clearly differs. Alcoholics that receive psychiatric therapy have already been typologically described (type I 18.53 %, type II 25.56 %, type III 31.74 %, type IV 24.15%). Sperling et al. have examined the distribu-

Fig. 51 Overview medication for alcohol dependence according to types

Summary of the pharmacotherapy according to the typology of Lesch

	Withdrawal treatment	Relapse prevention
Type I	Benzodiazepines,Clome thiazole	Acamprosate, Disulfiram, Cyanamid, Cave: D1-Antagonists
Type II	Tiapride, Cave: Benzodiazepines, Gamma-Hydroxy-Butyric Acid	Acamprosate, Cave: Benzodiazepines, Gamma-Hydroxy-Butyric-Acid, Clomethiazole, Meprobamate
Type III	Gamma-Hydroxy-Butyric Acid	Naltrexone, Antidepressants e.g. Milnacipran, Sertaline, Carbamazepine, Gamma-Hydroxy-Butyric Acid, Cave: D1-Antagonists, Topiramate ???
Type IV	Gamma-Hydroxy-Butyric Acid and Carbamazepine	Naltrexone, Nootropics, Gamma-Hydroxy-Butyric Acid, Atypical Neuroleptics, Ondansetrone ???

Lesch an Soyka, 2010

tion of types in regard to gender and found that type III prevails more frequently among women, whereas type IV is more frequent in men (Sperling W. et al. 1999).

The types also differ as regards sequelae, like the severity of liver disease or biological markers. Wirnsberger et al. examined 333 alcohol dependents (according to ICD-10 and DSM-IV) (172 men and 161 women) who were in-patients at the psychiatric hospital in Vienna. Liver damage was significantly severer in Type I and type IV than in type II and III (Wirnsberger et al. ESBRA 2007).

Our study of 509 alcohol dependents according to DSM-IV was not able to find a relationship between typology and exposure to alcoholism in the family (unpublished studies).

In her graduate dissertation, Barbara Koenig investigated the classification of types in prisons and was able to show that 49 % of type IV patients, 38 % of type III patients and 13 % of type II patients were detained in these prisons. No single type I patient was assessed in prison. Contrary to this, she showed that more type I-and type II patients than type III-and type IV patients were admitted to a specific inpatient addiction therapy centre (Anton-Proksch-Institute). Mainly type III patients were admitted to psychiatric hospitals. A German research group examined alcohol dependents that committed murder and found that offenders were mostly type II, type III and type IV patients. In this case, type II patients were usually first offenders, whereas type III and type IV patients had already previously committed criminal acts (Reulbach U et al. 2007). Today we are convinced that differences in therapy between various care institutions (emergency units, internal surgery departments, psychiatric departments, prisons,

Fig. 52 Gender distribution

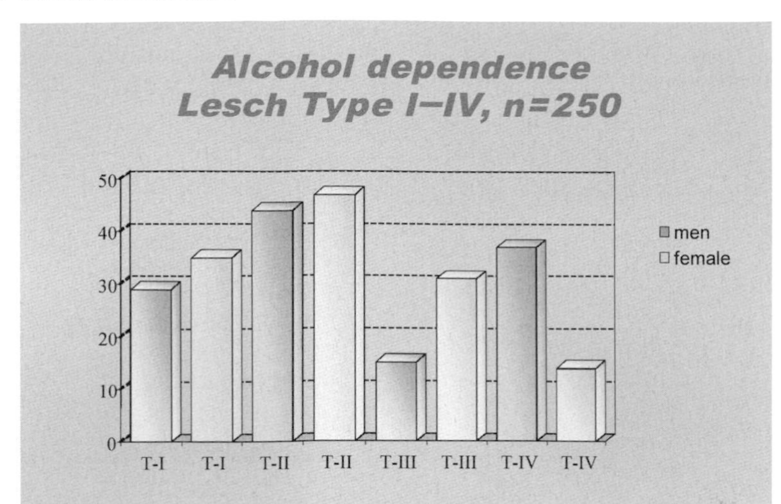

Fig. 53 Mean value of liver function and % CDT in regard to Lesch's typology

	GGT U/l	ALAT U/l	ASAT U/l	FIB mg/dl	CDT %
Type I	287,00	47,44	54,09	447,57	5,21
Type II	123,87	41,96	42,96	378,41	4,16
Type III	122,74	36,04	37,87	385,28	3,02
Type IV	221,25	54,00	37.87	379,60	4,25
Signifikance	p<0,01	p<0,05	p<0,05	p<0,05	p<0,05

n = 333

homeless shelters or specific addiction hospitals) are due to the fact that different subgroups of alcohol dependents, as defined by Lesch, are treated in different institutions. In his article, Wetschka Ch. discusses which sociotherapeutic concepts should be recommended for type IV and type III groups (see chapter 10).

6.3.8 Lesch's typology from an international comparative perspective

All typologies in alcohol dependents overlap to a certain extent. Typologies that differentiate two subgroups (e.g. Cloninger CR and Babor TF) are often described more precisely by typologies that define four subgroups. The onsetof an alcohol dependence, which Cloninger CR and Babor TF describe as a fundamental factor, does not play an important role in Schuckit's MA or Lesch's OM typology. The so called "primary alcoholism" according to Schuckit is represented by Lesch's type I and IV, whereas the "secondary alcoholism" according to Schuckit is in line with Lesch's type II and III. Figure 54 illustrates that those typologies which are divided into four subgroups, show a clear concordance. Mild and episodic disease progressions, as well as the progression accompanied by social problems, are mirrored by the respective types according to Lesch, namely type II (mild progression), III (episodic progression) and IV (negative progression). Lesch's type I, which is only defined by regular and high amounts of drinking with acute withdrawal symptoms and/or withdrawal seizures, has no matching typologies (US and England). Typologies originating from the US and England always include a group of polytoxicomanics. In those countries, Lesch's type I patients might fall into the group of polytoxicomanics. In Portugal, Cardoso showed a significant correlation between the Neter-typology and types II, III and IV according to Lesch, but he also defined a group of very young polytoxicomanics as a separate subgroup (Cardoso Neves JM et al. 2006; Prombo S et al. 2008). Alongside this typological classification, other factors play an important role. As depicted by many other studies, the onset of the alcohol addiction, genetic vulnerabilities and an antisocial personality disorder seem to be important factors, significant for therapy and progression. If, however, a pathway analysis is carried out on alcohol dependents in order to determine the factors which solely, or in interaction, cause a relapse, it shows that there are also other important dimensions (Fig. 55). Lesch developed a structured interview including all these important items. One page of this instrument is used for the assessment for Lesch typology (www.lat-online.at).

When factors described by the pathway analysis are linked to current literature on relapse prophylaxis, it becomes clear that social or family-related factors play an important role alongside the typologies. Our survey tool (PC-version) includes one page that exclusively tackles typology. All other pages deal with factors which have been described by the pathway analysis and in relapse prophylaxis literature (Fig. 55). For several years we have been carrying out research in which we use the PC-version of this survey tool and try to correlate other factors with the typologies.

The computerized survey tools (www.lat-online.at – Lesch Alcoholism Typology) for a precise assessment of alcohol dependents (according to criteria like onset of addiction, genetic vulnerabilities and typology) can be found in Appendix 1.

6.4 The relationship between alcohol dependent patients according to Lesch's typology and the severity of tobacco addiction

As alcohol and tobacco are often consumed in combination, it makes sense to use Lesch's Alcoholism Typology (LAT) together with the European Smoker Classification Scale. Our research group was able to show that the intensity of craving was significantly stronger when the individual was abusing both alcohol and nicotine than when only one

Fig. 54 Comparison of different typologies

Subgroups in Alcohol dependence

Lesch 1990	Zucker 1997	Del Bocka & Hesselbrock 1996	Windle & Scheidt 2004	Cardoso Neves et al, in A&A 2006
Type II	More mild course subtype	Low risk, low severity	Mild course cope with stressors	Anxiopathic - typifies an anxious functioning
Type III	Negative affect	Negative affect	Major depressive generalized anxiety	Thimopathic - typified by affective symptomatology
Type IV	Antisocial alcoholics	Chronic/ASP	Chronic/ASP	Sociopathic - characterized by disruptive behaviours under alcohol influence
Type I			Polydrug use?	Heredopathic - congregates familiar and genetic influences on alcoholism
Babor and Cloninger 2 Type solutions, personality traits of Cloninger fit very well to Lesch typology (e.g. harm avoidance Type II)				Adictopathic - isolates younger individuals who consume alcohol and other types of psychoactive substances

Fig. 55 Factors influencing relapse, presented by a pathway analysis

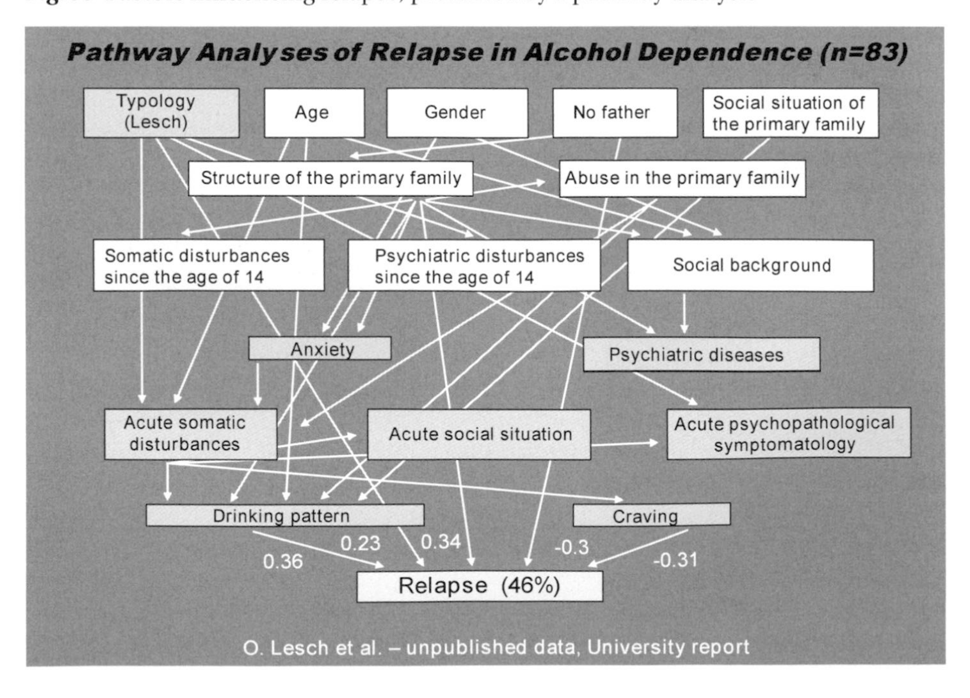

addiction was present (Hertling I et al. 2005). This increase in craving was found in all forms of craving. Alcohol dependent smokers showed depressive symptoms and sleep disorders significantly more often, whereas nicotine dependents who didn't abuse alcohol mainly smoked for weight control and to cope with stress. Especially type I, type III and type IV but not type II alcohol dependents with tobacco addiction score positive on the Fagerstroem-scale. We assume that tobacco ingredients are used as a drug substitute by type I and type IV alcohol dependents, whereas type III-patients use both alcohol and tobacco as therapy for their basic dysfunction. These considerations should furthermore be integrated into therapy.

7

Motives for alcohol-and/or tobacco addicted patients to seek medical help

7.1 Tobacco addiction

60 % of tobacco dependents describe themselves as "dissonant" smokers. They try temporarily or permanently to reduce their smoking or even try to quit. Knowing that smoking leads to sequelae, knowing their withdrawal symptoms, this group often needs an impulse from the social environment (partner, work place etc.) or somatic symptoms (shortness of breath, stomach pain, pregnancy etc.) to quit. By contacting a therapist, the dissonant smoker group shows that they have realized their nicotine problem. When these individuals get effective help, they are easy to motivate to reduce or even quit smoking.

About 40 % of tobacco dependents are "consonant" smokers. They perceive smoking as an important part of their life and think that every therapy deprives them of something pleasurable. This group starts therapy during a later phase of their dependence development. They never seek help voluntarily but only when forced by external factors (e.g. smoking ban at work or somatic sequelae that are connected to smoking: COPD, stroke etc.) to change their smoking habit.

In this group, education about the relationship between tobacco ingredients and their present diseases is extremely important. In the case of an actual disease, this disease should be treated primarily. The patient should feel that there is interest in his well-being and that there are people to help him get a better quality of life. This motivational work takes time and a number of appointments are required. The linkage to a therapy centre, a regular check-up at the practitioner's or with an appropriate medical specialist should be the first goal. After a therapist has been contacted, an exact date for the reduction or abstinence of smoking should be set and a clear goal should be formulated. The therapeutic procedure for reaching this goal should be accepted by patient and therapist and should be realistic. Withdrawal symptoms should be treated in order to cause as little brain damage as possible (nicotine substitution therapy e.g. with the right supplement at a well combined, sufficient dosage). Relapse prevention and withdrawal symptoms will be discussed in more depth in the section on therapy (Lesch OM. 2007).

7.2 Alcohol addiction

We assume that the majority of alcohol-addicted patients meet the diagnosis criteria for an alcohol addiction already during adolescence. We could show that, for example, 3.2 % of 18-year-old men have already "reached" the diagnostic for an alcohol addiction (Kapusta ND et al. 2006, 2007). As drinking is an accepted behaviour in wine producing countries, alcohol dependents drink many years before they notice that they have alcohol-related health problems or problems with the partner, or at work, or with their driving license. In the beginning high amounts of drinking are usually admired by the environment and it takes many years until it is realised that the alcohol dependent individual has a serious alcohol problem. The environment and also the employer usually react with control and rules, which the individual often can't follow. This process also lasts several years and only when health problems set in (sequelae, withdrawal symptoms or even withdrawal seizures) is the patient forced by the environment to consult a doctor, psychotherapist or psychologist. This means that at the initial meeting the patient expects "to hear new rules" which he knows he/she probably won't be able to follow.

The diagnostic process should be started immediately if the patient comes to treatment without any sequelae and no severe intoxication. The patient's history should also be explored in terms of whether there have been any lengthy periods of abstinence. If there have been, the patient should be questioned about what helped him to stay abstinent. This might represent a strategy, which could be followed again in therapy.

The severity of the expected withdrawal syndrome should be explored. The majority of patients have experienced several withdrawals without therapy and are able to describe this experience very well (see chapter 9.1). The primary therapy goal should be the reduction of drinking behaviour or, if accepted, an absolute abstinence until the next appointment (preferably no later than seven days). The possibility of relapses occurring during this time should also be discussed. The patient is asked to describe these relapses so that better therapeutic strategies can be offered. If these patients desperately want an in-patient admission, their wish should definitely be granted, but they should only be transferred to institutions that offer stable psychotherapeutic support after a short (up to 14 days) in-patient stay. It is recommended that one specific person or a selected team should be in charge of counselling before, during and after in-patient admission. The principle "out-patient care comes prior to in-patient care" is of course also valid for alcohol dependent patients. Rigid and lengthy therapy concepts and rules, which serve the institution rather than the patient, should be rejected.

If pressure from the closer environment enforce the treatment, the patient should primarily be treated outside of this environment structure. If problems with the partner play a pivotal role, it is important to first establish a trusting bond with the patient. Conversations and therapeutic concepts that incorporate the partner should be introduced later (e.g. five one-hour meetings with the patients and the sixth session with the partner on the patient's approval). In the case of pressure from the workplace, clear rules should be formulated regarding which information should be provided to the employer or to the labour union. The patient's consent is needed if the cost of treatment is covered by the employer, or if the employer requires regular therapy reports. Yet, defined rules have a positive therapeutic effect for this relationship (patient-doctor-employee). If the loss of a driving licence is the main reason for treatment, a prognosis can be made for alcohol dependents according to type after three or nine months and it is suggested that the driving licence be issued for a limited period of two years. Here the patient should provide a therapy report in order to be eligible to drive a car.

If the motivation for receiving therapy is influenced by sequelae, the procedure needs to be modified according to the severity of the sequelae. Decompensated liver cirrhosis or a metastasising carcinoma requires a different treatment procedure than slightly elevated liver functions or mild anaemia. It is suggested that therapy is carried out in the specific department which is treating the sequelae (e.g. individuals with a liver disease should receive gastroenterological treatment or heart patients cardiological treatment first). At these specialized departments, an addiction therapist or a psychiatrist who has a liaison with this department should be available.

At the clinical department for transplantation and the clinical department for gastroenterology and hepatology, in collaboration with the outpatient centre for alcohol related health problems, together with a ward for crisis intervention at the University Hospital for Psychiatry in Vienna, we were able to show that this type of provision leads to improvement and also to clearer indications for transplantation. In a few studies, we were also able to show that this concept not only improves abstinence rates, but also the quality of life of those affected with liver disease (Berlakovich GA et al. 1999; Baischer W et al. 1995).

When patients feel that their sequelae have been treated adequately, they are often also motivated to seek treatment for their alcohol dependence. Patient information and a clear therapy concept are beneficial in helping patients. If they are sent to another institution for treatment, patients often feel very disappointed and usually terminate therapy. For these patients, inpatient withdrawal therapy is usually not required. Often regular outpatient appointments and therapeutic strategies according to Lesch's typology are enough.

7.3 Sequelae that bring patients into therapy

7.3.1 Tobacco and sequelae

7.3.1.1 Introduction

Tobacco and its ingredients impair virtually all bodily functions and all fields of medical specialisation refer to the partial aetiology of "smoking". In 2007, we described these damages in more depth in a collection of essays but not all disciplines were considered. In Austria, 8 million inhabitants, around 14,000 deaths per year are related to tobacco abuse. The combination of tobacco and alcohol abuse with overweight and little exercise is in fact life shortening.

7.3.1.2 Tobacco and neurology

Smoking belongs to the most modifiable risk factors for diabetes mellitus or arterial hypertonia or alcohol abuse. When smoking, the risk of an ischemic stroke is doubled and a total of 25% of all strokes are directly or indirectly linked to smoking. Smoking potentiates the risks of other factors such as the consumption of oral contraceptives.

As passive smoking also increases the risks in a similar way to active smoking, it can be assumed that there is a "threshold" which increases the risk and that the dose response relationship is not linear. After a stroke, a smoke-free lifestyle significantly decreases the risk of another stroke. Giving up smoking is clearly more effective than prevention with aspirin. After as little as twelve months of abstinence, a 50% reduced vascular risk can be observed and, after a further five years without smoking, the risk for vascular diseases is almost as low as it is for a non-smoker. (Sander D et al. 2006; Goldstein LB et al. 2006; Wold PA et al. 1988).

7.3.1.3 Tobacco and internal medicine

7.3.1.3.1 Heart diseases and circulatory disorders

Everyone knows that smoking causes heart attacks and the commonly used term "smoker's leg" suggests that individuals are well aware that smoking causes peripheral arterial obstructive disease. The INTERHEART study shows that 36% of primary heart attacks are caused by smoking (Yusuf S et al. 2004). There are also clear gender differences. A man who smokes 20 cigarettes daily increases his risk of a heart attack by three times. Women between the age of 35 and 52 who smoke increase their risk of a heart attack by six times (Bolego C et al. 2002). The cigarettes smoked daily show a linear relationship to the frequency of heart attacks. The more cigarettes smoked, the higher the risk of an acute myocardial infarction (Yusuf S et al. 2004). At the Mayo Clinic, the influence of smoking and the risk of myocardial infarction and death after transdermal coronary intervention (PCI) were examined. After PCI and quitting smoking the risk had been completely normalised. In PCI-patients, smoking led to an increase of risk of myocardial infarction (MI) (+ 108%) and cardiovascular death (+ 76%) (Hasdai D et al. 1997). Similar studies exist for aortic aneurysm, peripheral arterial obstructive disease and for diabetes type II. In obesity research, the metabolic syndrome and the interaction between smoking, depression, alcohol and obesity plays a major role. A regular increase in weight in regard to age is linear. This linear curve increases with adverse life situations and severe stress causes episodic increases in weight (Melis T et al. 2007; Unachuku CN. 2006).

7.3.1.3.2 Pulmonary diseases

Tobacco withdrawal is the most important and the only effective pneumological therapy. In Austria, smokers face an average shortening of life by 23 years. In Austria in the year 2000, around 2,700 smokers died of a bronchus carcinoma and around 1,000 of COPD (Vutuc C et al. 2004). Since 1970, the bronchus carcinoma mortality rate in women has doubled. Even with acute COPD, quitting smoking significantly improves the progression. Patients might not fully recover their health but the process and worsening of the respiratory disease can at least be slowed down.

7.3.1.4 Oncological diseases

Besides the previously discussed bronchus carcinoma, smoking also significantly increases the risk for other carcinoma. This is the case for all kind of cancer (breast, prostate etc.) but clear data exists in particular regarding an increased risk for larynx, pharynx and mouth cancer. Smoking increases the risk for these carcinoma by 24 times and the risk for oesophagus by 7.5 times. A smoke-free life can improve the progression of these severe carcinoma.

7.3.1.5 Dentistry

Apart from the ugly smoker's plaque and periodontitis, smoking also plays a role in tooth transplantations (Ness L et al. 1977). The healing processes in the mouth area, are considerably slowed down by smoking (Tonetti MS et al. 1995; Trombelli L et al. 1999; AAP 2005). The increased risk for oral cancer has already been pointed out.

7.3.1.6 Psychiatry

Individuals with a schizophrenic psychosis often heavily abuse tobacco during neuroleptic treatment. Tobacco decreases the blood level of neuroleptics and is also effective against the extrapyramidal side effects of classic neuroleptics. Nicotine acts as a dopamine agonist and thus has antidepressant effects. Patients with a schizoaffective psychosis often smoke to elevate their mood.

7.3.2 Alcohol and sequelae

7.3.2.1 Introduction

Depending on duration of consumption and drinking behaviour (dosage, daily alcohol consumption, temporary binge drinking), alcohol damages all organs. Alcoholic beverages do not only consist of ethanol, but also of methanol and other alcohols. Methanol, in particular, seems to be an important factor in cerebral damage. Depending on the type of alcohol beverage, there are milligram or gram dosages of methanol in one litre (see Fig. 5).

Ethanol and other concomitant substances change haematopoesis, fat metabolism and also all other metabolism processes. An enlargement of erythrocytes, elevated blood lipids and elevated uric acid with retarded blood clotting and pathological liver functions are all related to alcohol. The human's immune system is weakened by alcohol abuse. In the literature, small amounts of alcohol are often considered healthy. This perspective is only valid for healthy patients who have never abused alcohol before or only temporarily. From our experience, we know that there are only very few individuals who do not drink increased amounts of alcohol over a longer period of time during adolescence or afterwards. The alcohol-related change in diet (lots of fat and meat, few vegetables and fruits) is an important factor in somatic damage (e.g. lack of thiamine). In an epidemiological study in Austria, we were able to show that 29% of all admissions to units for internal medicine abused alcohol, which could be objectified by an elevated% CDT. In the case of planned surgeries, 12% of patients admitted showed an elevated% CDT level (Lesch OM et al. 1996). This is also the fact when% CDT levels are measured at a surgical intensive care unit. In Berlin it was found that patients with elevated% CDT were more likely to develop somatic problems than patients with a low% CDT. Patients with increased% CDT also showed a doubled length of stay in hos-

Fig. 56 Number of alcohol abusers in general medical practice 2,000 patients
Lesch E et al., unpublished data

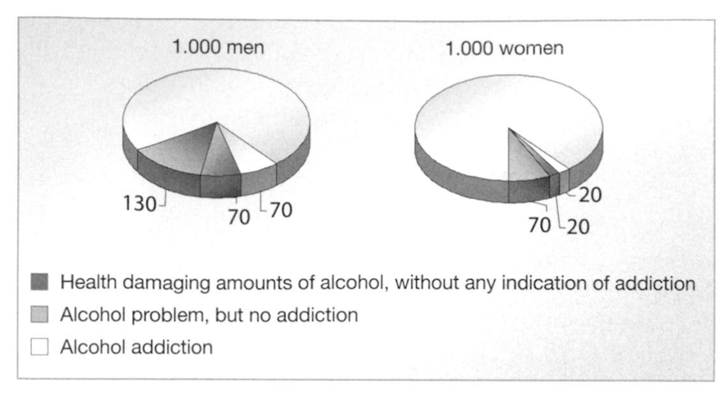

pital (Spiess C et al. 2000). A quarter of the patients seen by general practioners are treated for alcohol abuse, in which clear gender differences exist.

Alcohol dependent patients who don't change their drinking behaviour after an in-patient treatment (type III- and type IV progressions) need significantly more in-patient admission at a somatic ward than type I-or II course.

When alcohol dependent patients are compared to a healthy population, life expectancy in the former is shortened by 23.9 years. The control group was recruited from general practitioners. These patients were recruited from the same catchment area as the alcohol patients (see Fig. 44).

As already documented in the longitudinal study, twice as many type

Fig. 57 Alcohol study 1976–1982–1995

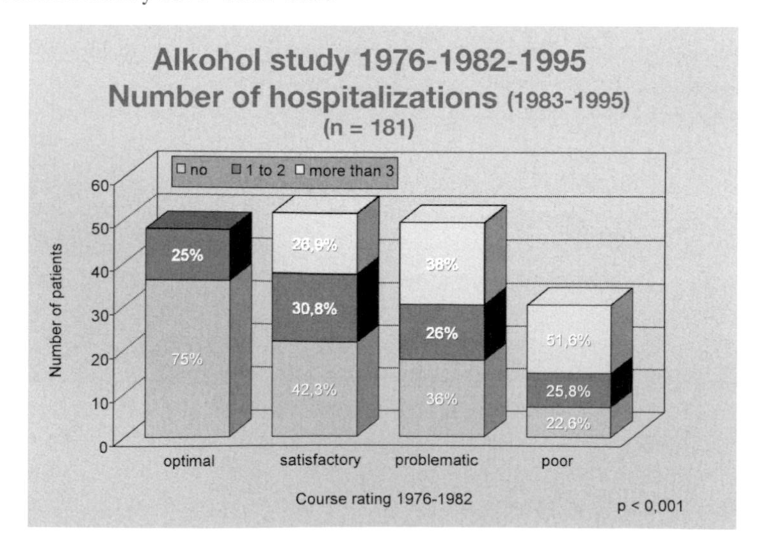

Fig. 58 Mortality and alcohol (illness course of 5,766 workers, with 1,643 persons dying within 21 years)

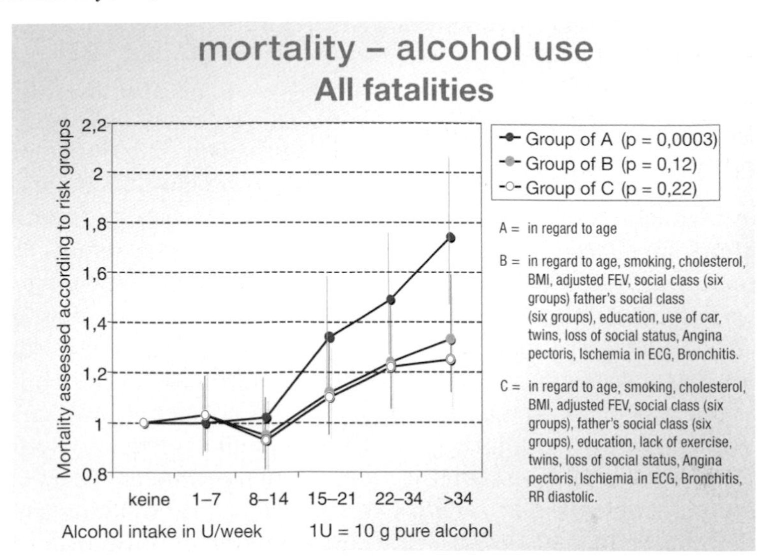

III-and type IV patients die as type I patients (see Fig. 43).

Alcohol increases mortality rates in a dosage dependent way. The increase in alcohol abuse especially with fuel or bootleg alcohols (e.g. in Russia) has lead to a clear reduction of life expectancies in Russia (Alcohol kills Russian working men, Haaga JV et al. 1997; Ogurtsov PP et al. 2001).

In a study on Scottish workers that considered educational levels and other risk factors, researchers were able to demonstrate that the total mortality rate was related to dosage in its progression. A very low dosage showed a levelled progression, but mortality rates increased with a dosage of three-eighths of a litre of wine daily or 21-eighths per week (factors Hart C et al. 2007; Smith D et al. 1998; Fig. 58).

In almost all somatic disciplines, it is highlighted that alcohol is a risk factor and when the term "alcohol" is entered as a search criterion into e.g. the "British Medical Journal" more than 2,700 publications are listed. There is virtually no medical journal which does not contain articles on alcohol. Due to the high number of publications, most textbooks concentrate on a few of the most important medical manifestations and we have had to do the same in this textbook although we are well aware that, in so doing, some very important aspects have been neglected. The European Society for Biomedical Research on Alcoholism (ESBRA, www.esbra.com), the International Society for Addiction Medicine and many others emphasize the importance of alcohol abuse and alcohol addiction in all medical disciplines and are attempting to create programmes that consider the sub-aetiology of alcoholism in most somatic diseases. In some disciplines, the diseases caused by alcohol have already been clearly described (Ranging from Wernicke's Encephalopathy, Alcoholic Amblyopathy, Alcoholic Cardiomyopathy to the Holiday Heart Syndrome, Johnson BA et al. 2003).

7.3.2.2 Alcohol's significance for neurology and psychiatry

As already highlighted, alcohol changes all functions in all cerebral circuits. Both intoxication and withdrawal impair the neuronal membranes. Neuronal damage is not only caused by alcohol and its aldehydes but also through malnutrition (especially vitamin deficiency) and craniocerebral injury. Previous cerebral damage (hypoxia during birth, cerebral traumata with neurological deficits, childhood epilepsies) sensitise the brain for alcohol. It is now known that severe mnestic disorders are frequent in groups with previous impairments (Lesch's type IV). Furthermore, the "symptomatic transitory psychotic syndrome"see page 7, 8 manifests in different forms during alcohol intoxication, depending on the amount, and rapidity, of alcohol drunk. Large amounts of alcohol consumed very quickly (drinking contests with e.g. 1 l Vodkas), can result in a loss of consciousness with different coma stages, which can be life threatening. A dimming of consciousness is not the dominant factor when alcohol is slowly resorbed. Here the significant factors are psychomotor changes and the concomitant symptomatic transitory psychotic syndrome (Wieck HH. 1956).

Chronic alcohol intoxication leads to a reduction of neuropsychological performance (different functions of intelligence, such as thinking, associating and memory performance). Psychopathological reactions might set in, depending on the severity of this reduced performance. Sensitivity to light and noise together with an emotional irritability (e.g. dysphoria in the morning after an alcohol overdose the night be-

Fig. 59 Progression of development and remission in steps

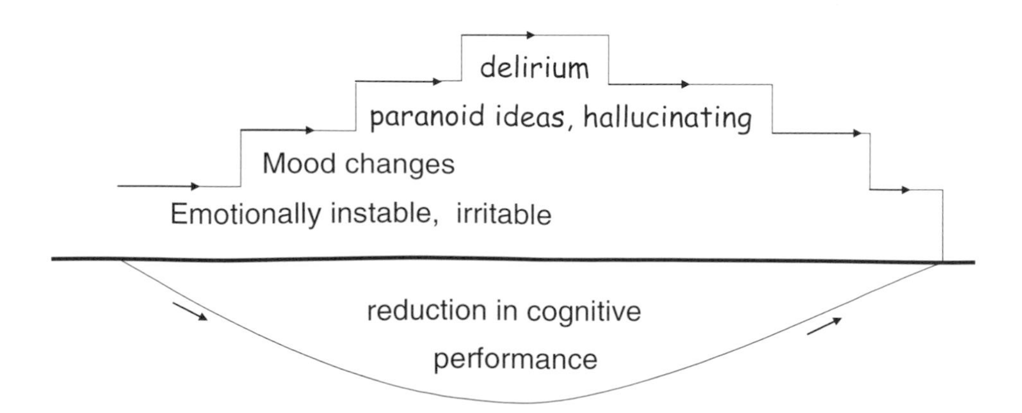

fore) occur. During severe impairment, virtually all patients react with affective symptoms which are characterized by dysfunctions in chronobiology (sleep disorders) and changes in drive and mood. If a reduction of performance due to intoxication or illness continues, the patient's perception changes and he might experience subjective delusional interpretations, often reflected by changing affectivity. These delusional elements often lead to a paranoid-hallucinatory syndrome. Hallucination may also manifest. If performance is furthermore reduced, confusion and severe anxiety with hallucinations can be observed. This condition is called "delirant symptomatic transitory psychotic syndrome", which is often complicated by vegetative syndromes and in 20% by epileptic seizures. Delirant syndromes without vegetative syndromes are not usually caused by alcohol but rather by other organic disorders. Further impairments lead to a clouding of consciousness up to the point of coma (all neurological levels). The recovery of these syndromes follows the same steps as the development of these symptomatic transitory psychotic syndromes. The recovery of delirant patterns that are caused by alcohol takes approximately six weeks until the point when no more psychopathological patterns exist.

7.3.2.3 Alcohol and psychiatric disorders

As already highlighted in chapter 6.1.1, other DSM-IV axis-I-diagnoses are often present in the course of alcohol dependence. Schizophrenic patients rarely regularly drink alcohol. 10% of these patients discover that alcohol has pharmacologically positive effects which help them to cope with their psychological symptoms. Patients with severe affective and cognitive "filter" dysfunctions suffer immensely from stimulus overflow and notice that alcohol helps them to tolerate this overstimulation. As alcohol changes the dopamine receptors, these patients are therefore more sensitive to neuroleptics that affect D2 receptors. Often severe extrapyramidal side effects occur. This patient group especially benefits from atypical neuroleptics which have GABAergic effects (e. g. Clozapine).

Fig. 60 Co-morbidity alcohol and depression based on gender

	Alcohol addiction		Alcohol abuse	
	Men	Women	Men	Women
Major depression	24,3 %	48,5 %	9,0 %	30,1 %
Dysthymia	11,2 %	20,9 %	3,6 %	10,1 %

*NCS (Kessler RC et al. 1996, 1997)

Fig. 61 Psychopathological relationships during in-patient admission

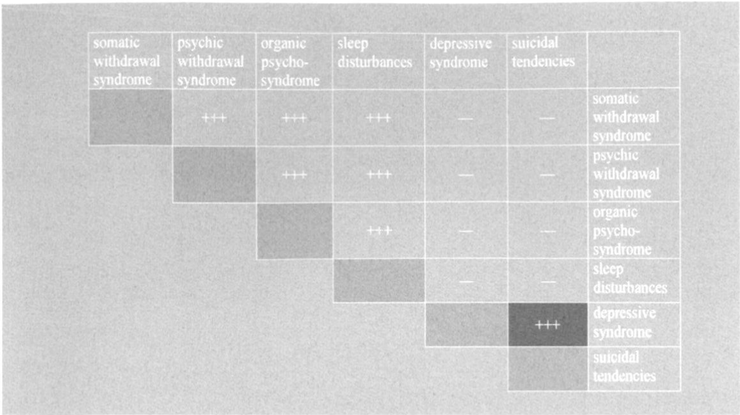

somatic withdrawal syndrome	psychic withdrawal syndrome	organic psycho-syndrome	sleep disturbances	depressive syndrome	suicidal tendencies	
	+++	+++	+++	–	–	somatic withdrawal syndrome
		+++	+++	–	–	psychic withdrawal syndrome
			+++	–	–	organic psycho-syndrome
				–	–	sleep disturbances
					+++	depressive syndrome
						suicidal tendencies

Fig. 62 Psychopathological relationships after twelve months in outpatient treatment (with same relationships showing at both times).

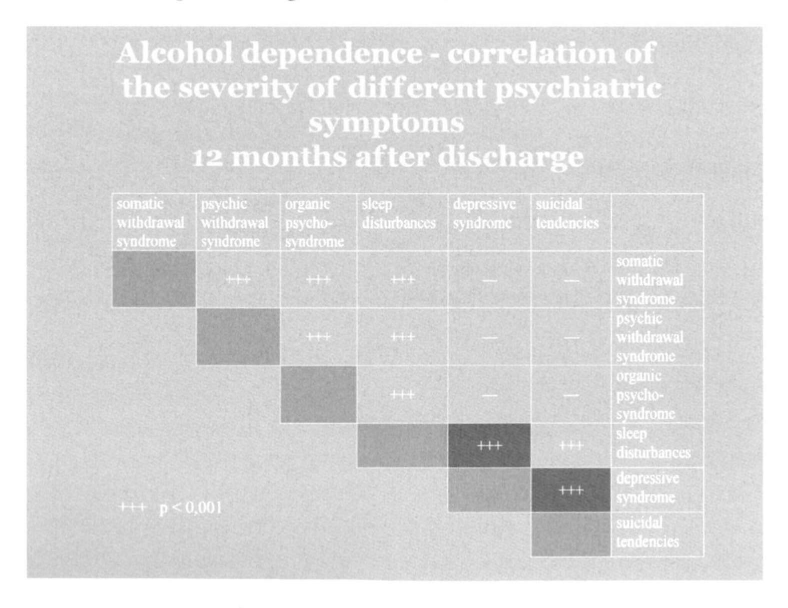

7.3.2.3.1 Alcohol and affective disorders

A large US epidemiological study which investigated the relationship between depression and alcohol addiction, found significant gender differences. It seems that women are more affected by affective disorders than men (Kessler RC 1997; Berner P et al. 1986; Driessen M et al. 2008).

In a prospective longitudinal study on alcohol dependent patients, Lesch OM 1985 examined the link between psychopathological symptoms during an in-patient admission at twelve months and four years after the admission into an outpatient setting (Lesch OM. 1985, Lesch OM et al. 1988; Figs. 61 and 62).

During admission mental symptoms like reduction of performance and sleep disorders significantly correlated with intoxication and withdrawal symptoms. Suicidal tendencies did not correlate with psychiatric syndromes and are likely to be caused by the difficult life situation of the affected at the time of admission.

A clearly differentiated pattern shows after twelve months or four years, which shows two evolving groups. One patient group showed symptoms that correlated with alcohol intoxication or withdrawal symptomatic. The other group showed chronobiological dysfunctions which correlated with affective symptoms, suicide attempts and suicides. These results clearly demonstrate that chronobiological dysfunctions can be defined as a major symptom of an affective disorder (comorbidity; Berner P et al. 1986; Dvorak A et al. 2003, Lesch OM et al. 1988).

In a prospective longitudinal study Angst et al. were able to show that mainly bipolar affective disorders lateron also meet the diagnostic criteria for an alcohol dependence, whereas there is no difference between patients with unipolar disorders and the normal population (the older the patients the more bipolar diagnoses, Angst J et al. 2006). The patient group which drinks alcohol to self-medicate their psychological disorder are classified into type III according to Lesch's typology. Depressive syndromes with sleeping disorders, linked to alcohol intoxication or alcohol withdrawal, should not have an axis-I-diagnosis (affective disorder) additionally. These symptoms are symptomatic transitory syndromes and subside after detox or with the diminishing of withdrawal symptoms without any therapy. Here the principle is: Alcohol addiction is treated first and if the psychiatric symptomatic still exists after two to three weeks of abstinence, then the (other) psychiatric axis-I-diagnosis should be treated (recommendation of the Plinius Maior Society, www.alcoweb.com).

7.3.2.3.2 Alcohol and Anxiety

Diverse forms of anxiety disorders show similarities in their longitudinal progression in that two thirds of patients with anxiety disorders develop alcohol or substance abuse. Only one third of anxiety patients reject medication, and also alcohol and tobacco consumption. An investigation of 100 anxiety patients with different forms of anxiety showed that anxiety patients who did not consume any alcohol had normal norharmane blood levels, while anxiety patients who temporarily abused alcohol had elevated norharmane levels even during abstinence (Leitner A et al. 1994). With regards to anxiety syndromes that later lead to abuse, it is important to first treat the abusing behaviour, which then enables therapy of the anxiety syndrome (therapy of alcohol dependents with anxiety or affective disorders should follow similar rules). Anxious or depressive symptomatic transitory syndromes (in connection with intoxication or withdrawal) should clearly be separated from real co-morbidities (anxiety disorders or affective disorders) (Wieck HH. 1967).

Basic disturbances of alcohol dependence and affective disorders are often due to pathological differences in temperament. The Temps scale was developed and has been validated in different languages and is able to assess the different temperament dimensions. (Erfurth A et al. 2005). Hyperthymic temperaments with different psychiatric diseases are often associated with positive outcomes. Cyclothymic temperaments (genetic or very early disturbances in brain development) influence psychiatric syndromes, increase co-morbidity rates and admissions to psychiatric wards and are often connected with poor outcomes and increased mortality rates. We were able to show in a sample of 116 alcohol dependent patients according to ICD-10 and DSM IV that Lesch type I patients have mostly a hypothymic temperament and Lesch type IV patients suffer from a cyclothymic temperament leading to very difficult social behaviours. These results fit very well with our prospective long term results showing that type I patients are often still sober after two years and type IV patients relapse very often.

These different temperaments also fit with a German study on persons who committed homicides showing that only Type II alcohol dependents have no criminal careers (Fig. 64). (Reulbach et al., 2007)

7.3.2.4 Alcohol and neurological disorders

If memory impairment is combined with a disturbance of time consciousness (the chronological organisation of events at certain times is not possible and the patient often confabulates) and additionally apathy, nystagmus and ataxia set in, the symptomatic is described as Wernick's encephalopathy. Besides the damage caused by alcohol, thiamine deficiency and genetic dysfunction of thiamine metabolism are discussed in the following paragraphs.

Rapid reduction of drinking can lead to epileptic "grand mal" withdrawal seizures. Haemorrhagic, embolic and also thrombotic strokes are very frequent in alcohol dependents. Often additional to these severe neurological

Fig. 63 Lesch typology and temperament

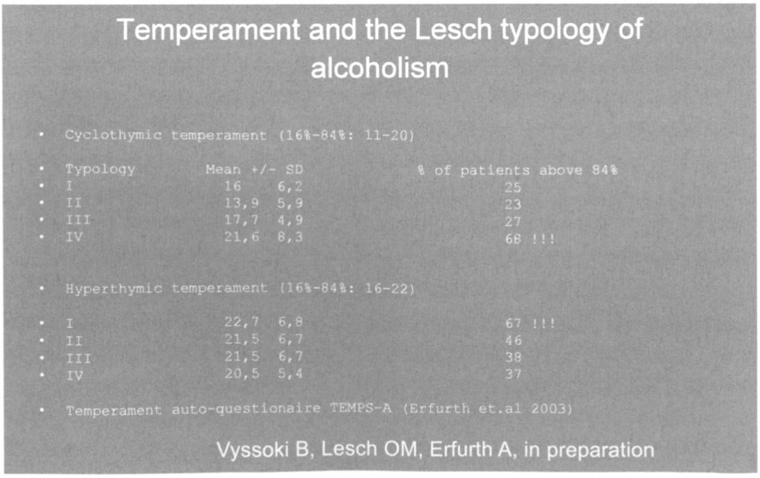

Temperament and the Lesch typology of alcoholism

- Cyclothymic temperament (16%-84%: 11-20)

Typology	Mean	+/- SD	% of patients above 84%
I	16	6,2	25
II	13,9	5,9	23
III	17,7	4,9	27
IV	21,6	8,3	68 !!!

- Hyperthymic temperament (16%-84%: 16-22)

Typology	Mean	+/- SD	% of patients above 84%
I	22,7	6,8	67 !!!
II	21,5	6,7	46
III	21,5	6,7	38
IV	20,5	5,4	37

- Temperament auto-questionaire TEMPS-A (Erfurth et.al 2003)

Vyssoki B, Lesch OM, Erfurth A, in preparation

Fig. 64 Homocide and alcohol dependence defined by Lesch's typology

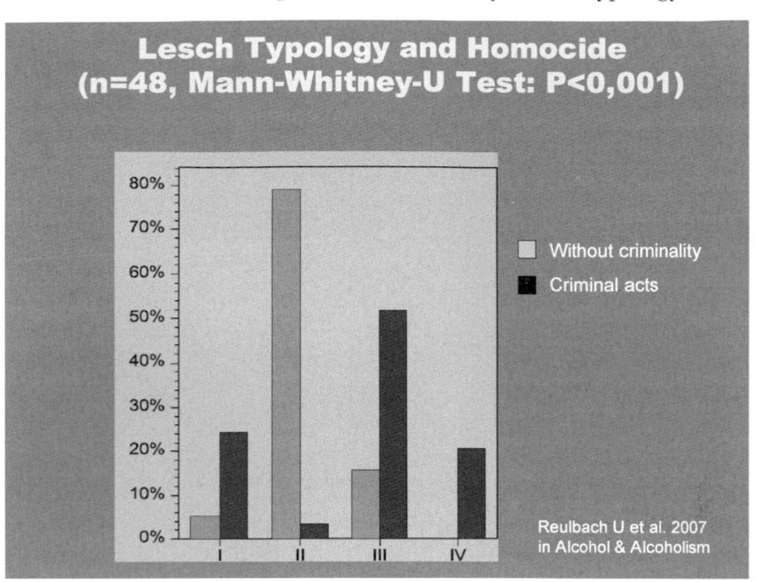

disorders are diabetes mellitus and hyperlipidemia with atherosclerotic disease and/or coagulopathy. Also alcohol and smoking increase the risk of suffering a seizure.

Around 1 % of alcohol dependents develop cerebellar diseases. Cerebellar cells are degenerated, coordination is increasingly impaired and severe ataxia of the legs is often observed. Arms are not as severely affected. A wide-legged style of walking with arms held at the side is characteristic in these patients. In 1999, a research group of the MUW (Medical University Vienna) showed that cerebral diseases, which were measured by platform posturography, significantly correlated with the duration of drinking behaviour (Woeber C et al. 1999). From a neurological perspective, this symptomatology can also be observed in Wernicke's encephalopathy (type IV alcohol dependents according to Lesch).

5 to 15 % of all alcohol dependents develop peripheral polyneuropathy that usually starts in the legs and can then shift to the arms. This symptomatic generally starts with paraesthesias which feel like the patient is wearing socks or gloves. Weakness, paraesthesias of burning character and pain are the prevailing symptoms. With the progression of the disease, atrophy and weakness of muscles are typically found in the peronaeus area. The Achilles reflex is alleviated or removed. Later the patella tendon reflex is also affected. A distal motor polyneuropathy, which primarily affects the legs, develops in later stages. Besides alcohol's effects, thiamine deficits are a topic of ongoing discussion. Alcohol dependents with severe polyneuropathy always show a poor type IV course and have a very slow ethanol and methanol elimination rate (see Fig. 6).

Alcohol induced psychotic disorders (Pathologischer Rausch), which can be caused by only small amounts of alcohol, are rarely seen and often interpreted as "partial epilepsy" or "dreamy states". During abstinence these patients show a normal EEG, during provocation (sleep withdrawal or alcohol), however, "Spike and Wave" patterns were observed in the temporal brain areas.

It is now proven that alcohol interferes with normal sleep pattern and that, as a result, individuals do not go through the healthy stages of sleep. If previous sleep disorders are present (e.g. nightly awakening in depression), alcohol aggravates these sleep disorders. Transitory depressive symptoms, caused by alcohol, or which set in during withdrawal, usually regress automatically after two or three weeks, with an improvement in the quality of sleep (Schuckit MA et al. 1997).

7.3.2.5 Alcohol and internal medicine

7.3.2.5.1 Gastroenterology

Alcohol impairs the entire gastrointestinal system. Oral inflammation and peptic oesophagitis are often a result of alcohol abuse. Acetaldehyde and formaldehyde seem to be the toxic agents within this damage. As acetaldehyde is also caused by smoking, these diseases are very numerous in smoking alcohol dependents (Salaspuro VJ et al. 2006; Salaspuro VJ and Salaspuro M. 2004). Alcohol causes anacide gastritis in the stomach which secondarily leads to dysfunctions in resorption, e.g. in vitamins. As around 40 % of alcohol is metabolized in the stomach, the breakdown of alcohol in the stomach is an important process for the liver and brain. Therefore individuals who had stomach surgery often don't tolerate as much alcohol as they did before. Diarrhoea after alcohol abuse is a sign of irritation of the large intestine. A portal hypertension might develop due to alcohol related liver damage and therefore internal and external haemorrhoids or oesophagus varices bleeding are often observed. As alcohol is metabolized by the liver in the so called "first pass effect", alcohol consumed over a longer period of time can damage the liver even in low doses (pure alcohol: 20g/daily for women; 40g/daily for men). Alcohol impairs gluconeogenesis and turns carbohydrate metabolism into fat production. According to the duration and amount of alcohol consumption, a fatty liver and alcoholic hepatitis can develop. Maintained over longer periods, this can lead to irreversible fibrosis and eventually to liver cirrhosis. Decompensated liver cirrhosis is characterized by a liver cell dysfunction in which portal hypertension with a splenomegaly, often with oesophagus varices and ascites, are present. Changes in hormone levels and weakness of the immune system with corresponding inflammations are often observable. At the onset of liver disease, ASAT is clearly higher than ALAT (positive de Ritis Factor) with a significantly elevated Gamma GT. In a fibrous reconstruction, the Gamma GT usually increases and at the same time ALAT gets on the same level or even higher than ASAT. Yet not all alcohol dependents develop liver cirrhosis. When all alcoholic dependents, treated at a psychiatric hospital, are examined for evidence of liver disease, it is apparent that especially type I and type IV patients according to Lesch are affected by severe liver damage. On gastroenterological wards treating primary liver diseases we could show that more than 50 % has been diagnosed as Lesch Type II patients. The rate of affective disorders and suicidal tendency were significantly lower in internal wards than in patients admitted with the diagnosis of alcohol dependence at psychiatric wards (Vyssoki B.et al. accepted in Alcohol and Alcoholism).

As a fifth of all elevated liver functions has an aetiology other than alcohol, it should be noted that either infectious diseases, cholostases or other rare diseases may be the reason for this elevation (see path diagnosis of the computer version of Lesch's typology (www.lat-online.at), Baischer W et al. 1995; Mihas AA et al. 2007; Maher JJ. 2007; National Institute of Health Consensus Development Conference Statement: management of hepatitis C. 2002). The mechanisms of how alcohol causes liver damage are not yet clear. The metabolising in the liver via hydrogenases and the MEOS-system or the catalase are likely to be involved, e.g. catalase deficiency damages liver cells. Genetic variants of the hydrogenases, but also diet and changes in vitamin levels especially B6, also seem to be crucial factors. Why some forms of alcoholic hepatiti later cause liver carcinoma is still unexplained. Genetic and biochemical models are discussed herein (Mihas AA et al. 2007). If the liver is so severely damaged that a liver transplantation is needed, preparation and aftercare with regards to drinking behaviour is just as important as surgery. The Vienna research group was able to show that in 97 alcohol dependents with liver transplantations, prognosis with regular psychiatric aftercare was very positive in regard to drinking behaviour (Berlakovich GA et al. 1999).

Pancreatitis only develops in a few patients. If the pancreas is affected, often a chronic pancreatitis develops (with a shortened life expectancy). This

Fig. 65 Liver transplantation and relapse rates

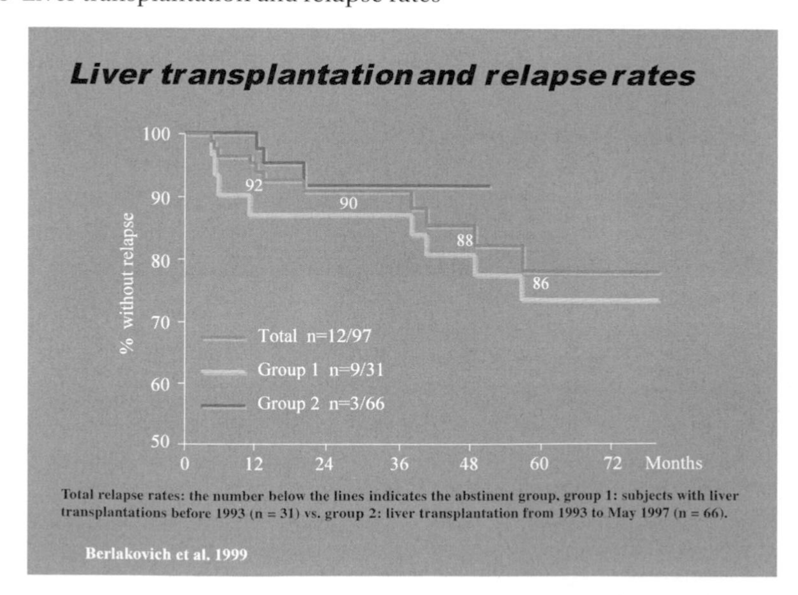

inflammation of the pancreas can lead to diabetes mellitus. Abnormal protein formation in the liver leads to dysfunctions in blood clotting and therefore haematoma can often be observed in these patients. Consequently, esophageal varices and haemorrhoidal bleeding become more difficult to treat and often cause death.

7.3.2.5.2 Cardiovascular system

Heart diseases like e.g. cardiomyopathy, heart rhythm dysfunction, coronary heart disease and blood pressure dysfunctions are more frequent in individuals who chronically abuse alcohol. Yet these underlying diseases can only be treated in a state-of-the art fashion if alcohol abuse is terminated or at least controlled (Preedy VR and Richardson PJ. 1994; Strotmann J and Ertl G. 2005).

7.3.2.5.2.1 Alcoholic Cardiomyopathy

In industrial countries, alcohol related cardiomyopathy is the primary form of secondary dilated cardiomyopathy. It is characterized by a dilating left ventricle (LV), an enlarged LV mass, a normal or decreased LV thickness and a dysfunction of ventricles with reduced secretion. A diastolic dysfunction is usually asymptomatic, while cardiomyopathy clinically manifests with a systolic dysfunction. The diagnosis is predominantly a diagnosis of exclusion inclusive of a long lasting alcohol anamnesis (Piano MR. 2002).

The progression of heart diseases is often reversible during abstinence. With further alcohol abuse a heart insufficiency develops, which clearly shortens life expectancy. Less than a quarter survive the following three years after diagnosis (Wynne J and Braunwald E. 2005).

7.3.2.5.2.2 Cardiac arrhythmia, "Holiday-Heart-Syndrome" and sudden cardiac arrest

Many studies have documented the relationship between increased alcohol consumption and cardiac arrhythmia (supraventricular arrhythmia like atrial fibrillation and ventricular arrhythmia; Rosenqvist M. 1998; Singer MV and Teyssen S. 2005). Chronic alcohol abuse leads to changes in the structure of the myocardium like fibrosis, hypertrophy, fatty infiltrations and a lowered resting membrane potential (Schoppet M and Maisch B. 2001). In acute cases, alcohol can lead to an increased release of catecholamines and an increase in heart

Fig. 66 Supraventricular arrhythmia in alcohol consumption

Rhythm	alcohol consumption					
	6 + (n = 1.322)		< 1 (n = 2.644)		Relative risk for 6+ vs. <1	p-value*
	%	Number	%	Number		
Atrial fibrillation	1,1	15	0,5	13	2,3	0,02
Atrial flutter	0,6	8	0,2	6	3,0	0,05
Supraventricular Tachycardia	0,4	5	0,1	2	5,0	0,03
Supraventricular Extrasystoles	3,3	43	1,3	32	3,0	<0,01
Fibrillation, fluttering or supraventricular Tachycardia	1,6	21	0,7	19	2,3	<0,01

*p-values for samples determined with McNemar-Test

frequency (Rosenqvist M. 1998; Huseyin U et al. 2005).

A case-control study showed that the relative risk for individuals who consume more than 420 grams/day of suffering from atrial fibrillation was 2.4x as high, as in the normal population (Ruigomez A. et al. 2002). Another study showed that the risk for men who consumed comparable amounts of alcohol was 1.46 times higher than in the normal population (Frost L. and Vestergaard P. 2004). The term "Holiday-Heart-Syndrome" evolved from supraventricular cardiac arrhythmia that was frequently observed at weekends and during holidays as a result of increased alcohol consumption (Singer MV and Teyssen S. 2005). Ventricular arrhythmia is associated with QT-lengthening in ECG, which points to an abnormal cardiac repolarisation. This form of arrhythmia is responsible for sudden cardiac arrest and is caused by the re-entry-mechanism with its circulating excitations in the heart (Rosenqvist M. 1998; Singer MV. and Teyssen S. 2005). Lengthened QT-intervals (Cuculi F. et al. 2006) and cardiac arrhythmia (Rosenqvist M. 1998) are also frequently observed in withdrawal.

Significantly more supraventricular, tachycardic arrhythmias were observed when 60 grams of pure alcohol were consumed daily in comparison to only 10 grams daily (cited by Singer MV. and Teyssen S. 2005).

7.3.2.5.2.3 Coronary heart disease and myocardial infarction

The relationship between ischaemic heart disease and alcohol has been controversially discussed in the literature.

Singer MV and Teyssen S. (2005) propose that a moderate consumption can actually protect the cardiovascular system. It is probable to suggest a U-formed progression. For example, Deev A. et al. found that level 1 drinkers suffer more from cardiovascular diseases than level 2-and level 3 drinkers, while the risk again increased for level 4 individuals (stronger drinkers) (Deev A. et al. 1998).

Results from a longitudinal Norwegian study which examined 40,000 participants over 40 years suggest that alcohol consumers are 2.5 times more likely to suffer from cardiovascular disease (Rossow I. and Amundsen A. 1997). Another study was not able to support the link between coronary heart disease (CHD) and beer consumption, although the risk of fatal heart attack was increased 6 times (Kauhanen J et al. 1997). Other studies have found a higher CHD risk in individuals who severely abuse alcohol (Overview by Davidson DM. 1989; Dyer A. et al. 1977; Malyutina S et al. 2002).

7.3.2.5.2.4 Hypertonia

According to the WHO, hypertonia is defined by a blood pressure value (RR) of 140/90 or above. Alcohol consumers are four times more likely to suffer from hypertension (Arkwright PD et al. 1982). Marmot MG et al. have found that the blood pressure value (RR) of men who consume more than 400 g of alcohol per week rises on average by 4.6/3 mmHg (Marmot MG et al. 1994). The RR in women who consumed more than 240 g per week increased by 3.9/3.1 mmHg. Contrary to the diastolic blood pressure, the systolic blood pressure strongly correlates with the amount of ethanol consumed ($p < 0.001$, Arkwright PD et al. 1982). The RR drops with the reduction of alcohol, with the systolic RR more strongly correlating than the diastolic blood pressure (Puddey IB et al. 1985). These effects of alcohol on blood pressure are independent of age, weight, smoking behaviour, exercise and salt secretion (Arkwright P.D et al. 1982; Puddey IB et al. 1985; Marmot MG et al. 1994).

7.3.2.5.2.5 Hypothesis on the aetiology of alcohol addiction and heart diseases

Additional to changes in lipid metabolism and the reduction of oxygen availability, we will also discuss the homocysteine metabolism in regard to both alcohol dependence and cardiovascular diseases. Numerous studies point to a connection between alcohol consumption and an increase of blood homocysteine levels (Hcy). Bleich S et al. showed that even with low amounts (30 g) of alcohol per day the Hcy significantly increased (750 ml beer or 3/8 wine; Bleich S et al. 2001). The homocysteine (Hcy) level already increased to 18 % after small doses over six weeks. Here the Hcy increased slightly more with red wine and spirit than with beer. A further study showed similar results, suggesting that homocysteine levels of alcohol dependents were twice as high as in an abstinent population (Cravo ML and Camilo ME. 2000).

Hultberg B. et al. observed higher homocysteine levels during alcohol intoxication, with normal levels in abstinence (Hultberg B et al. 1993). Kenyon S. H. et al. illuminated the link between alcohol abuse and hyperhomocysteinaemia by examining the influence of ethanol on homocysteine. The homocysteine metabolism can be portrayed as follows (Kenyon SH et al. 1998).

The influence of alcohol is best explained by the effect of acetaldehyde on methionine synthesis as acetaldehyde directly blocks this synthesis. As this enzyme depends on vitamin B12, the effect of B12 should also be considered (Hultberg B. et al. 1993).

Fig. 67 Intracellular homocysteine metabolism

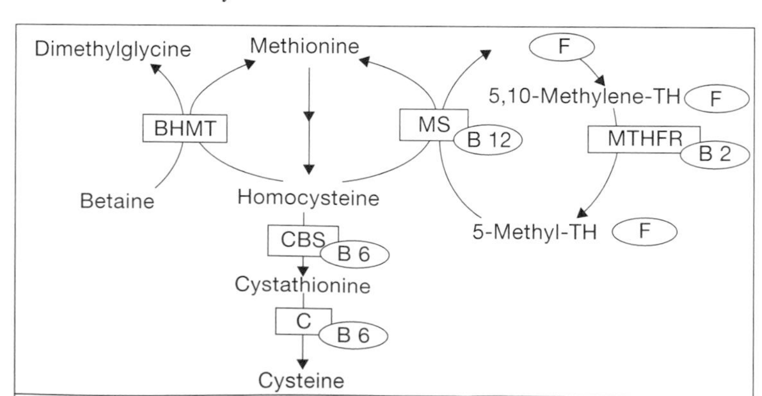

BHMT = Betaine-Homocysteine Methyltransferase, B2 = Vitamin B2, B6 = Vitamin B6, B12 = Vitamin B12, C = γ-Cystathioninase, CBS = Cystathionin-β-Synthase, F = Folic acid, MS = Methioninsynthase, MTHFR = 5,10-Methylentetrahydrofolat-Reduktase, THF = Tetrahydrofolicacid.

Blood vessel damage is very diverse and in the case of alcohol dependents, homocysteine metabolism has been suggested as playing a role (Stanger O. et al. 2003). Heart insufficiency and coronary heart diseases are also being discussed in regard to homocysteine metabolism (Hermann M et al. 2005; Vasan RS et al. 2003; Nygard O et al. 1997).

This relationship is also represented by the survival rates of patients with coronary heart diseases in regard to homocysteine levels (Nygard O et al. 1997).

7.3.2.5.2.6 Alcohol typology according to Lesch – Homocysteine level – Heart diseases

Bleich S and his research group showed that homocysteine levels are only elevated in Lesch type I alcohol dependent patients (Bleich S et al. 2004). 'Grand mal' epileptic withdrawal seizures seem to be an important indicator for high homocysteine levels. During abstinence in typeI patients, the homocysteine level regresses within one to two weeks. Type I alcohol dependents with withdrawal seizures showed significantly higher plasma-homocysteine

Fig. 68 Mortality rates and homocysteine level

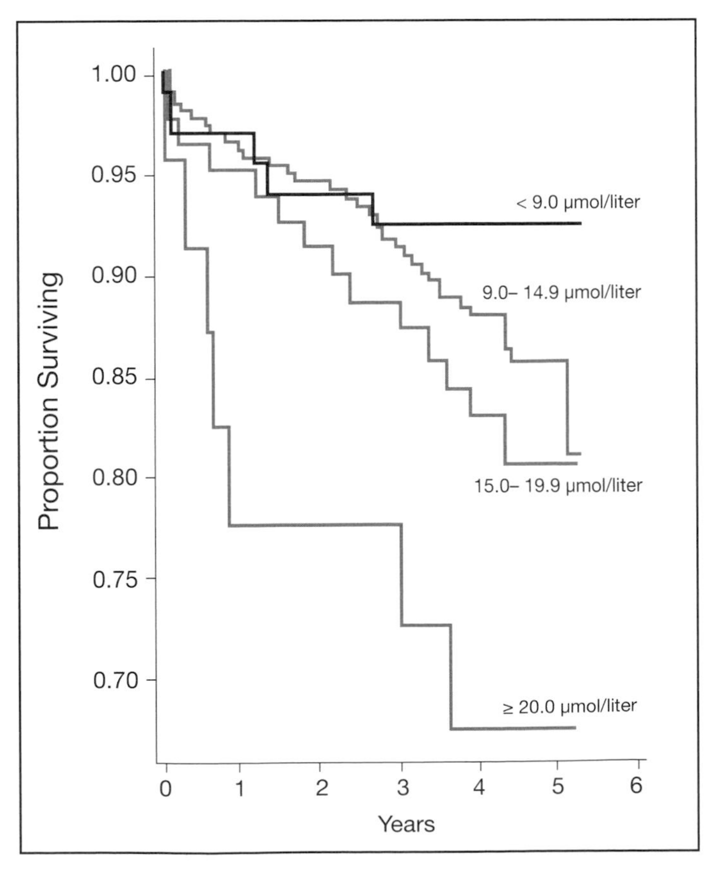

Fig. 69 Frequency of MTHFR genotypes and serum homocysteine level in alcohol dependents, classified according to Lesch's typology, in comparison to healthy control groups

	CONTROLS		LESCH TYPE I		LESCH TYPE II		LESCH TYPE III		LESCH TYPE IV	
	N	%	N	%	N	%	N	%	N	%
CC	35	**37,6 %**	10	**76,9 %**	5	**55,5 %**	30	**37,5 %**	11	**61,1 %**
CT	41	**44,1 %**	3	**23,1 %**	4	**44,5 %**	41	**51,3 %**	5	**27,8 %**
TT	17	**18,3 %**	0	**0 %**	0	**0 %**	9	**11,2 %**	2	**11,1 %**
N	93		13		9		80		18	
HOMOCYSTEINE M ±*SD* (μMOL/L)	**10,5** ± *5,9*		**21,8** ± *12,3*		**17,5** ± *7,0*		**18,1** ± *9,9*		**17,2** ± *11,9*	

Saffroy R et al. 2008

levels (55.8 ± 30.7 nmol/l) while type II, III-and IV patients had a homocysteine level of 39.7 ± 21.9 during intoxication. Furthermore, at admission type I patients showed significantly higher alcohol levels (Bleich S et al. 2004). As type I tend to consume the highest amounts of alcohol in regular doses throughout the day (Jellinek's delta-type), it is possible that the homocysteine level remains high for years. The complicated mechanism of homocysteine suggests that different substances but also different genetics correlate with the development of the subtypes of alcohol dependence and with blood vessel or heart disease.

Saffroy R. and colleagues examined alcohol dependent patients who they classified according to Lesch's typology and Babor's typology. Results showed that the methylentetrahydrofolate reductase gene, which influences homocysteine, is associated with type III according to Lesch. Furthermore, type B according to Babor showed a significantly lower frequency of the MTHFR-677TT gene (Saffroy R et al. 2004, 2008). Today we know how homocysteine is generated from methionine metabolism and how pyridoxine, folic acid, cobalamine and the homocysteine level are associated in the blood (Devlin AM et al. 2006, De Bree A et al. 2002, Stanger O et al. 2003.)

A German study showed that the MTHFR-393-polymorphism-CC-CA-AA is elevated in type IV according to Lesch and results also suggest that this polymorphism frequently occurs in type I (Boensch D et al. 2006).

The above-cited results from basic research highlight the different mechanisms of homocysteine metabolism. Yet the results in regard to subgroups of alcohol dependents are still to be interpreted with caution. From a clinical perspective, all aspects of this metabolism should be taken into consideration when examining the relationship between alcohol and heart disease.

The relationship between homocysteine level and survival rate in heart disease suggests that homocysteine has toxic effects on the heart and circulation. From an alcohol research perspec-

Fig. 70 MTHFR and the typology according to Lesch

Folic acid-producing reductase MTHFR
n = 134

MTHFR-393 polymorphism CC-CA-AA

		CC	CA/AA
Lesch I	n = 26	68 %	32 %
Lesch II	n = 65	86 %	13 %
Lesch III	n = 58	92 %	7 %
Lesch IV	n = 18	60 %	40 %

tive, the relationship between type I alcohol dependence, homocysteine and heart disease is important because clear therapeutic consequences can be derived from it. Homocysteine may be a biological marker for the effectiveness of acamprosate in alcohol abusing individuals with heart disease. This is supported by the fact that type I dependents are characterized by their high homocysteine levels and that an administration of acamprosate doubles abstinence rate.. If patients do not stop drinking, administration of folic acid could reduce homocysteine levels in (drinking) type I patients and will prevent cardiac sequelae.

7.3.2.5.3 Oncological diseases

Alcohol in combination with overweight and smoking increases the risk of various forms of carcinoma (Teschke R and Goeke R. 2005). With reference to the "Global Burden of Disease Project", the WHO indicates that every year 1.8 million people worldwide die from alcohol related cancer. These represent 3.2 % of all deaths per year. There are many forms of cancer associated with alcohol, but there is consensus that the cancer forms presented in Fig. 71 are linked to alcohol.

Every year, 5.2 % of men and 1.7 % of women are diagnosed with alcohol related cancer (Baan R et al. 2007; Bofetta P 2006a, 2006b). The link between amounts of alcohol consumed and the risk of developing a carcinoma is undisputed. The risk of suffering from cancer of the pharynx-gastrointestinal tract is already increased with a consumption of 50–80 g of alcohol per day. Elevated acetaldehyde levels, but also alcohol by itself irritates the entire mucous membrane of the mouth-stomach-intestinal tract. Therefore it is not surprising that 85 % of patients with mouth-pharynx carcinomas are diagnosed as alcohol dependent. Alcohol reduces salivation and increases the secretion's viscosity. This impairs the mechanical cleansing of the mucous membrane and the teeth and weakens the immune system. Pathogenic germs then cause an inflammation of the mucous membrane (e.g. gingivitis and paradontitis). These conditions increase the vulnerability to carcinogens. Acetaldehyde activates these carcinogens. The damaged mu-

Fig. 71 Alcohol-Tobacco: sites of tumours (Seitz HK and Stickel F 2007)

Associations between chronic alcohol and/or tobacco consumption and malignant tumours of different organs.
(-) no association; (+) possible association; (+) additive effect;
(+++) potentiating effect; + significant association

Sites of tumours	Increased risk of carcinom		
	Alcohol	Tobacco	Alcohol + Tobacco
Oral cavity	+	+	+++
Pharynx	+	+	+++
Larynx	+	+	+++
Lungs	(+)	+	++
Oesophagus	+	+	+++
Stomach	(+)	+	+++
Small intestine	-	?	?
Colon	+	-	?
Rectum	+	-	?
Liver	+	+	+++
Pancreas	(+)	+	++
Mamma	+	-	?
Thyroid	(+)	-	?
Skin	(+)	-	?
Prostate	(+)	-	?
Urinary bladder	-	+	?

cosa stimulates cell regeneration via genetic changes (acetaldehyde has multiple mutagenic effects on the DNA) and dysplasia, leukoplakia and eventually carcinoma develop (Seitz HK and Stickel F. 2007; Hoermann K and Riedel F. 2005). Adequate pre-and postoperative support of alcohol dependent cancer patients significantly reduces complications and halves the duration of in-patient admissions. Abstinence not only decreases the risk for carcinoma, but is also important for the prognosis of a cancerous disease.

Alcohol clearly increases the risk for breast cancer in women and in men abuse of alcohol is associated with prostate cancer (Terry MB et al. 2006). The heightened risk for liver cell carcinoma has been described in numerous studies, although additional infections (hepatitis B and C) have not sufficiently been considered (Petry W et al. 1997). Although alcohol by itself represents a moderate risk only, in combination with hepatitis B the risk for a primary liver cell carcinoma significantly increases. As already emphasized, alcohol metabolism, in particular aldehyde plays an essential role in the genesis of carcinoma. Alcohol related carcinoma of the oesophagus is linked to Aldehydedehydrogenase-2*2(ALDH-2*2)-allele. Besides these alleles, it has been argued that other genetic variants like alcohol dehydrogenase 1C*1(ADH-1C*1)

Fig. 72 Alcohol and carcinoma: possible pathways

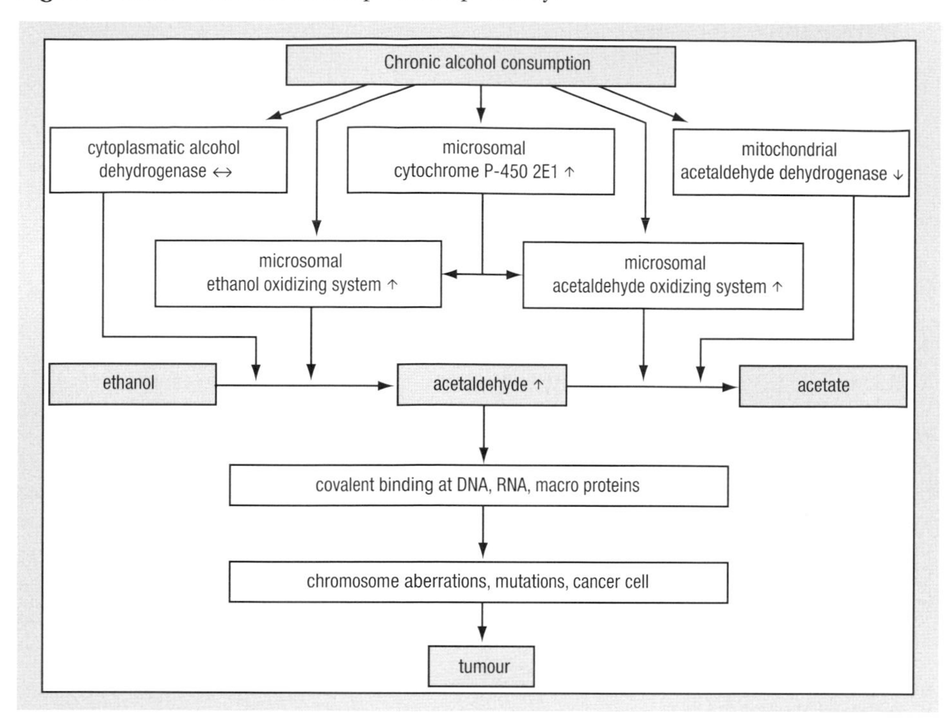

homozygotes and methyl-tetrahydrofol reductase (MTHFR)-677CT variants, increase the alcohol related risk for carcinoma. Variants of MTHFR have been examined in regard to the alcohol typologies according to Lesch and Babor and it is interesting to see whether Barbor's type B or Lesch's type III have a higher risk for cancer. Yet research on this issue is still lacking(Seitz HK and Stickel F. 2007; Saffroy R et al. 2004).

Teschke R and Goeke R have introduced a concept which considers different factors that can cause a tumour. The above findings should be integrated into this concept (Teschke R and Goke R. 2005).

The role of alcohol should not be underestimated with regards to therapy and the progression of carcinoma because e.g. alcohol related alterations in metabolism can change the effects and side effects of chemotherapeutics.

7.3.2.6 Alcohol and medication for sequelae

Depression and anxiety in particular are treated by psychopharmaceutical agents and the fact that most of these medications interact with alcohol is rarely considered. In the chapter on oncology (7.3.1.4) we have already pointed out to this interaction. Today, we differentiate between the impact of an acute alcohol intoxication on the effects of different medications and the influence of chronic alcohol intoxication on the pharmacological aspects of medication. Principally, an acute alcohol intoxication increases the effective levels of medication, while chronic intoxication leads to enzyme induction, which clearly reduces the effectiveness of medications (Ramskogler K et al. 2001).

These two figures only show the most prevalent interactions. Ultimately every medication which is eliminated by the cytochrome P450 metabolism or that has effects on cerebral functions whose vulnerability has been changed by alcohol, is influenced in its effect. For example, alcohol sensitizes the dopamine receptor and this is why classic neuroleptics or antiemetics often cause severe extrapyramidal sequelae.

Fig. 73 Acute Alcohol abuse and medication

Medication	Type of interaction	Clinical effect
NSAIDs	Activity reduction of ADH	Increase in plasma level of ethanol and pharmacon
Psychopharmaca (benzodiazepines, barbiturates, tri-and tetracyclic antidepressants, clomethiazole)	Competition with ethanol on the binding receptor at the cytochrome P 450	Synergistic effect with increase in sedation and deterioration of psychomotoric functions
Antiepileptics, oral antidiabetics, anticoagulants, antihypertensives, paracetamol	As above	Lengthening of half live time with a risk of over-dose and related complications
Disulfiram, antidiabetics (sulfonyl carbamide-type) antibiotics	Inhibition of ALDH	Flushing- facial rash, blood pressure problems, nausea and vomiting

Ramskogler et al. Wiener klinische Wochenschrift 2001

Fig. 74 Chronic alcohol abuse and medication

Medication	Type of interaction	Clinical effect
NSAIDs	Activity reduction of ADH	Increase of plasma level of ethanol and pharmacon
Psychopharmaca, antiepileptics, oral antidiabetics, anticoagulants, antihypertensives, rifampicine	Accelerated metabolism of substances via the induced cytochrome P450 (especially 2E1)	Shortening of half life time with reduced clinical effect
Anaesthetics, isoniacid, phenylbutazone, paracetamol	As above	hepatotoxic metabolites increased

Ramskogler et al. Wiener klinische Wochenschrift 2001

8

Detection of alcohol and tobacco addiction

8.1 Recommendations for the first contact

Clinician's dialogue regarding alcohol addiction

85 % of all adults in central Europe drink alcohol more or less regularly and this is why the question "do you drink alcohol" is almost always answered with "yes". But this answer does not provide any information about the interaction of psycho-social-biological problems caused by alcohol and therefore this question should be avoided. Abusers and dependents know their problem, which they experience as failure, and for which they often feel guilt or shame. Antoine de Saint-Exupery has brilliantly described this situation in the 12th chapter of his book "The Little Prince" (1943), Fig. 75.

The patient is afraid that his alcohol abuse will be discovered and at the same time he knows that he can only be helped if his alcohol consumption is addressed. This strong ambivalence leads to a change of behaviour in the patient. There are times when patients are more easily motivated and times

Fig. 75 Shame and alcohol abuse

The next planet was inhabited by a tippler. This was a very short visit, but it plunged the little prince into deep dejection.

"What are you doing there?" he said to the tippler, whom he found settled down in silence before a collection of empty bottles and also a collection of full bottles.
"I am drinking," replied the tippler, with a lugubrious air.
"Why are you drinking?" demanded the little prince.
"So that I may forget," replied the tippler.
"Forget what?" inquired the little prince, who already was sorry for him.
"Forget that I am ashamed," the tippler confessed, hanging his head.
"Ashamed of what?" insisted the little prince, who wanted to help him.
"Ashamed of drinking!" The tippler brought his speech to an end, and shut himself up in an impregnable silence.

And the little prince went away, puzzled.

"The grown-ups are certainly very, very odd," he said to himself, as he continued on his journey.

when motivation towards a lifestyle change is in fact impossible. The nature of interaction between therapist and patients is therefore of great importance. The guidelines for therapeutic dialogue should always be considered. Basic conditions like a comfortable atmosphere (a quiet room without a telephone) and sufficient time (the initial meeting should last at least 35 minutes) are necessary. Clinicians should definitely be aware of transference and countertransference issues. Like in any other psychotherapy, the therapist starts with open questions, which show the patient that there is an interest in him as a person and that there is someone to help him. Every question, which could be interpreted as senseless curiosity, should be avoided. In this conversation, the relationship between problems, wishes, feelings, thoughts, fears and the effect of alcohol should be elaborated gradually. Ambivalences should be amplified. Positive factors concerning drinking (e. g. drinks taste good and eliminate negative feelings) and negative factors, which argue for a reduction

Fig. 76 The following questions may be asked to find out about the perceived value of alcohol:

- Do you like the taste of alcohol or do you drink alcohol because of its effects?
- If yes, what effects do you wish for (to get drunk, changes in mood, to cope with anxiety etc.)?
- Describe any positive effects of alcohol. Can you also think of any negative effects and consequences of alcohol?
- Is there any link between the problems, for which you consulted me and the discomforts caused by alcohol ?
- When you stop drinking for a few days, does your condition improve or deteriorate?
- Are there any other ways to alleviate your (psychological or physical) complaints?
- Does drinking alcohol help? If yes, how much do you drink to alleviate your complaints? How much alcohol can you handle?
- When you have had too much alcohol at a party, do you have alcohol-related symptoms the next day (headache, circulatory problems, unrest, agitation)? Do you then drink again to alleviate these symptoms? How much alcohol do you need for this?
- When taking medication for your symptoms, were you able to reduce or even terminate alcohol consumption? If you weren't able to reduce drinking, what were the reasons for this? (e. g. withdrawal symptoms, psychological or social problems etc.)?
- Did you feel better when you didn't drink over several months? What helped you to stay abstinent? Why don't you try this again?
- Are there any places or situations, in which you find it very difficult not to drink (so-called "hot spots"), and are there places and situation, in which you never drink any alcohol (so-called "Cool Spots")?

and termination of drinking (reinforcement of problems, psycho-social reasons etc.), should be clearly discussed (Fig. 76).

The aim of the initial meeting is to determine factors that provide information about the value that alcohol has for the patient's well-being. Every objectification of the drinking behaviour or alcohol sequelae is helpful, e. g. severity of liver disease, assessment of withdrawal syndrome and objectification of the intoxication (e. g. via a breathalyzer). If the therapist observes during the initial meeting that the value attributed to alcohol is consistent with an abuse or addiction, the aim of this meeting is the planning of further meetings. These meetings should be conducted by the therapist who conducted the initial meeting or with experts who have relevant psychotherapeutic and pharmacotherapeutic competencies. Patients can quit treatment at any time and it is recommended that the therapeutic location be changed as seldom as possible. The aetiology and diagnostic of alcohol dependence and the link to medical conditions can only explicitly be made after several meetings. If the patient is strongly intoxicated during the initial meeting (blood alcohol or breath alcohol level above 1.5 mg), the meeting should be brief, but if possible another meeting, taking place within the next 24 hours, preferably in the morning, should be offered. If the patient mentions developing acute delirium over night or urgently wanting to drink alcohol in the morning, an adequate medication for his withdrawal symptoms (see chapter 9) should be prescribed, before drinking can be reduced.

Once the interaction between alcohol intake and the medical condition has been elaborated, the next step is to clarify whether alcohol abuse or dependence is present. For this the ICD-10 or DSM-IV (see chapter 5) should be used. As general practitioners often have too little time for this diagnostic, there are instruments available that enable an objectification by using only a few questions. Within medical practitioner or non-psychiatric medical specialist settings, four questions have prevailed, as summarized by CAGE (Fig. 11, Ewing JA. 1984).

If one of these questions is answered with "yes", patients almost always meet the diagnostic criteria for alcohol abuse according to DSM-IV or ICD-10. If two or more questions are answered with "yes" then a DSM-IV or ICD-10 diagnosis of alcohol dependence is very likely (Chan AW et al. 1994; Liskow B et al. 1995; Bradley KA et al. 2001; Saremi A et al. 2001). If the diagnosis is made according to ICD-10 or DSM-IV, Lesch's survey tool can be used for a more specific diagnosis (see Appendix 1). This computer programme assesses most of the important criteria that should be employed for the treatment and prognosis of alcohol dependents (e.g. alcohol-positive family anamneses, onset of acute alcohol abuse etc). Only one page of this survey tool is concerned with the classification of the typology. Adequate withdrawal treatment and relapse prevention can only be commenced after a classification has been made (Lesch OM et al. 1990, the typology computer programme can be found at www.lat-online.at).

8.2 Assessment of drinking behaviour by using biological markers

Markers for a predisposition and for an early detection, as well as markers which objectify an existing alcohol use or abuse, and markers which are associated with alcohol dependence, have been differentiated (Overview Fig. 77).

8.2.1 Trait markers

All these markers differ between alcohol dependent patients and the normal population (Pettinati HM et al. 2003; Koob GF and Le Moal M. 2006; Lalemand F et al. 2006). In the last year, these markers have also been further investigated in regard to Lesch's subgroups, personality dimensions and Cloninger's types. Significant differences were found in these subgroups (genetic differences as well as differences in alcohol metabolism and amino acids). The differences in Lesch's typology illustrate that these types seem to have different enzyme equipments (Fig. 6, Hillemacher T and Bleich S. 2008).

8.2.2 State markers

State markers provide information about drinking amount and drinking profile. Acute intoxication is best measured by identifying the type of alcohol and its degradation products (breath and blood alcohol). Nowadays breath measurements for assessing the alcohol level in unconscious persons are available. If the last intoxication dates back a few days, metabolites of alcohol in the blood and urine can provide information, e.g. ethyl glucuronide (Wurst F, et al. 2010). The drinking behaviour of the last 14 days is best measured by %CDT but with only 63% sensitivity. Even with a massive increase of alcohol consumption (more than 80g of pure alcohol daily for more than three weeks) 37% don't show an elevation of %CDT. Liver parameters and MCV are able to detect longer periods of alcohol abuse. If ASAT is twice as high as ALAT, an alcohol abuse is very likely (De-Ritis-Quotient, Singer MV and Teyssen S. 2005; Renz-Polster H et al. 2007). If ALAT is above 200 or slightly higher, the elevation of ASAT is usually also caused by

Fig. 77 Trait markers, state markers and markers associated with alcohol dependence (according to Koller G and Soyka M. 2001)

- **Trait markers**
- Monoaminooxidase
- MAO-B
- Dopamine receptor genetics
- Dopamine Beta Hydroxylase
- Endocrine parameter like ACTH, cortisol, prolactine, TSH, TRH
- Alcohol dehydrogenase (ADH2, ADH3)
- Aldehyde dehydrogenase (ALDH2, ALDH3)
- Adenylate cyclase
- Induced potentials
- Tryptophan hydroxylase (5-HIAA)

- **State markers**
- Blood alcohol level
- Acetaldehydes and formaledehyde condensation products
- Acetate
- Ethyl glucuronide
- Methanol
- Alkaline phosphatase
- Blood and urinary beta-hexoaminidase
- MCV
- ASAT; ALAT; GAMMA GT
- % CDT

- **Associated markers**
- Blood groups (MMS-blood group)
- HLA Antigens
- Transcetolases

Fig. 78 Overview biological state markers of alcohol abuse

Biological markers that indicate alcohol abuse

	Sensitivy	Specificity	Normalisation in abstinence
Breath alcohol	100 %	100 %	Hours
Ethyl glucuronide	100 %	100 %	Days
MCV & GGT	63 %	80 %	1–10 Weeks
% CDT	65 %	96 %	2–4 Weeks

- Cut-off-points:
- Breath alcohol = ≥ 2,5 ‰. chronic abuse
- ASAT > ALAT = Alcohol; ALAT > ASAT = liver disease
- Gamma-GT = >1,3-times the upper standard value
- MCV = > 95, suspected alcohol abuse
  = > 98, alcohol abuse
- % CDT = ≥ 2,6 % (new cut-off; without trisialo)

Lesch OM, Walter H, 1995

other liver diseases. 20 % of all elevated Gamma GT levels are not caused by alcohol and a third of all heavily drinking alcohol dependents show normal liver function tests. MCV above 95 indicates alcohol abuse and in 80 % of patients a MCV above 98 indicates a massive and lengthy alcohol abuse. The degradation of liver function tests often takes several weeks and very high Gamma GT values (e.g. > 300) often don't completely degrade despite abstinence (e.g. only a value between 60 and 80 is reached). The degradation of MCV usually takes even longer than degradation of liver function tests.

8.2.3 Associated markers

A connection between these markers and alcohol abuse can be expected. These markers aim especially at giving information about the etiological causes of alcohol abuse. Although primarily of scientific interest, they are investigated by only few research centres (Wurst FM. 2001).

8.2.4 Practical suggestions for the use of biological markers for forensic purposes

8.2.4.1 Blood alcohol measurement

Alcohol is absorbed by the mucous membrane of the gastrointestinal tract, mainly by the stomach, metabolised by the liver and only minor quantities are eleminated by respiration. Therefore alcohol can be measured in the blood and also in the breath. The absorption depends on many factors (weight, diet, speed of drinking etc.). The elimination depends on liver functioning and alcohol degradation is accelerated by liver enzyme induction. If other medication which takes the same degradation path (P450 etc.), is taken in addition to alcohol, it leads to severe interactions (see chapter 7.3.2.6) and consequent changes in blood levels. It is assumed that persons without a genetic vulnerability for alcohol dependence (e.g. no alcohol dependent father or mother), who rarely drink alcohol, eliminate around 0.12 ‰ alcohol per hour, while patients with a genetic vulnerability who regularly drink alcohol are able to eliminate up to 0.25 ‰ of alcohol per hour. The severity of a liver disease (e.g. decompensated liver cirrhosis, child B or C) clearly changes these elimination rates.

The analytical procedure consists of four single measurements with two different measuring methods (gas chromatography, ADH process, Widmark process). The mean value of these four single values, rounded to two decimals, adds up to the blood alcohol concentration (BAC).

The maximal tolerance between these single values may only be 10 % of the mean value. Precision and accuracy of these measurements are permanently monitored by commercially produced control samples with known content. Intercomparison programmes regulate external quality control.

Procedures which do not include four values with two measurements are controversial, e.g. in persons who have an accident, whose blood is only tested by using the ADH process.

8.2.4.2 Blood alcohol concentration (BAC)

The alcohol amount in venous blood is indicated by g/l or per mille (1 g/l = 1 ‰).

For forensic purposes it is often necessary to count back from a specific value, for which the following options are often used. All these assessments are based mainly on the Widmark formula.

Fig. 79 BAC retrograde calculation

The following procedures enable the intoxication to be calculated backwards to a point of time in the past:
- Widmark's formula
- Widmark's procedure
- Vidic's procedure
- Fous's formula
- Watson's formula

The Widmark formula forms the basis of all these procedures and is internationally accepted. It allows a retrograde calculation of the alcohol concentration.

8.2.4.3 Widmark Formula

By calculating the maximal BAC c from alcohol consumed amount A in grams and the body weight p, the alcohol amount can be measured according to the formula $c = A/(p*r)$ as proposed by Widmark in 1932 (with r=reduction factor). As alcohol is water soluble, it does not disperse to the bones and to the fatty tissue and therefore these body dimensions are not included. The mean value for men is $r = 0.7$, whereas the mean value in women is $r = 0.6$ as they have more fatty tissue. New approaches, e.g. by Watson, consider size, age and gender additional to body dimensions. In modified form, these formulas are the basis of all calculation programmes.

8.2.4.4 Breath alcohol

Blood alcohol is released from the alveolae of the lung to the inhaled air, whereby alcohol is measured during exhalation (0,4 mg/l = 0,84 ‰). This ratio is not constant and changes with time, a process in which individual factors, especially body temperature, plays a role. During the absorption phase, the alcohol distribution between arterial and venous circulation also has powerful effects on the balance of dispersion of blood/breath alcohol. Therefore all attempts to accurately (fluctuation at 0.1 mg/l) calculate blood alcohol concentration via conversion from measured breath alcohol concentration have principally failed. Yet for clinical purposes and for approximate evaluations in road traffic situations, the breath alcohol value is absolutely sufficient.

The present generation of breath alcohol analysers which are recalibrated every six months (so called "approved instruments"), analyze two independent breath samples in brief consecutive order with an infrared optical and an electro chemical measuring system, with an additional standardization of breath temperature to 34 °C. This virtually excludes all sources of error like residual alcohol in the mouth, manipulation of breathing technique, cross sensitivity for other substances like acetone etc. If both processes show consistent values, the results are directly written in mg/l respiration air.

8.2.4.5 Products of alcohol metabolism

8.2.4.5.1 Ethyl glucuronide

In 1967, "activated" glucuronic acid (Uridin-5-diphospho-ß-glucuronic acid) was detected in human urine for the first time. This acid is generated like a direct alcohol metabolite and its existence can be proven over a relative long period (around 80 hours) in the urine or serum.

Quantitative analysis via GC/MS as trimethylsilyl ether (fragments: 160, 261, 405) with d5-ethylglucuronide is an internal standard (Wurst F. 2001; 2010 Hartmann S et al. 2007).

Alcoholic beverages don't only consist of ethanol, but also of methanol and long-chain alcohols. When drinking alcohol, both ethanol and methanol

Fig. 80 Elimination of ethanol (BEC) and methanol (BMC)

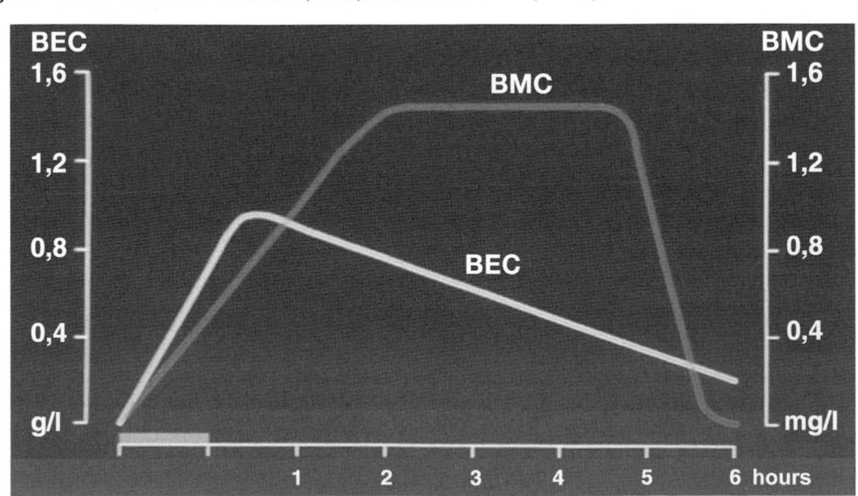

are absorbed and ethanol is more quickly eliminated than methanol. Methanol is not eliminated until a level of 0.4 g/l ethanol is reached.

Additional to the normal degradation pathway, alcohol dependents activate the MEOS system and catalase for the degradation of methanol in order to eliminate methanol despite a high ethanol level (alcohol dependent patients who continuously drink alcohol don't reach less than 0. 4 g and therefore have too much methanol in their bodies). Lesch's types, however, differ in terms of degradation speed (Fig. 6).

By summarizing these results, we can see that by analysing both, methanol and ethanol, we can draw conclusions about the acute or chronic use of alcohol, and partially also about the consumption behaviour of alcohol dependents.

Alcohol intoxication in patients who are normally abstinent, elevates the ethanol level, but the methanol level remains low.

If a patient is continuously intoxicated, methanol levels are elevated (a methanol level often above 10 mg/l)) additional to the elevated ethanol level (Sprung R et al. 1988; Bonte W. 1987; Leitner A et al. 1994).

If these measurements are repeated after one hour and the patient does not only eliminate ethanol but also eliminates methanol despite the elevated ethanol level, we can conclude that the MEOS and catalase systems are activated. This suggests that the patient metabolises alcohol differently than healthy individuals. These patients almost always meet the diagnostic criteria for an alcohol dependence according to DSM-IV and ICD-10.

8.2.4.5.2 %CDT (Carbohydrate-deficient-transferrin)

In 1976, a transferrin variant was discovered in the serum of alcohol dependent patients. In the following years, transferrin research showed that the carbohydrate deficient transferrin (%CDT) is more specific than all other markers. Serum transferrin has a polypeptide structure with polysaccharide side chains. The absence of such side chains

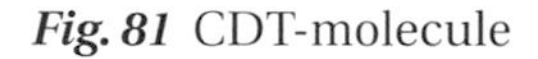

Fig. 81 CDT-molecule

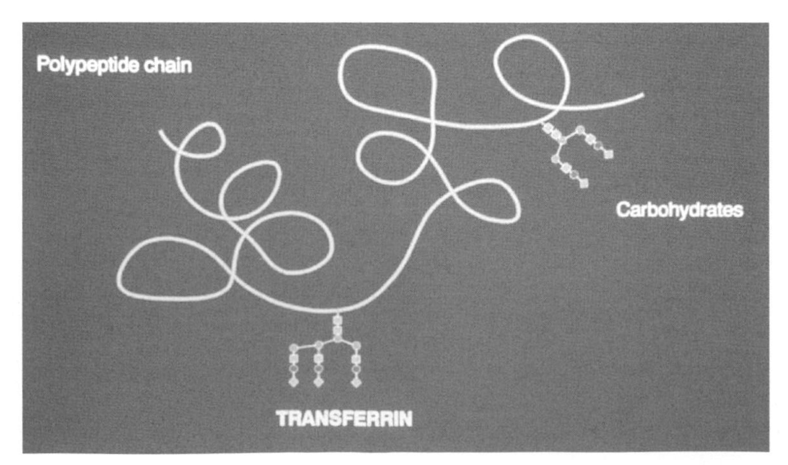

has been pinpointed as a consequence of the effects of alcohol.

The specificity is high, between 75% and 98% (Stibler H and Borg S. 1986).

The sensitivity is reported mostly between 63% (Lesch OM et al. 1996) and 80% (Litten R and Allen J. 1992) (Review by Walter H et al. 2001). In Europe, the sensitivity in studies which have included clinical alcohol dependents according to DSM-IV, is almost always indicated around 63%.

We were able to examine %CDT of healthy participants in a drinking experiment and results showed that even a daily amount of 80 gram of pure alcohol over three weeks does not elevate the %CDT in healthy persons (Lesch OM et al. 1996). 63% of alcohol dependent patients showed an elevated %CDT during intoxication, which degraded after two to three weeks of controlled abstinence. The %CDT value didn't correlate with the amount or duration of drinking, suggesting that different sensitivities are influencing the %CDT value, independent of drinking behaviour.

Those patients who react sensitively to alcohol with %CDT (which means that they had already reached an elevated %CDT value previously) show an increase in %CDT even after the consumption of low amounts. Our therapy studies showed that %CDT can be used as a biological marker of relapse. After three weeks of absolute abstinence patients reach an individual basis value. The basis value correlates with relapse if its value is increased by 0.8% within the standard value. The %CDT is not influenced by other diseases (e.g. diabetes etc). Only in severe liver diseases, which lead to a significant reduction in blood coagulation assessed by normotest, the %CDT value correlates with the severity of the liver

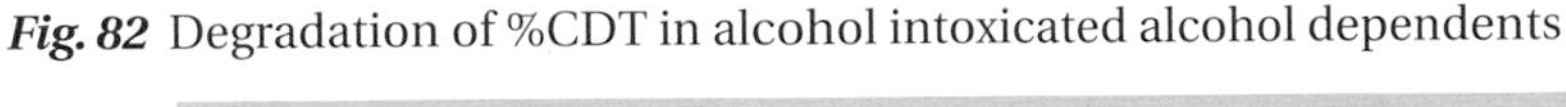

Fig. 82 Degradation of %CDT in alcohol intoxicated alcohol dependents

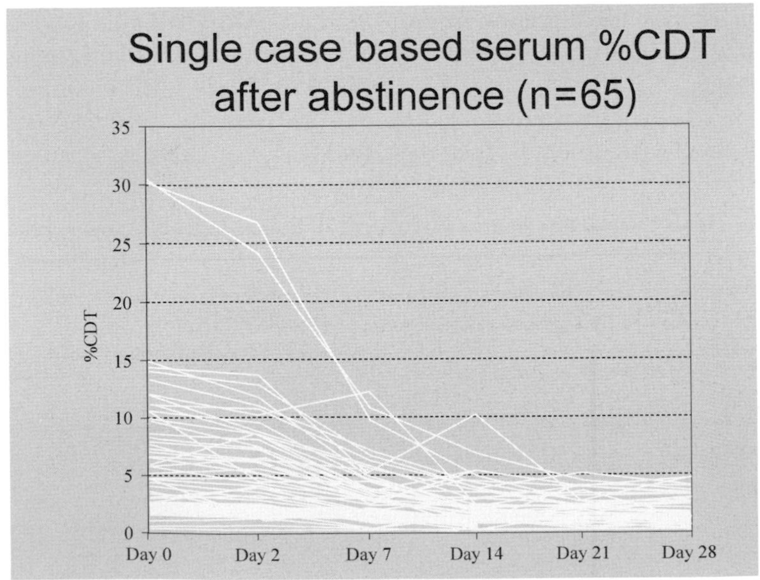

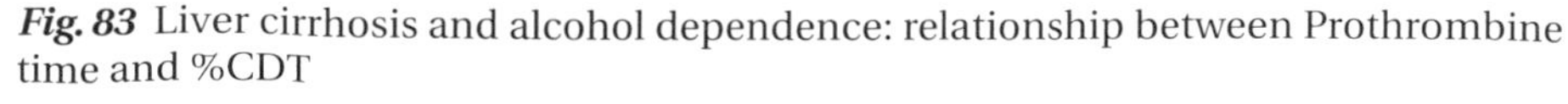

Fig. 83 Liver cirrhosis and alcohol dependence: relationship between Prothrombine time and %CDT

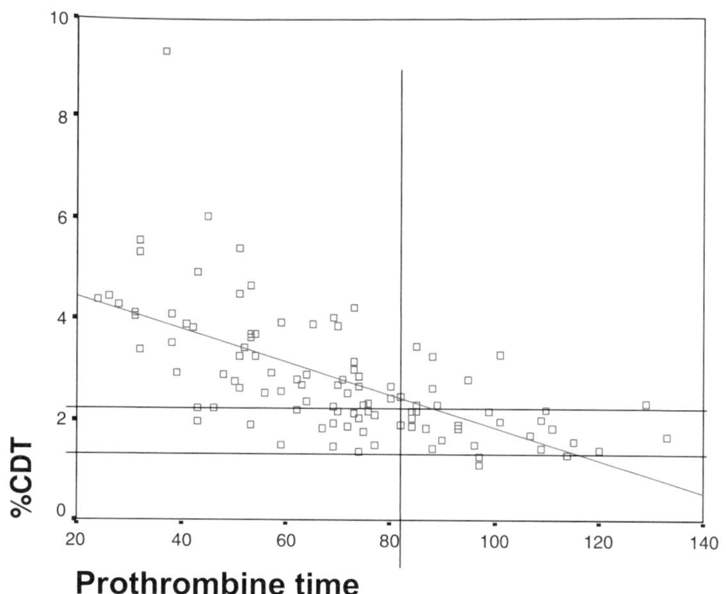

damage and not the drinking behaviour.

If blood coagulation is so severely impaired that the normotest is below 75 %, the %CDT loses its significance as a marker because the elevation of the %CDT now depends on the severity of liver damage.

After a liver transplantation, the %CDT is able to document further abstinence (Berlakovich GA et al. 1999).

In the long term course after liver transplantation percentage CDT shows a sensitivity of 92 % and a specificity of 98 % according to alcohol intake.

As most alcohol dependents smoke, the %CDT has been examined in regards to smoking and it has been shown that it can be used as a marker for ac-

Fig. 84 %CDT as control for abstinence in alcohol dependents with liver transplantations

n = 97	Alcohol dependence		Sensitivity % = (11/11 + 1) x 100 = 92 %
%CDT	Relapse	No relapse	Specificity % = 83/2 * 83) x 100 = 98 %
Positive	11	2	
Negative	1	83	Berlakovich G et al. 1999

tive drinking in alcohol dependents who smoke (Whitfield JB et al. 1998).

Additional to these very specific markers for drinking behaviour, indirect markers are available which mirror alcohol-related changes. Obviously these changes might have other causes too. Hepatitis, e.g. or choleostasis can elevate liver levels in the same way. Such acute chronic diseases change the haemogram, like for example the MCV. The advantage of these markers is the fact that they are still detectable after a period of abstinence (weeks up to months). As blood clotting is of eminent importance for surgical intervention and alcohol dependents with liver damage often have blood coagulation disorders, these markers can be used to confirm long-term abstinence (over weeks). The combination of these markers increases sensitivity at the costs of specificity. Liver parameters are clinically the most common markers today (ASAT, ALAT, de Ritis Factor, Gamma-GT, as well as the MCV and the %CDT). The sensitivity of these different markers is also influenced by genetic and other causes. The relationship between these markers is still unclear. This influence can be seen by the fact, that the different markers do not correlate to each other (Fig. 85).

8.3 The clinical dialogue in tobacco addiction

In essence, similar rules apply for tobacco dependents as for alcohol dependents, although stigmatisation and shame play a less important role. Smoking should be directly tackled as a risk factor for health and the relationship between problems and smoking should be the focus of exploration. The distinction between abuse and dependence and a precise diagnosis of smoking dependence are the next steps. An objec-

Fig. 85 The relationship between different markers (n = 56) in alcohol dependent patients

males	RIA AXIS	ELISA AXIS	RIA PH	ELISA PH	DSM Score	Malt F	Malt S	Malt	MCV	Gamma GT	ASAT	ALAT
RIA AXIS	1.000											
ELISA AXIS	.920	1.000										
RIA PH	.860	.893	1.000									
ELISA PH	.864	.885	.941	1.000								
DSM Score	-.064	-.006	-.045	-.053	1.000							
Malt F	.022	-.045	.021	.063	.174	1.000						
Malt S	.170	.198	.131	.078	.438	.179	1.000					
Malt	.124	.097	.098	.092	.396	.776	.759	1.000				
MCV	.024	.037	-.069	-.032	-.217	-.095	-.374	-.303	1.000			
Gamma GT	-.181	-.216	-.177	-.130	.209	.143	.057	.131	.093	1.000		
ASAT	.095	.096	.056	.101	.078	.113	.115	.148	.086	.022	1.000	
ALAT	.052	.078	-.008	.003	.096	-.044	.235	.121	-.091	.321	.775	1.000

tive evaluation of the number of cigarettes smoked and the expected withdrawal syndrome, as assessed by using a Smokerlyzer (measuring the level of carbon monoxide in respiratory air), is helpful for the motivational dialogue. Spirometric findings document the direct impact of smoking on respiration (Lesch OM. 2007). Diagnosing and addressing tobacco dependence significantly increases motivation to reduce or quit smoking.

9

Therapeutic strategies in alcohol and tobacco addiction

9.1 Motivation for therapy in different settings

If an alcohol and/or tobacco problem forms part of the clinical picture of the patient, it is important to initiate therapeutically available strategies that meet the patient at the point that feels subjectively "right" to him i.e. the demands made on the patient should be modest at the beginning. This will vary according to setting. One can easily imagine that the therapeutic options available at the general practitioner's are different to those in a homeless shelter or in a specific addiction treatment centre.

9.1.1 Motivational interviewing at the general practitioner's

Somatic problems are the most frequent reason why alcohol and tobacco dependent patients consult a practitioner. Patients seldom seek assistance for social problems at the general practitioner's and only a small minority regularly request a medical check-up. Most patients have a relationship of trust with their practitioner, who is the pivotal element in every course of treatment. A medical specialist is rarely consulted. Only in exceptional cases, can patients be motivated to consult a psychiatrist or to seek admission to a detoxification centre. In this case, these patients who are highly motivated to undergo specific therapy should be sent without delay to specialists (e.g. detoxification centres). These institutions should possess a therapeutic chain (outpatient – inpatient – outpatient) and should offer outpatients a psychotherapeutic setting with the option of brief inpatient admission. The duration of an inpatient admission depends on the psychiatric and somatic symptoms and typology.

Patients who consult a medical practitioner because of somatic problems,, but deny their alcohol problem, should be confronted with their problem by using the guidelines of the Plinius Maior Society (www.alcoweb.de). These guidelines describe mechanisms to raise the patient's awareness of his drinking behaviour and offer motivational strategies to change drinking behaviour. Absolute abstinence is an acceptable goal, but also dosage reduction as well as the reduction in the duration and severity of drinking episodes, are acceptable therapy goals.

If one of the above therapy goals is accepted, withdrawal treatment or a reduction of drinking ("Cut down drinking" according to the method of Sinclair D) can start. The goal of withdrawal treatment is to make the first phases of abstinence easier and to reduce the craving for tobacco and alcohol. An inpatient withdrawal treatment should only be recommended if it is the patient's explicit wish and/or if severe withdrawal or sequelae are diagnosed. Suicidal patients and patients with very adverse circumstances (e.g. the homeless) should be admitted immediately.

If the patient can't be motivated towards an inpatient admission or if none of the points above apply, withdrawal therapy can be carried out at home. Besides adequate medication, simple recommendations on self-care are very helpful for withdrawal. It is crucial that regular check-up appointments are made at short intervals.

9.1.2 Motivational interviewing in internal medicine

In essence, this procedure is not very different to the motivational dialogue at the general practitioner's. These patients more often have acute somatic problems, sometimes even life-threatening (e.g. bleedings in liver cirrhosis, dyspnoea in COPD etc). Therapy of the somatic disease is pivotal and the situation should be used to start a withdrawal therapy. In this situation patients are often more approachable and more likely to accept a therapy setting that offers relapse prophylaxis over a longer period of time. The interaction between withdrawal medication, required medication for the somatic disease, withdrawal symptoms and the actual somatic disease needs to be considered. After the withdrawal symptoms subside, it is appropriate to set up an ambulant therapy setting which offers different options according to typology. Lesch's type I patients should be further treated by an internist, while type II-and type III-patients need a psychotherapeutic-psychiatric-setting. Type IV patients can be cared for by social workers qualified in addiction, together with an internist.

9.1.3 Motivational interviewing during pregnancy

As it is already known that not only tobacco but also alcohol damages the unborn child, the gynaecologist should tell every woman not to smoke nor drink alcohol during pregnancy. If a woman smokes and/or drinks alcohol during pregnancy, the motivating dialogue should address the topic of abstinence. The Viennese research group showed that this talk motivates most women to quit smoking and drinking. Only those who are not able to reduce smoking despite these recommendations should take part in a withdrawal programme. As passive smoking is also an important topic for pregnant women, their families should also be invited to join these programmes.

9.1.4 Motivational interviewing in psychiatric settings

As expected, most patients primarily enter a psychiatric setting because of mental symptoms like anxiety or depression. They usually expect to receive psychopharmacological treatment, e.g. anti-depressants. As far as this group is concerned, it is important to address the tobacco and alcohol problem and to make the patient aware that the first important step in therapy of the psychiatric symptoms is either to reduce consumption or to become abstinent.

In the case of abstinence, the patient needs adequate withdrawal medication. Therapy for the psychiatric symptoms should be started after fourteen days of abstinence. If antidepressants, e. g. tricyclics are administered in an early phase of withdrawal, the symptomatology of the transitory psychotic syndrome (see page 8) might be aggravated and could lead to delirant states or epileptic seizures. Reducing smoking often changes psychiatric symptoms (anxiety disorder is ameliorated, but in some cases depressions might get worse).

If the patient is suicidal, admission to a stable setting is recommended. Regular short-term outpatient appointments are absolutely categorical and different styles of motivation and psychotherapeutic behaviour should be used depending on the specific subgroup.

While Lesch's type I-and type IV-patients require education and a behaviourally oriented therapeutic approach, type II patients need stabilisation (and often meet the criteria of a dependent personality). It is common for the partner, who is usually powerful, to want to "put" the patient into therapy (image: like a car into service). Type II patients need protection, support, rewards and realistic short-term therapy goals.

Performance-oriented, type III-patients have usually already informed themselves about the therapeutic process by reading books or using the internet. Mostly they want to cut down their drinking. They are very often quite resistant to changing their lifestyle (and their subjective convictions of having to be perfect). The aim of motivation in Lesch's type III patients is to help them learn to understand the pathogenic process, which often takes several months to up to half a year. "Therapeutic abstinence" during the first months is extremely important. A calm and patient way of listening is needed. One must wait until a stable emotional basis has been formed between patient and therapist. Approaches that structure too early might be successful in the short run (several months), but do lead to relapse if no changes are made in lifestyle and in the mechanisms to deal with adverse situations and stress (alcohol for relief). Depressive symptoms and feelings of guilt often follow. This often leads to the patient stopping therapy. Inpatient therapies with rigidly structured procedures and without continuing therapy after discharge often lead to a severe suicidal crisis in relapsed patients. The commitment of the patient to a stable outpatient relationship (crisis concept) after inpatient treatment is essential.

Certain detoxification centres employ very rigid therapeutic concepts which serve the organisation of the institutions but rarely the patients. These concepts are often divided into four stages which include: (1) detoxification (2) motivation (3) activation and (4) planning of long-term treatment.

There are institutions which only offer stage 2 and stage 3 for usually six to eight weeks in an inpatient setting. Some wards only offer stages 1–3, so that detoxification is included in the eight-week inpatient admission. Few institutions have sufficient programmes for all stages. Ideal would be a programme in which the therapist, or the therapeutic team, assists the patient before inpatient admission, is responsible for him during inpatient admission, and is also in charge of a two-year outpatient therapy after discharge. Outpatient therapy should help to ameliorate problems by offering regular psychotherapeutic sessions (individual) and specific pharmacological therapy. Relapses should be a cause for modifying the therapeutic concept, but should never be a reason for terminating therapy.

9.2 Pharmacotherapy of alcohol and tobacco addiction

Biological principles of pharmacotherapy (see chapter 3.4)

9.2.1 Alcohol addiction

Acute Alcohol consumption activates GABA-A, blocks NMDA-receptors, stimulates ß-endorphin and dopamine release and activates the serotonin system (Tabakoff B and Hoffman PL. 1991). Higher concentrations of serotonin are caused by either an increase in release, or partial blockade, of the presynaptic reuptake (Le Marquand D et al. 1994). This is what causes the sedating and euphorising effects. Another acute effect of alcohol is the activation of subunits alpha3beta2 and alpha3beta4 of the nicotine receptor (Cardoso RA et al. 1999).

Chronic consumption, however, leads to the opposite effects. In order to maintain homoeostasis, GABA-A-receptors are functionally changed and glutamate receptors and opiate receptors are increased in numbers. Dopamine is gradually reduced and, only after abstinence, does the dopamine system slowly recover. Also the sedating and euphorising effects decrease. More alcohol needs to be consumed to attain the original effects (increase in dosage).

As alcohol dependents/abusers consume alcohol in large amounts over a long period of time, they can be viewed as chronically intoxicated. Standard alcohol not only contains ethanol but also methanol, propanol, butanol and other ingrediants. All of these are resorbed in the gastrointestinal tract. Stomach and liver functions are very important as a large proportion of these

Fig. 86 Effect of acute alcohol consumption on transmitter systems

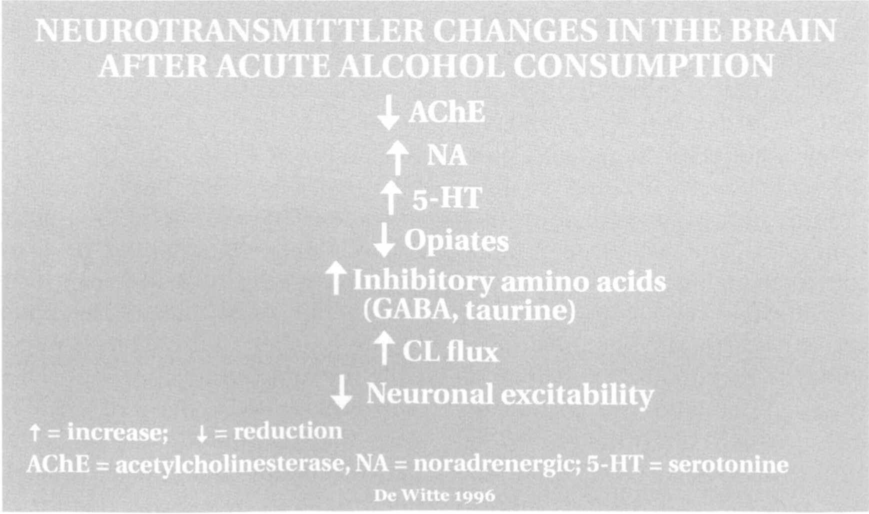

NEUROTRANSMITTLER CHANGES IN THE BRAIN AFTER ACUTE ALCOHOL CONSUMPTION
↓ AChE
↑ NA
↑ 5-HT
↓ Opiates
↑ Inhibitory amino acids (GABA, taurine)
↑ CL flux
↓ Neuronal excitability
↑ = increase; ↓ = reduction
AChE = acetylcholinesterase, NA = noradrenergic; 5-HT = serotonine
De Witte 1996

Fig. 87 Changes in transmitters after chronic alcohol consumption

↑ AChe muscarinic receptors
↑ ß-NA receptors
↓ 5-HT
↑ Opiates (sensitive to encephelines)
↑ Excitatory amino acids (glutamate aspartate)
↑ Ca entry
↑ Neuronal excitability

↑ = increase; ↓ = reduction
AChE = acetylcholinesterase, NA = noradrenergic; 5-HT = serotonine

DeWitte P 1996

alcohols is already inactivated by these organs. Stomach function impairments, reduced intestinal functions (e.g. stomach surgery, Billroth II) and acute disturbances in liver function significantly increase the alcohol content in the blood and brain.

The effects of alcohol on the brain are not only inhibitory and, for this reason, alcohol is used not only as a tranquilizer or a sleep-inducing agent, but is also consumed for its mood altering effects and its ability to affect drive. Today it is known that chronic alcohol consumption changes neurotransmission in practically all systems (activating, but also inhibiting).

Besides, aldehydes, the first degradation products, combine with dopamine to form THBCs or the so-called tetrahydroisoquinolines (TIQs). The binding of aldehyde with indolamines produces beta-carbolines. Both condensation products change brain functions over time. TIQs, in particular, occupy the opiate receptor. There has been discussion about whether this mechanism can partly explain the so-called "endogenous craving" for alcohol (Bonte W. 1987; Sprung R et al. 1988; Musshoff F et al. 2005). However alcohol also stimulates the release of ß-endorphin-like peptides and met-encephaline in the hypothalamus and striatum. Chronic alcohol consumption leads to an elevated availability of binding sites (receptors).

Early onset of drinking or traumatic disorders (mental or somatic trauma) interferes with normal brain development. This leads to an increased vulnerability and to an aggravation of the existing brain impairment. Also early consumption and prenatal effects of alcohol lead to long-term learning disabilities. When patients with high alcohol consumption were compared to abstinent individuals, the former groups' hippocampus was reduced in size, suggesting that less tissue is available for the neuronal network that is responsible for learning and memory (Beresford et al. 2006). From an aetiological perspective, this result can be linked to high cortisone levels (Beresford TP et al. 2006a).

Addiction memory is activated and addiction-related information is stored in the limbic system. The limbic system is involved in pleasure, emotion, experiences, drive and also supports cognitive functions. Chronic stimulation activates the dopaminergic reward system (ventral tegmental area – nucleus accumbens), which leads to an adaptation of this system. The neurotransmitter dopamine controls the extrapyramidal motor function (impairment of these functions is visible in intoxicated individuals). An over-activation of this transmitter leads to psychotic states. A deficiency leads to motor dysfunctions like M. Parkinson. When alcohol is consumed occasionally, dopamine is released, lifting the mood and sometimes even causing euphoria. Chronic dependence leads to dopamine depletion and to typical motor dysfunctions (therefore, not every motor dysfunction has polyneuropathic causes). In interaction with noradrenalin, dopamine controls the activity of the cholinergic system. Acetylcholine is important in connection with smoking as nicotine receptors are cholinergic receptors.

Studies which have tried to reduce craving by classical neuroleptics antagonising the dopamine receptor, have mostly failed (Wiesbeck G et al. 2001; Walter H et al. 2001). More recent studies on topiramate, which controls dopamine release, seem to be more promising, especially since the dopamine antagonistic effect is connected with GABA-agonistic and glutamate-antagonistic effects (in particular an AMPA-[alpha-amino-3-hydroxy-5-methylisoxazole-4-propionic acid] and a kainate-receptor-antagonism) (Nguyen SA et al. 2007; Johnson BA. 2004; Johnson BA et al. 2004). It has been shown that this effect profile is successful in reducing symptoms of nicotine withdrawal (Ait-Daoud N et al. 2006).

Glutamate is an activating neurotransmitter with various sub-receptors (NMDA, AMPA and Kainate). Alcohol primarily binds to the N-Methyl-D-Aspartate subreceptors (NMDA). The ability to bind with NMDA receptors, blocks activity and can be linked to the analgesic effects of alcohol. Through this blockage, the number and sensitivity of NMDA receptors increases in order to compensate. Thus there is more stimulation in the CNS and more GABA activity is required. This leads to an increase in dosage to avoid withdrawal symptoms. Furthermore, this glutamate activation is associated with cell loss and corresponding cerebral sequelae like cognitive dysfunctions, Korsakov's dementia etc.

The glutamate system influences the nucleus accumbens via afferents. Next to topiramate, acamprosate has positive pharmacotherapeutic effects in alcohol dependence and works by reducing corticomesolimbic glutamate activity. Acamprosate antagonises NMDA and the Kainate receptor subtype 5 (mGlur5; De Witte P et al. 2005). Studies on conditioned alcohol cues showed that acamprosate works by reducing autonomous reactions to these cues, while the mμ-opiate antagonist naltrexone could reduce craving overall (Ooteman W et al. 2007). Ooteman et al.

did not find that these medications had any effect on cortisol. This is contrary to other authors who found that naltrexone activates the HPA-axis (hypothalamic-pituitary-adrenocortical-axis), as a result of which they suggested that naltrexone is more effective in women (Kiefer F et al. 2005). If patients are divided into subgroups, clinical effects are more clearly distinguishable. For example, it was found that acamprosate had better abstinence rates in type I and II according to Lesch (Lesch OM et al. 2001). These results have been replicated for type I (Kiefer F et al. 2005a). In this study, the abstinence rate in the placebo group of type II, even after three months, was so good that neither acamprosate nor naltrexone was able to show any effect. In this study, Kiefer showed that naltrexone significantly improved abstinence rates in types III and IV (Kiefer F. et al. 2005a). These results can be supported by data from basic research, since if treatment runs smoothly, acamprosate reduces craving mainly during abstinence, while naltrexone is able to reduce the amounts and the duration of drinking (Volpicelli JR et al. 1997; Garbutt JC et al. 2005; O'Malley SS et al. 2007).

Studies with the NMDA-antagonist neramexane were not able to produce an increase in abstinence rates (unpublished data).

A hypofunction of NMDA-receptor subtypes of cortical limbic afferents has recently received attention from schizophrenia research and has been linked to the high prevalence (85%) of indirect glutamate activating substance abuse (stimulants) in schizophrenic patients (Coyle JT. 2006).

Endocannabinoids influence GABAergic and glutamatergic synapses and interact with dopamine and acetylcholine. CB-1-and CB-2-receptors have been researched and CB-1-receptors were mainly localised in limbic brain areas. The CB-1-antagonist, rimonabant, has been discussed as a very promising alternative to current pharmaceutics for nicotine dependence (Cohen C et al. 2005), alcohol dependence and overweight (Simiand J et al. 1998). Alcohol related dopamine release is antagonised by CB-1-blockers, whereby no positive emotional reinforcement occurs. Animal experiments showed that CB-1-antagonists reduce the amounts of alcohol drunk (Colombo G et al. 1998). Later studies demonstrated a relationship between CB-1-receptors and opiate receptors and pointed to a possible clinical combination of opiate antagonists and CB-1-antagonists (Colombo G et al. 2005; Cohen C et al. 2002; Anthenelli R. 2004; Klesges RC et al. 1997, 1989; Soyka M et al. 2008)

Serotonin stimulates dopamine release in mid brain (VTA) and therefore advocates the subjectively pleasurable, so called "reward effects" of alcohol (Lovinger DM. 1997). Clinical observations of the frequent co-morbidity of alcohol dependence with anxiety and depression (van Praag HM et al. 1991; Virkkunen M et al. 1994, 1996) or impulse control disorders (Linnoila M et al. 1983; Virkkunen M et al. 1997) suggest a dysfunction of the serotonin system. Alcohol related heightened serotonin release seems to play a role in "relief drinking" (drinking to reduce anxiety and depression) (Cooper ML et al. 1995; Markou A et al. 1998). However, it must be noted that experiments with animals showed more positive results than later clinical studies with SS-

RIs (Heinz A et al. 2001; Johnson BA. 2000; Lovinger DM. 1997; LeMarquand D et al. 1994; Naranjo CA and Knoke DM. 2001; Pettinati HM et al. 2003; Garbut JC et al. 1999; Johnson BA and Ait-Daoud N. 2000; Kranzler HR et al. 1996; Litten RZ and Allen JP.1998). These studies probably failed because comorbidities were excluded and no subgroups were used and possible effects on subgroups could not therefore be observed. Lovinger's work points to an elevation of reuptake (Lovinger DM. 1997). Genetic studies on serotonin transporters show an unclear picture (Caspi A et al. 2003; Hill EM et al. 2002; Kranzler HR et al. 2002). Patients with an early onset of drinking, in particular, show dysfunctions of the serotonin system (Benkelfat C et al. 1991; Buydens-Branchey L et al. 1989; Demir B et al. 2002; Javors M et al. 2000; Krystal JH et al. 1994; Swann AS et al. 1999; Virkkunen M and Linnoila M. 1997). When patients had an early onset of drinking, their subjective reasons for doing so are often that they could tolerate alcohol "well". Schuckit MA et al. (2006) showed that this patient group is especially at risk. This alcohol tolerance might be connected to a serotonergic hypofunction, which might be caused by genetic or previous social stress factors (Caspi A and Moffitt TE. 2006). This tolerance apparently reduces the GABAergic effects of alcohol and individuals are less sedated than those with no genetic vulnerabilities. This suggests a genetic disposition for excessive alcohol consumption.

In alcohol dependents with an early onset of drinking, alcohol modulates the 5-HT-3 receptor. Also ondansetrone, a 5-HT3-antagonist, is effective in reducing the quantity and frequency of drinking in patients with an early onset of drinking (Johnson BA. 2004). Reduced MAO activity has also been found by several researchers (Anthenelli RM et al. 1995; Demir B et al. 2002; Rommelspacher H et al. 1994; Sullivan J et al. 1990). Pettinati has emphasized that multiple dysfunctions in the serotonin system play a role in dependents as well as in excessive drinkers. Yet it is likely that the original acute effects of alcohol are merely restored by a simple increase of serotonin in the synaptic cleft (e.g. with SSRIs). Clinically, this could also be the case as SSRIs could potentially promote a relapse when no other medicine is administered (Pettinati HM et al. 2003).

In animal experiments, reduced pre-synaptic noradrenalin reuptake (in the locus coeruleus) has been linked to alcohol consumption (Hwang BH et al. 2000). Due to fact that research has focused a great deal of attention on the dopamine reward system, the noradrenergic reward system has been relatively neglected and is only now gradually beginning to receive more attention (Weinshenker D and Schroeder JP. 2006).

9.2.2 Tobacco addiction

Tobacco contains about 4,800 pharmacologically active substances. Together with the mono-amino-oxidase-system, nicotine seems to be the most fundamental substance for the development of an addiction. Nicotine activates nicotinic acetylcholine receptors. These are ionic channels whose walls are made up of five protein chains. Acetylcholine binding changes the structures in the cell membrane so that sodium and/or calcium can enter the neuron. The formation of the protein chains that build up the wall of the receptor varies and is characteristic of specific organs and functions. For example, the receptors in the brain are made of α4β2- or α7-subunits. A relatively large amount of calcium can pass these cells and because of this, they are very suitable for the formation of memory. In fact, animal experiments showed that nicotine promotes memory formation. Furthermore, it was shown that memory formation plays an important role in tobacco dependence.

Smoking stimuli are therefore especially "effective" because memory has been intensively channelled by nicotine. In animal experiments, this channelling was still present after months of abstinence.

Nicotinic receptors stimulate mesolimbic-mesocortical dopaminergic neurons in the ventral tegmentum. These effects explain why a partial α4β2-receptor antagonist like e. g. varenicline can be used as an anti-craving substance in relapse prevention. Nicotine substitutes are also active via this mechanism. Varenicline stimulates receptors slightly to moderately, but blocks the stimulation of nicotine. The dopaminergic neurons are stimulated also by endorphinergic and endocannabinoidergic neurons. This is very important for treatment with the μ-opioid receptor-antagonist, naltrexone, and the cannabinoid-1-receptor-antagonist, rimonabant, respectively.

Findings from positron emission tomography, an imaging technique which makes visible nicotinic receptors in the brain are very surprising (Brody AL et al. 2006). A single drag from a cigarette already leads to the occupation of nicotinic α4β2-receptors for around three hours in several brain regions. After one cigarette, around 90 % of receptors are switched off for at least two and a half hours, after two or more cigarettes receptors are switched off even longer. Researchers have concluded

Fig. 88 Nicotinic acetylcholine receptor (nAChR)

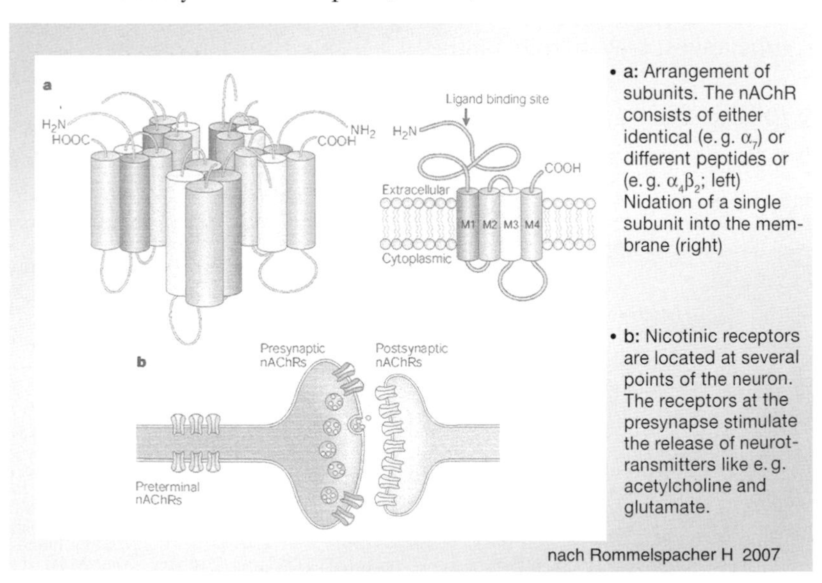

- **a:** Arrangement of subunits. The nAChR consists of either identical (e. g. α_7) or different peptides or (e. g. $\alpha_4\beta_2$; left) Nidation of a single subunit into the membrane (right)
- **b:** Nicotinic receptors are located at several points of the neuron. The receptors at the presynapse stimulate the release of neurotransmitters like e. g. acetylcholine and glutamate.

nach Rommelspacher H 2007

that a smoker who smokes 20 cigarettes a day, for example, does not have any α4β2-receptors available. Experiments with cell cultures showed that these receptors are inactivated by nicotine only a few seconds after stimulation (down-regulation by phosphorylation). These studies on dosage dependence also showed that craving only diminishes when more than 75% of receptors are occupied. It was concluded from these data that the avoidance of craving is a central motive for continuing to smoke. This also explains why the dependence potential and risk for relapse in tobacco smoking is so high in comparison to other addictive substances. It is very difficult for an ex-smoker to avoid cues about his tobacco dependence (cigarette automat, remembering the feeling of relaxation after a cigarette etc.)

How is it possible that smoking can still have desirable effects despite these conditions? In order to explain this, it must be acknowledged that tobacco smoke contains around 4,800 substances (German Cancer Research Centre Heidelberg, 2006). Thus, many other substances play a role in the stimulation of the mesolimbic dopaminergic neurons. In in-vivo microdialysis experiments with animals, it was found that the application of β-carbolines (norharmanes und harmanes) leads to the release of dopamine in the nucleus accumbens and therefore changes the central relay stations in the reward system (Sallstrom-Baum S et al. 1995, 1996). Although β-carbolines can be found in low concentrations in the body, they are formed from tryptophan via pyrolysis and then inhaled. They accumulate in the brain, with regions like the substantia nigra and the ventral tegmentum showing levels of norharmanes with an almost thirty times higher concentration. This relationship is schematically portrayed in the following figure (Rommelspacher H et al. 2007).

Conclusion

- Nicotine and alcohol consumption have much in common and, from a biological perspective, two directions in regards to anti-craving-effect and relapse prophylaxis are currently apparent :

Fig. 89 Changes caused by chronic smoking and rebound phenomena

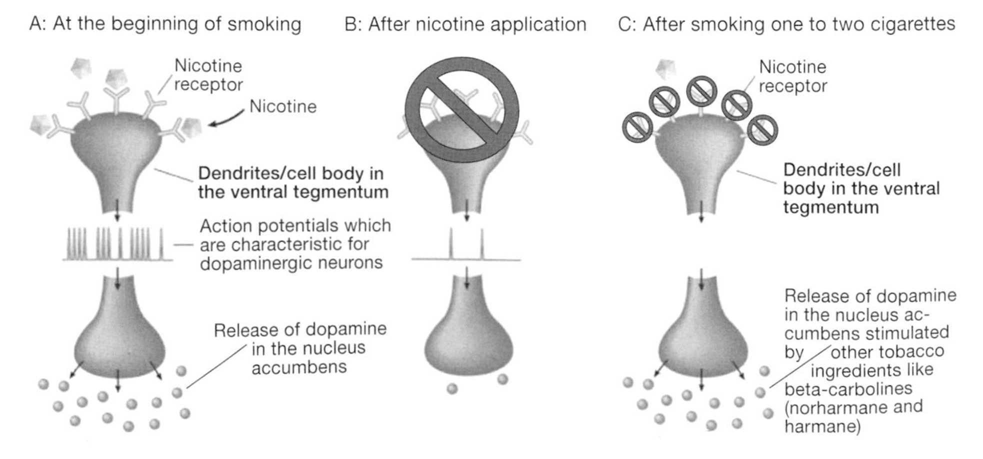

- Opioid/dopaminergic effects are associated with rewards and need an opiatantagonistic, a CB-1-antagonistic and partly also a glutamatantagonistic profile for pharmacological therapy.
- Serotonin and GABA/Glutamate are associated with reliefs (relief drinking, relief smoking) and require pharmacological treatment with antidepressants, anxiolytics and anti-glutamatergic drugs.

9.3 Pharmacotherapy of alcohol withdrawal

9.3.1 Withdrawal syndrome

Chronic alcohol consumption up-regulates the glutamate system, GABA-stimulation is terminated and an excitatory clinical picture of varying strength develops. Withdrawal symptoms usually set in after alcohol consumption is decreased or completely terminated.

In severely dependent patients, who are admitted with more than 2,5 ‰ breath alcohol, the withdrawal symptoms usually set in at two per mil breath alcohol. There are somatic and psychological withdrawal symptoms. The CIWA-Ar-scale is suitable for measuring somatic and psychological withdrawal symptoms (Stuppaeck CH et al. 1994; Pittman B et al. 2007), Fig. 90.

Typical withdrawal symptoms are tremor, sweating, anxiety and agitation.

9.3.2 Therapy of withdrawal states

Withdrawal can be carried out in an outpatient or inpatient setting, depending on the severity of the withdrawal symptom and the somatic-medical situation.

The primary goal of the therapy is the specific therapy of withdrawal symptoms. Medication should be chosen and dosed according to the severity of the intoxication, the severity of alcohol sequelae (e.g. a liver damage changes the metabolising of most medicaments) and the nature and severity of withdrawal symptoms. Withdrawal medication should meet the following criteria:

- Prevention of withdrawal symptoms (early start of therapy, high doses at the start)
- Avoidance of secondary damages caused by the medication (aggravation of liver damage; cave: cardiac arrhythmia, cave: seizures)
- The medication should not disturb the motivation process (heavy sedation does not allow a motivational dialogue)
- No polypragmasy needed

Goals should be defined according to withdrawal symptoms, which are different for each of Lesch's types.

In type I, the withdrawal symptoms usually subside after five days, while it takes 14 days to subside in type II and III. The withdrawal symptoms in type IV are a combination of previous cerebral damage and cognitive dysfunction with symptomatic transitory psychotic syndromes and these symptoms can set in over months again and again. Therefore goals and medications are different for each group and need to be defined accordingly (see chapter 9.3.3).

The duration of treatment depends on the typology. If the symptomatic does not develop according to a typical course type, often other factors (combinations with tranquilizers) or other somatic diseases need to be defined as causes of this atypical sympto-

Fig. 90 Clinical Institute Withdrawal Assessment of Alcohol Scale, Revised (CIWA-Ar) (Sullivan J T 1989)

Alcohol Withdrawal Assessment Scoring Guidelines (CIWA – Ar)

Vital Assesment

Nausea/Vomiting – Rate on scale 0–7 0 – None 1 – Mild nausea with no vomiting 2 3 4 – Intermittent nausea 5 6 7 – Constant nausea and frequent dry heaves and vomiting	Tremors – have patient extend arms & spread fingers. Rate on scale 0–7. 0 – No tremor 1 – Not visible, but can be felt fingertip to fingertip 2 3 4 – Moderate, with patient's arms extended 5 6 7 – severe, even w/arms not extended
Anxiety – Rate on scale 0 – 7 0 – no anxiety, patient at ease 1 – mildly anxious 2 3 4 – moderately anxious or guarded, so anxiety is inferred 5 6 7 – equivalent to acute panic states seen in severe delirium or acute schizophrenic reactions.	Agitation – Rate on scale 0–7 0 – normal activity 1 – somewhat normal activity 2 3 4 – moderately fidgety and restless 5 6 7 – paces back and forth, or constantly thrashes about
Paroxysmal Sweats – Rate on Scale 0–7. 0 – no sweats 1– barely perceptible sweating, palms moist 2 3 4 – beads of sweat obvious on forehead 5 6 7 – drenching sweats	Orientation and clouding of sensorium – Ask, "What day is this? Where are you? Who am I?" Rate scale 0–4 0 – Oriented 1 – cannot do serial additions or is uncertain about date 2 – disoriented to date by no more than 2 calendar days 3 – disoriented to date by more than 2 calendar days 4 – Disoriented to place and/or person
Tactile disturbances – Ask, "Have you experienced any itching, pins & needles sensation, burning or numbness, or a feeling of bugs crawling on or under your skin?" 0 – none 1 – very mild itching, pins & needles, burning, or numbness 2 – mild itching, pins & needles, burning, or numbness 3 – moderate itching, pins & needles, burning, or numbness 4 – moderate hallucinations 5 – severe hallucinations 6 – extremely severe hallucinations 7 – continuous hallucinations	Auditory Disturbances – Ask, "Are you more aware of sounds around you? Are they harsh? Do they startle you? Do you hear anything that disturbs you or that you know isn't there?" 0 – not present 1 – Very mild harshness or ability to startle 2 – mild harshness or ability to startle 3 – moderate harshness or ability to startle 4 – moderate hallucinations 5 – severe hallucinations 6 – extremely severe hallucinations 7 – continuous hallucinations
Visual disturbances – Ask, "Does the light appear to be too bright? Is its color different than normal? Does it hurt your eyes? Are you seeing anything that disturbs you or that you know isn't there?" 0 – not present 1 – very mild sensitivity 2 – mild sensitivity 3 – moderate sensitivity 4 – moderate hallucinations 5 – severe hallucinations 6 – extremely severe hallucinations 7 – continuous hallucinations	Headache – Ask, "Does your head feel different than usual? Does it feel like there is a band around your head?" Do not rate dizziness or lightheadedness. 0 – not present 1 – very mild 2 – mild 3 – moderate 4 – moderately severe 5 – severe 6 – very severe 7 – extremely severe

matic (e.g. diabetes mellitus, cerebral bleeding).

According to current research, withdrawal medication should have the following characteristics:

- Effects of medication should improve the underlying biological dysfunctions that are caused by giving up alcohol
- The medication's effects set in quickly and are controllable
- The medication does not cause any long lasting cognitive impairment
- The medication has a low addiction potential
- The medication shows a low liver toxicity
- The medication has few side effects and there is no vital risk when relapsing (cave: interactions)

Besides oral administration, the medication should also be available in a parenteral form so that no medication change is needed during the treatment.

The dosage should be adequately high at the beginning of withdrawal. The amount of dosage depends on the quantity and nature of the addictive drug(s) consumed, and the frequency at which it is consumed, and needs to be modified according to age, somatic impairments (e.g. decompensated liver cirrhosis, renal damages due to abuse of analgetics, cardiac arrhythmia). When determining the correct dosage, it is helpful to ask the patients how much alcohol they normally need to cope with their withdrawal symptoms.

Important elements of a withdrawal therapy are education about symptoms and the withdrawal progression, and the creation of an environment in which the patient feels safe and secure.

As mentioned most of the cases can be treated in an outpatient setting, but in figure 90 some situations are listed when inpatient treatment is needed.

Patients who feel informed and comfortable and who have a carefully scheduled activity programme require significantly lower amounts of with-

Procedure:

1. Assess and rate each of the 10 criteria of the CIWA scale. Each criterion is rated on a scale from 0 to 7, except for "Orientation and clouding of sensorium" which is rated on scale 0 to 4. Add up the scores for all ten criteria. This is the total CIWA-Ar score for the patient at that time. Prophylactic medication should be started for any patient with a total CIWA-Ar score of 8 or greater (ie. start on withdrawal medication). If started on <u>scheduled</u> medication, additional PRN medication should be given for a total CIWA-Ar score of 15 or greater.
2. Document vitals and CIWA-Ar assessment on the Withdrawal Assessment Sheet. Document administration of PRN medications on the assessment sheet as well.
3. The CIWA-Ar scale is the most sensitive tool for assessment of the patient experiencing alcohol withdrawal. Nursing assessment is vitlly important. Early intervention for CIWA-Ar score of 8 or greate provides the best means to prevet the progressio of witdraa.

Fig. 91 Recommondations for inpatient withdrawal treatment

- In case of the home environment being unsupportive in regards to the patient's abstinence and animating the patients towards drinking
- In case of previous withdrawal seizures or delirium tremens
- In case of polytoxikomania
- In case of strong tremor and tachycardia in present intoxication
- In case of orientation difficulties or hallucinations
- In case of suicidal tendencies
- In case of jaundice, liver cirrhosis or other signs of physical weakness and acute malnutrition
- In case of several home-based withdrawals having failed in the past
- In case of the patient preferring an inpatient admission

drawal medication. Furthermore, these patients have fewer critical incidents than patients in different conditions (e.g. accident victims with high levels of aggression in a hospital corridor with stressed staff). If withdrawal therapy is done at home, as it is in the majority of cases, it is important to inform patients about the danger of combining medication and alcohol. They should also be told not to drive a car or handle domestic appliances (mixer, electric knife, iron etc) or dangerous machinery. Simple advisory brochures can be very helpful (www.alcoweb.com).

Fig. 92 Recommendations for home-based withdrawals

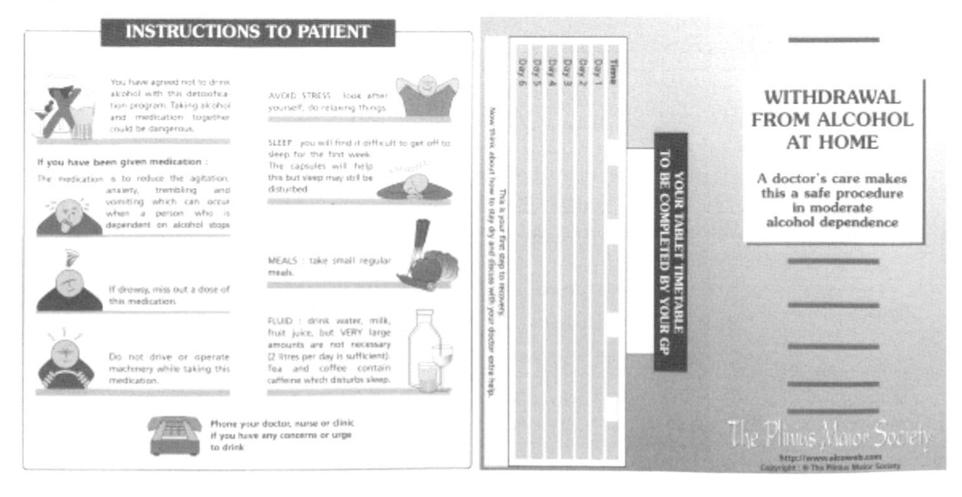

9.3.3 Therapy of the withdrawal syndromes according to Lesch's typology

9.3.3.1 Management of detoxification in Lesch's type I alcohol dependents

Withdrawal symptoms
Type I patients are often highly intoxicated when coming to the first therapy meeting (> 1.2 mg/l). Withdrawal symptoms can already set in after reducing the alcohol amount: three-dimensional tremor, heavy perspiration and vegetative instability (blood pressure and pulse fluctuations, instable cardiovascular system). The existing sleep onset and sleep maintenance insomnia lead to higher levels of anxiety and agitation (very high scores on the items tremors, anxiety, and agitation of the CIWA-Ar-scale, Fig. 90).

Patients are familiar with these symptoms from previous experiences and therefore know that the first three days are usually the most difficult. They fear these symptoms and have tried to combat them with alcohol in the past. Around 20% are at risk for developing complications: grand mal seizures can occur on the first or second day after reducing the amount of alcohol. Often patients report a history of previous seizures. Delirium tremens can set in together with, or independent of, grand mal seizures. This delirium tremens is characterized by heavy respiration, high suggestibility, a loss of orientation and optical hallucinations of small objects (micropsia).

Aetiology
This group uses alcohol as a medication to ameliorate withdrawal symptoms. A biological vulnerability has been hypothesized (elevation of acetaldehyde levels even during abstinence). Withdrawal should be perceived as a rebound phenomenon (GABA-hypersensitivity, GLUTAMAT-GABA-imbalance). Furthermore a depletion of the dopaminergic system has been observed.

Duration
Acute withdrawal symptoms are present for approximately three to five days. After that, symptoms are very mild or non-existent.

Withdrawal therapy
From the start, benzodiazepines with a good antiepileptic profile should be administered in high doses, e.g.: oxazepam, diazepam or chlordiazepoxide. Instead of waiting until acute withdrawal symptoms set in, symptoms should be treated as early as possible (severity of liver damage must be considered when titrating the dose). If there is a history of withdrawal seizures and/or delirium tremens, medication has to be dosed high enough. In order to specify the dosage, the patient should be asked, how much alcohol he/she normally needs, in order to eliminate withdrawal symptoms. If very high dosages of benzodiazepines are needed, they should slowly be reduced over a period of 10 to 14 days. When transferring the patient (inpatient to outpatient, intensive unit to normal unit), it is important to continue following exactly the medication reduction programme which has already been devised. Abrupt termination of medication can lead to grand mal epileptic seizures. If there is a high risk for grand mal seizures, antiepileptic therapy can be added. In sufficient dosage, benzodiazepines do have sufficient antiepileptic effects.

For strong alcohol craving despite sufficient benzodiazepine therapy, we suggest administering caroverine 60–120 mg daily, an anti-glutamatergic substance which reduces alcohol craving. Acamprosate (relapse prophylaxis) is started immediately to reduce the intensity of craving. Thiamine is administered parenterally in doses between 150–300 mg to improve cognitive performance.

Further important factors are:

- Fluid and electrolyte substitution
- Monitoring in case of severe vegetative instability
- Cave: no parenteral administration of beta-blocker (risk for cardiac arrest)!
- Anti-dopaminergic neuroleptics can increase later on relapse rate

Motivation

These patients have an impaired alcohol metabolism with dysfunctions in neurotransmitter interaction. Type I patients suffer from withdrawal symptoms and severe alcohol craving. There is no history of psychiatric illness. Adequate explanation of the medical causes of the problem, as is the case with every chronic, somatic illness, e. g. diabetes mellitus, is of paramount importance. After reaching an understanding of the subjective intolerance of alcohol (like an "allergy"), motivation for an abstinence lasting for at least several months can be achieved. Abstinence is only attainable if withdrawal states are treated sufficiently (no abstinence attainable without enough medication and enough motivational work).

During abstinence, the motto is "protect and support". When speaking to clients, it is important to use simple, clear sentences which are easily understandable; short-term goals should be agreed upon (no long-term plans at this stage). During withdrawal, patients suffer, above all, from disturbances of concentration and memory. Therefore the contents of what has been discussed will need to be repeated again and again. If patients do not feel they have a supportive environment at home and that abstinence won't be possible, a short inpatient treatment (10–14 days) might be suggested.

Therapy goals

Total abstinence is central to a solution and can be achieved if the above-mentioned therapy is followed.

9.3.3.2 Management of detoxification in Lesch's type II alcohol dependents

Withdrawal symptoms

During the course of treatment, patients of this group usually show low blood alcohol levels and alcohol consumption is interrupted by more frequent but shorter periods of abstinence. During withdrawal, anxiety, emotional instability and sleeping disorders (difficulty falling asleep) frequently occur. Patients feel tense, woebegone and are seeking help. Crying alternates with aggressive outbursts, especially when drunk. Blood pressure and heart rates are increased. Acute sweating of the palms and mild sweating of the trunk are present. A fine, two-dimensional tension tremor only shows when patients are asked to stretch both arms forward. In the case history, no severe withdrawal symptoms are reported, with no seizures and no polyneuropathy. The withdrawal is a mixture of mild alcohol withdrawal and a basic anxiety disturbance.

Aetiology
Alcohol is used like an anti-anxiety medication, especially in situations of conflict (abused for relief of tension). It is assumed that an increased activity of the MAO system (mono-amin-oxidaser) is the cause of the biological vulnerability.

Duration
Withdrawal symptoms last for 10 to14 days. If some symptoms last for a longer time, then either they don't originate from alcohol but from a basic disturbance, or they might be caused by a longer intake of benzodiazepines or other hypnotics.

Withdrawal therapy
Non-benzodiazepine anxiolytic substances work best. We recommend e.g. tiapride, trazodone or doxepine. Dosage should be according to the severity of the anxiety states as well as the severity of the sleep onset insomnia. In most cases, 150 to 300 mg tiapride or trazodone are sufficient. There is no need for antiepiletic treatment.

Benzodiazepines and sodium oxibate should not be used because the patient is in great danger of shifting his dependence from alcohol to these compounds.

Withdrawal medication with benzodiazepines is only carried out in cases of concomitant abuse of tranquilizers. In such a case, withdrawal therapy is then conducted according to the criteria for benzodiazepine withdrawal (saturation with benzodiazepines until the patient is free of symptoms, followed by a slow reduction over the course of several months and gradual adjustment to anti-depressants).

Motivation
All that promises support and protection is helpful in this group of patients because of their primary low selfesteem. They don't feel safe and secure. The aim of motivation is to make the patient understand that psychotherapy is crucial to enhancing self-worth. Furthermore, it is important that the following topics are tackled in psychotherapy: coping with anxiety, aggression and stress; separation strategies and reciprocal and balanced relationships with others.

Another responsibility of motivational work is to educate the patient about the relationship between the effects of alcohol and their insecure personality and inadequate strategies to cope with stress. It is also essential to define factors that perpetuate alcohol consumption and factors that promote abstinence. These different factors represent the patient's inner ambivalence, which can be used to motivate him towards long-term abstinence.

Therapy goals
The most important therapy goal is the strengthening of the ego and the acquisition of adequate separation strategies, which on the one hand enhance coping skills for dealing with stress, but can also prevent stress from developing in the first place. The patient's drinking behaviour is not a central aspect of therapy. During psychotherapy minor relapses ("slips") are to be expected. These "lapses" are of short duration and usually don't involve any loss of control.

9.3.3.3 Management of detoxification in Lesch's type III alcohol dependents

Withdrawal symptoms

This group consists of patients with very different degrees of intoxication. Sometimes type III patients are actually completely abstinent when coming to the initial meeting.

Withdrawal symptoms: elevated blood pressure and heart frequency; heavy hand perspiration, light trunk perspiration; a two-dimensional tremor is only observed in patients holding up an arm. Patients are usually very strained and show suicidal tendencies. They often suffer from feelings of guilt, perceive themselves as a failure and show instable, but also incontinent mood (as manifested by e.g. crying fits during intoxication). Furthermore, patients suffer from sleep onset and sleep maintenance insomnia. The case history shows low to medium withdrawal syndromes, mostly without withdrawal seizures, and severe polyneuropathy is absent.

Aetiology

Alcohol is abused because of its mood lifting and sleep inducing effects. Although alcohol might induce sleep, it still has disturbing effects on the architecture of sleep and most chronobiological functions such as drive, mood and sleep).

Limbic system dysfunctions and disturbances in the hypophysis-thyroid axis are signs of a biological vulnerability. The symptoms can be described as a combination of alcohol withdrawal and depressive disorders

Duration

Detoxification lasts 10 to 14 days. Possible symptoms which occur later, usually originate from personality disorders or concomitant consumption, e.g. of benzodiazepines.

Withdrawal therapy

Anxiolytic substances that don't belong to the benzodiazepine group are used for withdrawal therapy in this group. Gammahydroxybutyric acid or trazodone are predominant. An antiepileptic therapy is usually not necessary.

Suggestion for dosage of gammahydroxy butyric acid: four times 7.5–10 ml per day (1 ml contains 175 mg sodium oxibate). On no accounte should this dosage be increased. Effects are reported very shortly after intake. If this dosage does not positively affect the withdrawal symptoms, benzodiazepine abuse is to be expected. If this is case, withdrawal therapy is then conducted according to criteria for benzodiazepine withdrawal (saturation with benzodiazepines until the patient is free of symptoms, followed by a slow reduction over the course of several months and graduate adjustment to anti-depressants).

Motivation

When educating patients, it should be noted that they have probably already sought information about the disorder from popular scientific literature. Be prepared to meet a partially informed patient. Patients may have already tried to apply some methods that were recommended by magazines.

The first step in therapy is to elucidate the relationship between the effects of alcohol as a buffer for a performance-oriented and controlled life ("Tellenbach personality") and the interaction between the effects of alcohol and the lack of experience-related and pleasurable activities. If type III patients manage to remain abstinent for 14 days, they are very likely to continue this abstinence for a few months. During these months, normal "functioning" is reported by the individual and the people in his/her social environment, without any therapy, and patients are only marginally willing to change their lifestyle. During therapy it is important to use the first months to clarify the ambivalence in regard to drinking and lifestyle.

It is also important that the therapist refrains from giving any advice. If therapy is structured too early, the patient might not allow any fundamental changes to his/her perception and behaviour despite managing to stay abstinent. The psychotherapeutic process should start slowly in order to avoid patients reacting with their learned performance-oriented mechanisms. This behaviour may change over the course of therapy. Due to narcissistic tendencies, the patient often perceives and judges therapy in a comparative way.

Therapy goal

Important therapy goals are both the reduction of heavy drinking episodes after months of abstinence and the treatment of the patient's personality disorder (Tellenbach personality). This is crucial because these personality traits cause psychological strain in patients and their social environment, which leads to severe changes in mood regardless of a relapse.

Further therapy goals are the reduction of relapse duration and frequency and severity of depressive symptoms (Cave: suicidal tendencies).

9.3.3.4 Management of withdrawal in Lesch's type IV alcohol dependents

Withdrawal symptoms

Patients show different degrees of intoxication when starting therapy. Withdrawal symptoms: fine tremor (like a lithium tremor), sweaty hand palms (at times no signs of perspiration during withdrawal = "dry withdrawal"), normal blood pressure, stable cardiovascular system.

Significant cognitive impairment to the point of orientation problems or confusion is a predominant symptom.

Light-induced activation and/or professional personal attention can often re-orientate the patient. However, during nights, deam-light and with no professional support, an orientation dysfunction may turn into complete confusion. False memory and even hallucinations can set in. Patients are very suggestible and often present an amentiell picture which is marked by helplessness and affective and/or paranoid symptomatic transitory psychotic syndromes. Due to severe cognitive dysfunctions, long-term therapy plans are impossible to make in the beginning. It is recommended that short sentences be formulated with clear short-term assignment of tasks. Anxious or agitated states are conditioned by orientation dysfunctions and misinterpretations of interactive processes.

Often epileptic seizures, which occur independently of alcohol consumption and withdrawal, were recorded in the case history. If such seizures have been recorded, it is important to be aware of the fact that GM seizures can set in at later stages of abstinence (after the tenth day of abstinence) or even later.

Often patients have a gait disturbance which is both cerebellar and due to severe polyneuropathies. When sedated, sometimes a "delirium in dorsal position" develops in patients with specific somatic problems, e.g. pneumonia. This can quickly turn into a vital risk.

Aetiology

Due to premature cerebral damage (before the age of 14, before brain development is complete) and its consequences, patients start consuming alcohol because they can't withstand the social pressure of our society to drink. Alcohol is merely a complicating factor within a bigger picture(adverse socialisation and cognitive impairments). The severity of performance reduction and psychopathological changes mainly correlate with previous cerebral damage and only secondarily with alcohol amounts consumed. Performance reduction is mainly caused by lack of ability and/or cerebral damages prior to the age of 14. Patients find it difficult to organise and add sense to everyday life. Furthermore, retarded alcohol elimination is a sign of a biological dysfunction, which causes damages that are predominantly caused by the alcohol per se than by its aldehydes.

Duration

As the causes of these symptoms are due to organic brain dysfunctions, regression of symptoms often takes weeks even months despite absolute abstinence. In some patients, no significant decline in symptoms can be observed.

Withdrawal therapy

For these patients, activation by light and personal counselling is more important than any medication (most suitable is one-to-one support)

Biologically active light and, if possible, brightly illuminated rooms with different sensomotor activities improve symptoms. As no cardiac and vegetative instability is at hand, patients should be mobilized as quickly as possible, possibly by including their families.

Nootropics to improve cognitive performance and anticonvulsive medication (e.g Carbamazepine) are recommended. Dispersion time needs to be taken into account due to a high risk of seizures. On average the dosage of Carbamazepine should not exceed 900 mg per day.

Sodium oxibate's effects are anxiolytic. Furthermore, it does not have any sedating properties with a dosage of four times 10 ml, does not significantly reduce cognitive performance, does not have any toxic effects on the liver and reduces alcohol craving. The short half-life time of sodium oxibate makes this medication well controllable. From our experience, patients of this group who take sodium oxibate are more easily motivated to start withdrawal therapy. As sodium oxibate is not an antiepileptic, it needs to be combined with common antiepileptics (e.g. Carbamazepine).

All medications which negatively influence cognitive performance, aggravate symptoms. Therefore sedating substances, like benzodiazepines, are contraindicated.

Benzodiazepines lead to confusion, noopsychological impairment and symptomatic transitory psychotic syndromes.

Atypical neuroleptics can be administered at short notice, e.g. quetiapine, olanzapine in case of productive syndromes and unrest at night (without vegetative symptoms).

Motivation
Motivational strategies should take account of impaired performance. Patients have difficulties following complicated matters and often tend to forget the things said. Only uncomplicated sentences, without multiple statements, should be used in conversation with these patients. Motivational work should be short and carried out regularly over several times a day. It is important to work on a structure for everyday life. Patients should be encouraged to include more and more activities when structuring their day.

Therapy goals
As patients are easily influenced by people in their social environment who also drink, and are reduced in their ability to give and receive criticism, severe relapses are not only to be expected but are rather the norm.

Therapy goals:

- Reduction of severity and frequency of relapses ("the aim is to survive")
- Relief from severe somatic problems
- Extension of abstinence periods
- Creating a daily structure

9.3.4 Complications in alcohol withdrawal

9.3.4.1 Withdrawal seizures (Grand mal)

Grand mal seizures can induce delirium tremens, but can also set in within the context of this condition. Therefore 20% of patients require anticonvulsive adjustment. This pharmacological adjustment should be effected when severe craniocerebral injuries have been recorded by case history or when seizures are already known from previous withdrawal therapies. Seizures in type I patients should be viewed as rebound phenomenon. In type III patients, this could be a rebound, mainly caused by benzodiazepines, while seizures in type IV should be viewed as a provocation of well-known seizure occurrences.

Therapy
When treating these disorders with the according antiepileptic medication (e.g. hydantoin, valproic acid, carbamazepine and others), we have to be aware that according to pharmacodynamics, these medications need time to reach effective dosages. Seizures setting in after day five suggest that these seizures are not only caused by alcohol withdrawal. Reasons could be a too rapid reduction of the withdrawal medication, but also epileptic occurrences independent of the alcohol dependence. Benzodiazepines, with their antiepileptic effect, are suitable for the treatment of type I and III patients. If benzodiazepines are dosed sufficiently, in most cases no further antiepileptics are needed. Seizures of type IV patients should primarily be treated with antiepileptics.

9.3.4.2 Delirant and associated states (meta-alcoholic psychosis)

In DSM-IV, these psychopathological syndromes are separated into psychotic, mood or anxiety disorders.

A fundamental factor in the genesis of this condition is a dopamine receptor hypersensitivity. Meta-alcoholic psychoses are in line with Wieck's symptomatic transitory psychotic syndromes (Wieck HH. 1967; Fig. 59, see explanation page 102f.). Its gradual progression of development and degradation corresponds with the deficits and recovery of single neuronal circuits (Glutamate-Dopamine-Endorphin, agitation-mood-reward-relief).

Delirium tremens (in type 1 patients, infrequently type III patients)

Delirium tremens usually sets in on the first or second day after abruptly changing or terminating alcohol use. Thus, it is suggested that a precise case history be taken covering especially alcohol, withdrawal symptoms and alcohol sequelae. The use of biological markers that indicate chronic abuse, even if patients are admitted for non-psychiatric reasons (e.g. admission into a surgery unit), are recommended. Established factors in surgery preparation are: MCV above 98 fl., gamma GT that is 1.3 times higher than the highest standard value, ASAT twice as high as ALAT (De-Ritis-quotient) and especially the %CDT (carbohydrate-deficient transferrin).

Precursors of these conditions are already apparent weeks before acute symptoms manifest. Frequent signs that have been reported are depressive or/and anxious mood, unrest and jumpiness. Patients often report insomnia with colourful and vivid dreams, which they experienced as very real and they find it difficult to separate dreams from reality.

Symptoms

Disorientation or erroneous orientation (delirious impairment of orientation, e.g. patient in hospital believes he is at the workplace), motor disturbance with optical (mostly micropsia) or tactile hallucinations, fumbling with blanket, false memory, high suggestibility, heavy perspiration, rough three-dimensional tremor. The severity of withdrawal can be measured through palpable muscular fibrillations which can be felt by slightly gripping the thenar. Cardiovascular instability and an electrolyte shift are life threatening (rapid changes in blood pressure, increase and decrease in heart frequency, arrhythmia). If delirium tremens does not set in until the third day of abstinence, there are more causal factors than pure alcohol withdrawal. For example, abrupt discontinuation of withdrawal medication or previous consumption of non-prescribed tranquillizers could play a role.

Therapy

Besides psychiatric symptoms, cardiovascular conditions, electrolyte metabolism and vegetative lability need to be considered. Therefore cardiac monitoring is a standard measure in these internist psychiatric emergencies (Lesch OM et al. 1986). Arrhythmia and ventricular fibrillation are the most common causes of death in delirium tremens (Cave: parenteral beta-blockers can lead to cardiac arrest). For the treatment of dehydration, it is recommended that liquids be infused with an electrolyte substitute and B vitamins (B 1, B 6 and B 12). Hypokaliaemia in plasma should be carefully substituted, because often an intracellular hyperkaliaemia exists, which could be worsened by enforcing potassium substitution. Tranquilizers in sufficient doses and in rare cases antiepileptics are needed. Neuroleptics should not be administered because they firstly lower the seizure threshold, secondly lead to severe extrapyramidal conditions and thirdly have adverse effects on long-term progression (Walter H et al. 2001).

Alcohol paranoia
(mostly type IV patients)
The reduction of mental performance caused by long-term alcohol dependence and by an adverse family situation often causes conflicts in the family. In some patients these can develop to the point of delusions (e.g. delusional jealousy). Often the female partner or the parents are the targets of such paranoid delusional interpretations. Aggressive attacks often might be directed at these persons. Aggressive individuals need to be admitted into inpatient care, because they can become dangerous for their environment.

Therapy: absolute alcohol abstinence; withdrawal therapy according to typology (see above). The delusional disorder often needs specific neuroleptic therapy (e.g. quetiapine). As in type IV, treatment requires long-term concepts within a stable setting.

Alcoholic hallucinosis
(mostly type IV patients)
Cerebral reductions in performance and reduced inhibition mechanisms lead to both acoustic and optic hallucinations without interpretations. If vegetative signs are weak, anxious conditions with denouncing voices, mainly in the second person, are very frequent. Suicidal tendencies are also frequent. Orientation is normal.

Therapy: absolute abstinence and neuroleptic therapy. Inpatient admission is often unavoidable.

Alcohol-induced Wernicke-Korsakow Syndrome (type I, III or IV patients)
This symptomatic is caused by chronic thiamine deficiency. Diet is often very poor, as patients predominantly "live on" alcohol. This behaviour causes severe nutritional deficiencies (e.g. folic acid and vitamin E deficiency, insufficient trace elements etc.).

Symptoms: motor ophthalmopathy (e.g. horizontal nystagmus), ataxia, polyneuropathy, frontal signs positive (palmo-and policomental reflex), disorientation, sometimes delusions (Korsakov psychosis).

Time and location based orientation is often deferred to the past and patients are highly suggestible. Misinterpretations of normal perceptions produce euphoric but also anxious conditions. Memory gaps are often filled with imaginary stories (confabulations). This symptomatic may be irreversible and can turn into a Korsakow-like dementia. Progression evaluation is possible six months after absolute controlled abstinence at the earliest and only within intensive rehabilitation programmes.

Therapy
Absolute abstinence, vitamin supplementation, with mainly thiamine parenterally in high dosage over three days. Nootropics, inpatient admission (thorough examination: such symptoms often have other additional causes).

9.4 Alternatives to withdrawal

Animal experiments support clinical observations that even higher amounts of alcohol (and tobacco) are consumed after temporary abstinence (Spanagel R and Hoelter SM. 1999). It has been observed that animals that didn't receive any alcohol for several days, consumed significantly more amounts of alcohol with higher alcohol content after abstinence. If severe withdrawals are expected, gradual reduction of alcohol amounts should be considered as an alternative (Sinclair JD. 2001).

9.4.1 Gradual reduction of drinking amount, "Cut down drinking", method according to David Sinclair

The so-called "extinction-method" (David Sinclair) is an alternative treatment for alcohol dependence. It reduces alcohol craving with opiate-antagonists (naltrexone) and, together with cognitive therapy, thus slowly weakens the learned process that has caused the alcohol dependence ("pharmacological extinction") (Hernandez-Avila CA et al. 2006). The association of stimuli "alcohol consumption-pleasurable feeling, positive reward" is gradually uncoupled, because no pleasurable feeling and feelings of reward set in due to the effects of opiate-antagonists ("pharmacological extinction"). Alcohol dependents should be in their normal environment (in which the dependence has developed) and should experience that alcohol doesn't have the "old", familiar effect anymore. This is due to the absence of endorphin effects caused by an mμ-receptor blockade. The association between alcohol consumption and pleasurable sensation is gradually loosened over a period of three months. The keeping of a drinking diary can visualize the success and regular dialogues (according to so-called "counselling standards") support the reduction of drinking amounts. This method is employed by so-called "ContrAL clinics" in the US and Europe.

The FDA already certified this method in the US in 1994. International acceptance of this method has evolved slowly and sporadically, probably due to possible competition with established therapy institutions and self-help groups. In the project "Combine", it was shown that Naltrexone worked on its own and that additional, specialised "counselling" did not lead to further improvement (Anton RF et al. 2006). In contrast, Chick et al. found that naltrexone is especially effective in combination with regular therapeutic conversations (Chick J et al. 2000).

A disadvantage of this method is the up-regulation of opioid receptors. A further disadvantage is that not all patients respond to naltrexone. Around 10% of patients are not able to reduce the amount they are drinking despite naltrexone intake. Reducing alcohol intake improves depressive symptoms, lowers the usually heightened blood pressure, reduces cardiovascular problems and lowers high cholesterol levels and elevated liver function tests. In some cases, naltrexone can't be administered. This applies to (infrequent) allergic reactions, concomitant use of opiates and severe liver damage.

A variation of the extinction method can be employed during standby periods before inpatient admission. By gradually reducing drinking amounts with naltrexone and arranging check-up appointments (every two days), waiting time is used in a meaningful way. At present this method is offered as pre-treatment at the Medical University of Vienna, Department of Psychiatry and Psychotherapy to a limited extent. In some patients this pre-treatment was so successful that the planned admission was no longer necessary.

Other patients were able to reduce their drinking by up to two thirds, which facilitated withdrawal. Less withdrawal medication was needed and the withdrawal period was significantly shortened. This does not only save costs but also prevents possible cerebral damage, which can be caused by withdrawal (Crews FT et a;. 2004). Neurotoxic damage caused by withdrawal is especially dominant in women (Hashimoto JG and Wiren KM. 2008).

From personal and clinical experience, this therapy is suitable for Lesch's types I, II and IV. The time before withdrawal is used in a meaningful way (waiting time before inpatient admission) by motivating patients, sensitising them to watch the amounts they are drinking and might positively integrate partners and prevents the patient from experiencing severe withdrawal and sometimes even avoids the need for inpatient admission. The application of this concept also prevents the conditioning of external stimuli and withdrawal symptoms

9.4.2 Case study: "Cut down drinking"

Accompanied by her partner, a patient, aged 48, comes to the "outpatient centre for individuals at risk of alcohol related illness" of the Medical University of Vienna, Department of Psychiatry and Psychotherapy. She is a housewife and has two adult sons. She states she is afraid of nearly everything (especially of the dark). She has been drinking to cope with her anxiety and, for the past two years, has also been drinking to alleviate her stomach pain (she also takes H_2-blockers) and arthritic knee pain. Knee surgery was successfully carried out this year, which reduced the pain. Nevertheless, she still keeps on drinking without a break (almost always associated with a loss of control). She shows a 40-year long concomitant use of beer, wine and hard liquor and mentions an insatiable craving for alcohol. She reports that she has been drinking increasingly more than she did previously, especially during the last two years. The patient suffers from feelings of guilt about not being able to stay abstinent and hopes that an inpatient admission will help her with this. The accompanying husband is supportive and does not put any pressure on the patient.

A type IV alcohol dependence was diagnosed in exploration. There are no occurrences of alcohol dependence or psychiatric disorders in her family. Alcohol dependence started after the age of 25 ("late onset"). The drinking amount is indicated at around 200 g daily and a withdrawal syndrome, like the one observed in type I patients, is identified. An inpatient admission is arranged and the patient is likely to be admitted in three to four weeks.

Naltrexone is prescribed as preliminary therapy at the first appointment. The patient receives the following information about the programme:

1. Daily intake of naltrexone; she is told that she is allowed to consume alcohol, but she should try to manage with the lowest required amount. In any case, she should drink the amount of alcohol that is needed to prevent withdrawal symptoms.
2. She should keep a drinking diary: one column each for wine, beer and hard liquor. Every eighth of wine, beer (0.3) and shots is to be

written down in the specific column.
3. At the beginning, a check-up appointment is arranged on every second day, which is cut down to every third day by week three.

Further, the patient is informed about the effects of naltrexone (fewer pleasurable feelings, gradually lessened craving for alcohol) and possible side effects (slight nausea, possible allergies). The patient starts with half a tablet on the first day, which is increased to one tablet a day from the second day onwards. An appointment for the next day is arranged.

The patient is to bring the drinking diary to this appointment. The recorded drinking amounts are discussed and consideration is given to when it would be easiest for her to abstain from drinking.

The drinking diary shows a daily consumption of 2.5 litre beer, five sixths of brandy and five eighths of wine (reduction to 150g pure alcohol daily).

Naltrexone is well tolerated and the drinking amount is reduced by 30 % over the next nine days. Light perspiration and trembling diminished within the next eight days. Blood sample: elevated liver function tests, cholesterol 332 mg/dl, %CDT 2.8 %, MCV 106 fl. The patient's %CDT is sensitive, which makes it very suitable for controlling abstinence (a possible increase of 0.8 % indicates a relapse). Marginal values are of secondary importance in this long-term monitoring.

The patient is encouraged to first abstain from brandy and then wine, so that only beer remains. After three weeks the patient has reduced consumption of brandy to one sixth, wine to two eighths and beer to 1.5 litres. She decided to continue without inpatient admission, because she wants to continue with this programme.

Three months after the start, the patient shows a daily alcohol consumption of 1.5 litres of beer. Another two months, she has replaced this with three bottles of alcohol-free beer, which she reduces to two bottles per week nine months after the start of the "cut down drinking" programme.

After eleven months, the patient wished to terminate the intake of naltrexone. This was discussed and implemented. To this day, 14 months after the beginning of therapy, the patient is still drinking two bottles of alcohol-free beer per week. No dosage increase was needed and the patient did not relapse. A test of biological markers confirmed abstinence (%CDT = 0.77 %, cholesterol 206 mg/fl, MCV: 93 fl, liver function tests in normal range). She still regularly attends the therapy meetings with her husband.

9.5 Pharmacotherapy of tobacco withdrawal syndrome

By addressing the smoking behaviour and offering individual advice, the amount of cigarettes smoked is significantly reduced in 20 to 30 % of tobacco abusing cases. A reduction of smoking behaviour reduces the number of sequelae and improves long-term progression of these diseases (e. g. COPD; Fiore MC et al. 2000). Regular follow-up meetings, in which the smoker is consulted, clearly improve results and are more important than shortterm pharmacotherapy (also see Lesch OM. 1985; 2007). The keyword "advice is effective" has internationally and repeatedly been supported (Fiore MC et al. 2000, 2008;

US Department of Health and Human Services; World health Organization 2003; Henningfield JE et al. 2005).

Different pharmacotherapy can even improve (sometimes even double) abstinence rates in tobacco abusers who don't meet the diagnostic criteria for dependence according to ICD-10 (Henningfield JE et al. 2005). Nevertheless, there is a large group of smokers who don't change their smoking behaviour despite taking anti-craving substances. This should make therapists aware of the fact that often several therapy meetings are needed to attain success. Patient support often marks the beginning of enduring improvements in smoking behaviour.

9.5.1 Symptoms of the tobacco withdrawal syndrome

The definition of the tobacco withdrawal syndrome is still controversially discussed, but the following symptoms have been agreed upon (see also Widiger T et al. 1994):

Fig. 93

- shift in mood
- irritability
- depressive mood
- nervousness and agitation
- higher vulnerability to stress
- heightened aggression
- impatience
- insomnia
- strong nicotine craving

Nicotine abuse and strong nicotine craving are not part of the tobacco withdrawal syndrome. Strong nicotine craving is however the most important reason for relapse. Yet this craving should not be evaluated as merely a withdrawal symptom because it has very different qualities, e. g. craving due to adephagia and the patient not wanting to gain any weight, or strong craving experienced when in the places and situations in which one used to smoke ("hot spots"). Symptoms of nicotine withdrawal syndrome are much more difficult to distinguish from the mechanisms of craving, which are important for relapse prophylaxis, as is the case in alcohol dependence.

In a study with 330 tobacco dependents according to ICD-10, we were able to show that only 55 patients (16.7 %) had severe withdrawal symptoms, while 128 patients (38.8 %) described mild withdrawal symptoms. The remaining 147 patients reported no withdrawal symptoms. Changes in mood, impatience and strong craving are essential withdrawal symptoms. Many patients only had specific withdrawal symptoms, the combination of two withdrawal symptoms was common and only 20.6 % of patients experienced all symptoms listed above (Lesch OM et al. 2004), see Fig. 94.

The duration of the withdrawal syndrome varies. It has been suggested that it lasts up to three months, but there is not enough scientific evidence to support this.

The Fagerstroem test correlates well with the severity of withdrawal symptoms and sequelae.

Today, nicotine withdrawal therapy in patients with Fagerstroem scores of five or above is carried out with nicotine supplements or varenicline.

Fig. 94 Constellation of tobacco withdrawal symptoms

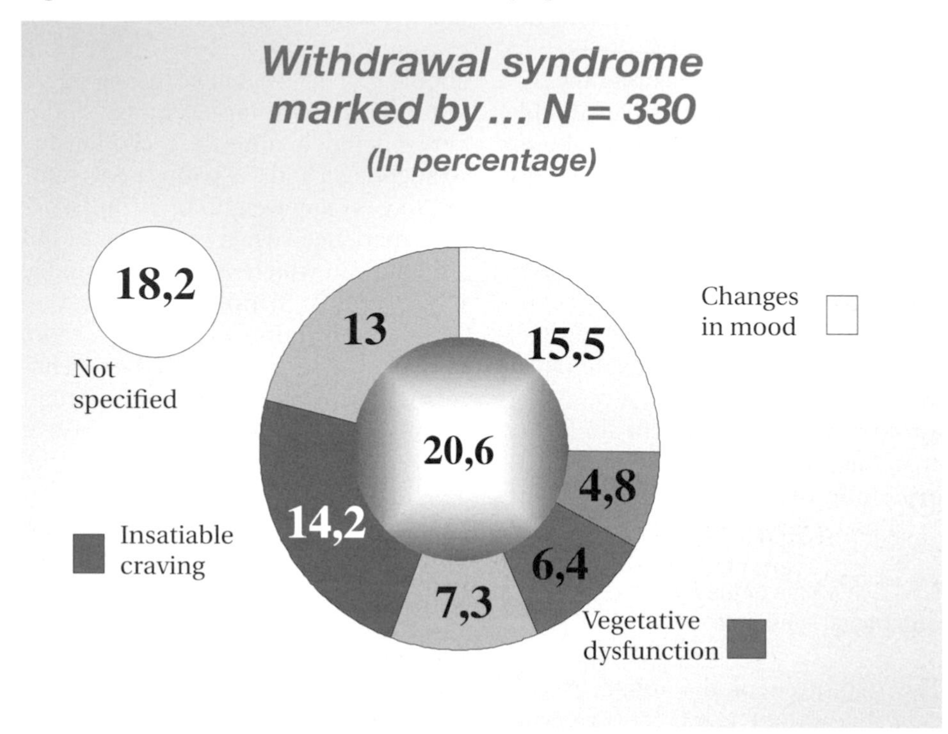

9.5.2 Therapy of the tobacco withdrawal syndrome

9.5.2.1 Withdrawal therapy of tobacco dependence with Fagerstroem ≥ 5

Nicotine supplements
Nicotine should be substituted in adequate doses (chewing gum, patches, inhaler and others).

Level-smokers should use nicotine supplements which provide a continuous nicotine supply, e.g. nicotine patches. Peak smokers, who smoke lots of cigarettes over a short period of time depending on the situation, might require high amounts of nicotine supplied very quickly (e.g. inhaler). Withdrawal symptoms and craving lasts for several weeks and often the administration of nicotine supplements is terminated too early. We recommend a continuous therapy of at least three months. From our perspective, there are not enough high quality studies on the duration of nicotine supplement therapy. Nicotine supplement is often combined in order to mix basis doses with rapid diffusion times (e.g. nicotine patches and inhaler).

Varenicline
Varenicline is a partial agonist of the $\alpha_4\beta_2$ subtype of the nicotinic acetylcholine receptor. In addition it acts on $\alpha_3\beta_4$ and weakly on $\alpha_3\beta_2$ and α_6-containing receptors. A full agonism was displayed on α_7-receptors. This selectivity sug-

gests that some smokers respond better than others: smokers, in whom different subunits of receptors play a role, profit less. Clinical studies have shown doubled abstinence rates and thus varenicline 1 mg twice daily can be recommended for nicotine withdrawal and craving (Fagerstroem 5 or above, Tonstad S et al. 2006; Zierler-Brown SL and Kyle JA. 2007; Oncken C et al. 2006; Williams KE et al. 2007; Coe JW et al. 2005; Gonzales DH et al. 2006; Cochrane Review Cahill K et al. 2007). Due to its effects, varenicline is recommended as a withdrawal medication, yet studies on dosage titration for withdrawal medication are still lacking in quality. Many patients complain about feelings of nausea.

9.5.2.2 Withdrawal therapy of tobacco dependence with Fagerstroem ≤ 4

These withdrawal symptoms can be treated with nicotine supplements or varenicline, but bupropion is also suitable. In this group, bupropion can be used for relapse prophylaxis and no readjustment of medication is needed.

The extent to which antidepressants, new CB-1-antagonists and clonidine can be used as a medication for withdrawal symptoms should be further investigated.

9.6 Medical strategies for relapse prevention

9.6.1 General guidelines for relapse prevention

The goal of withdrawal therapy is to maintain abstinence and a drug-free life. Of central interest is the therapy of basic dysfunctions, which have led to tobacco-and alcohol consumption. The therapy plan in this phase should be straightforward. Patients should feel secure and should be helped to see that abstinence means an enhanced quality of life and not merely the loss of an addictive drug). Withdrawal therapy and relapse prophylaxis should be based on a well-connected therapy chain (outpatient, semi inpatient, inpatient). This enables quick and efficient interventions in case of relapses. Medical/biological, psychotherapeutic and sociotherapeutic competencies are needed in therapy. Teams should be well staffed, with stable personnel that are easily approachable for patients. Only organisations like this can guarantee long-term therapy which runs efficiently. Obviously this requires more cost expenditures than commonly available for addiction therapy, but also saves money by reducing inpatient admissions (e.g. severe withdrawal with acute admissions to intensive units, more frequent admissions due to sequelae). Early interventions made by the counselling team, reduce the severity and duration of relapses. Merely providing short-term outpatient or inpatient crisis intervention, without a concept of what the next steps are, is insufficient.

Realistic and attainable therapy goals need to be agreed upon in which abstinence, the ultimate goal of therapy, should not be neglected even if only a reduction of substance consumption can be attained at first. Some patients require long-term substance substitution therapy despite all therapy options. Substitution therapy (sodium oxibate in type IV alcohol dependents, morphine supplements in opiate dependents) promotes social stabilisation and

Fig. 95 Cornerstones in relapse prevention

- Availibility and stability of the therapeutic team
- Individual pharmaco- and psychotherapeutic offers
- Earliest possible start of treatment and
- Modification of withdrawal treatment according to the underlying basis dysfunction (e.g. different treatment according to Lesch's typology)
- Incorporation of (stabilising) family members and treating possible co-dependencies (e.g. brochures for the affected and their family members – "Alcohol relapse, what next?" etc.)

permits other therapeutic/psychotherapeutic interventions. Changes in dosage of maintainance therapy should be made carefully and slowly. Even with withdrawal therapy, some patients can't come off addictive substances. In some cases, therapy is aimed at improving secondary complications and sequelae. Alcohol dependence is a disease with a recurrent progression and it is well known that at least 50 % of patients relapse during the first three months. Early and quick detection and flexible handling of relapses (e.g. medical adjustment, psychiatric and psychotherapeutic intervention, short inpatient admission) are one of the most important goals.

9.6.2 Goals for relapse prevention

Definition of a realistic therapy goal: absolute abstinence or reduction of addictive substance or "only" supporting the patient, which was shown to reduce mortality rates.

If the patient is still abusing the addictive substance, one goal might be to at least reduce secondary complications (e.g. risk for infections, road safety). It is important never to give up and to ensure that this feeling is passed on to the patients and the team. One relapse is often succeeded by another, and then followed by long-lasting abstinence.

Motivational work in therapy: Every alcohol dependent has different personality traits, which require the implementation of appropriately suited motivational methods (e.g. more imperturbability and calmness in Lesch's type II; the freedom to choose, the freedom not to have to do something in Lesch's type III and type IV).

Some patients are faced with a legal situation which requires them to have psychotherapy (inpatient or outpatient). These forms of therapy, with their stipulations about specific treatment approaches, are scarcely welcomed by patients or therapists. However, positive progressions have often resulted from these therapies.

Psychotherapy in relapse prevention differentiates between the therapy of those psychological disorders which perpetuate substance consumption, and therapy of those disorders which form the basis of addictive substance consumption (e.g. personality disorders).

Despite diverse psychopharmatherapeutic approaches, there is no single standardized therapy for withdrawal and relapse prevention worldwide. Throughout the world, the difference between wishing to combat negative emotions and wishing to enhance well-being is acknowledged

9.6.3 Medication against so-called "positive" craving (= desire for pleasurable, rewarding effects of the addictive substance)

9.6.3.1 Alcohol

Dopamine antagonists (neuroleptic substances) don't have any relapse inhibiting effects (Wiesbeck G et al. 2001). In therapy, 5-HT2A antagonists have been used as atypical neuroleptics. Quetiapine was shown to have positive effects in Babor type B patients (early onset, severe progression of alcohol dependence), but not in Babor type B (late onset, mild progression) (Kampman KM et al. 2007). Animal experiments showed that the CB-1 antagonist rimonabant prevents nicotine-associated alcohol relapses (Lopez-Moreno JA et al. 2007).

The mμ-opiate antagonist Naltrexone has repeatedly been shown to reduce the amount of drinking and the effects of relapse (Volpicelli JR et al. 1992; 1997). All studies on the effects of naltrexone point to a reduction in the amount and duration of drinking.(Volpicelli JR et al. 1997; Petrakis IL et al. 2004; O'Malley SS et al. 2007). With this pharmaceutical, a gradual dosage reduction can be considered as an alternative to alcohol withdrawal (Pettinati HM et al. 2006). There is also discussion about the possibility of directed dosing (only in the case of relapse) instead of daily dosing (Hernandez-Avila CA et al. 2006).

The established pharmaceutical, disulfiram, which inhibits the breakdown of acetaldehydes, is clinically effective. Yet one limitation is the patient's frequent lack of compliance regarding intake, which is typical in the case of aversive medication. From experience, this medication has positive clinical effects, but data shows a different picture (Blanc M and Daeppen JP. 2005). More recent studies, with a controlled intake of medication, suggest disulfiram to be more effective than naltrexone (De Sousa A and De Sousa A. 2004). Disulfiram, the inhibitor of dopamine beta-hydroxylase, which is important for noradrenalin biosynthesis, is a further indicator of the importance of the reward system (Weinshenker D and Schroeder JP. 2006). The necessity of regular monitoring of liver functions during disulfiram therapy is emphasized. (Chick J. 2004).

As already mentioned, topiramate inhibits dopamine release, but at the same time also has partial GABA agonistic and glutamate antagonistic effects and thus suggests a new future direction (Ma JZ et al. 2006).

Partial CB-1 antagonists have been and will be developed because the endocannabinoid system plays an important role in craving. Therefore, it has been assumed that a blockade of this system reduces craving and balances activity of the endocannabinoid systems (in regard to increased appetite and overweight) (Xie S et al. 2007). Up until now, the partial CB-1 antagonist, rimonabant, has been approved in Europe as a medication for the metabolic syndrome. It may also be effective in relapse prophylaxis or in reducing drinking amounts (Colombo G et al. 1998; Lopez-Moreno JA et al. 2007). The stress reducing effects of tricyclic antidepressants (effects on the HPA axis), in particular, seem to be entirely or at least partly moderated by the endocannabinoid system (Hill EM et al. 2002).

9.6.3.2 Tobacco

There have been positive results for varenicline as well as nicotine supplements and partly positive results regarding rimonabant (Reid RD et al. 2007). A CB-1receptor antagonist seems to be more suitable for this group of patients as the partial nicotine agonist varenicline leads to dopamine release (Cahill K and Ussher M. 2007). The CB-1 antagonist, rimonabant, was shown to inhibit pharmacologic peak releases of dopamine that are induced by addictive substances (Cheer JF et al. 2007). The warning that depressive symptoms in rimonabant treated tobacco dependent patients is increasing, should be investigated in prospective controlled studies. Also naltrexone has been tested as an augmentation of nicotine substitution (O'Malley SS et al. 2006).

9.6.4 Pharmacotherapy against the so-called "negative" craving (= desire for addictive substances to relieve negative mood and anxiety)

9.6.4.1 Alcohol

The required pharmacologic profile needs to have antidepressant, anxiolytic, calmative and anti-glutamatergic effects. Gaba-A effective medications, like diazepam, are used in withdrawal worldwide but need to be reduced and/or terminated early enough because of their own addictive potential. Gaba-B receptors also influence the effect of alcohol on cells, namely via the influence of protein kinases. An examination of baclofen showed that it was able to reduce the alcohol associated up-regulation of alpha subunits in protein kinase (Lee HY et al. 2007).

Antidepressants that go beyond a pure re-uptake inhibition can be suitable (e.g. dual anti-depressants, tricyclic antidepressants, partly also SSRIs, Pettinati HM. 2001). 5HT-1A has protective effects against stress-induced hippocampal changes (Joca SR et al. 2007). Antihistaminergic substances have calmative and sleep-inducing effects. The central alpha-2-adrenergic agonist clonidine is especially effective against vegetative overstimulation during withdrawal (Schnoll RA and Lerman C. 2006).

Acamprosate seems to be the most well-known substance with anti-glutamatergic effects that has been properly investigated by alcohol research (Lesch OM and Walter H. 1996; Withworth AB et al.1996; Spanagel R and Zieglgansberger W. 1997; Chick J. 1995; Lesch OM et al. 2001; Mann K et al. 2004; Verheul R et al. 2005).

Caroverine, oral or as an infusion, has proven to be clinically effective for withdrawal (Koppi S et al. 1987), but has not been further tested. Positive effects on withdrawal have been found in lamotrigine (inhibits glutamate release), memantine and the AMPA/kainate antagonist, topiramate (Krupitsky EM et al. 2007).

Against all expectations (Hoelter SM et al. 1996; Danysz W et al. 2002; Nagy J. 2004), relapse prevention studies on the glutamate antagonists, memantine and neramexane, have only produced negative or no continuous positive effects on abstinence (Evans SM et al. 2007).

Animal experiments showed that the nicotinic acetylcholine agonist, varenicline, is successful in reducing drinking amounts (Steensland P et al. 2007). Also CRF (corticotrophin releasing factors) antagonists (Heilig M and Koob GF. 2007) could be used as medication in relapse prophylaxis in the future.

9.6.4.2 Tobacco

Nicotine is hypothesized to have antidepressant effects. Therefore, nicotine supplements may be suitable for the period following the termination of smoking. For nicotine withdrawal and its negative craving symptoms, the antidepressant bupropion is an approved medication. During and after nicotine withdrawal, dysphoric mood, irritability and even depressive symptoms set in frequently. The continuation or restart of smoking could be prevented by these antidepressant effects, especially in combination with nicotine supplements (Covey LS et al. 2007). Yet there are also studies on bupropion that show negative results (Simon JA et al. 2004; Stead L and Lancaster T. 2007). Dopamine antagonists, opiate antagonists and CB-1 antagonists are not expected to be effective in this group of patients. Partial nicotine agonists like varenicline might have positive effects in the above mentioned group (Rollema H et al. 2007).

9.6.5 Pharmacotherapy in relapse prevention in dependent patients

9.6.5.1 Alcohol

The information in the above paragraphs has underlined the complexity of the neuronal and neuron-modulating relationship of different therapy approaches. Accordingly, and in practice, medication, which is effective in different ways, has been introduced for relapse prophylaxis of alcohol and tobacco dependence. These have been proven to be effective in subgroups of alcohol and tobacco dependents, see Fig. 96.

These different mechanisms of action require a more precise diagnostic than recommended by ICD-10 and DSM-IV for the diagnosis of dependence. Therefore, the establishment of subgroups of tobacco and alcohol dependents is essential for specific pharmacotherapy. There is sufficient data on the specific therapy of alcohol dependence (see chapter 6). Several typologies have been shown to be clinically relevant, with the following frequently used in therapy studies: within the two cluster solutions, especially the typology according to Cloninger (Cloninger et al. 1988) with type 1 (anxious, passive-dependent, rapid tolerance development) and type 2 (antisocial personality, patients seeking the euphorising effect, early onset of drinking) as well as the typology according to Babor (Type A: late onset, mild progression; type B: more risk factors in childhood, positive family anamnesis regarding alcohol, early onset of drinking, more psychological dysfunctions). Within the four cluster solution, Lesch's typology has been used in therapy studies. Leggio published 2009 the medications having accepted data for subgroups of alcohol dependent patients (see Fig. 97).

9.6.5.2 Tobacco

Relapse prevention in tobacco dependence show also very different treatment approaches and some medications are

Fig. 96 Pharmaceuticals and their effects in relapse prevention of alcohol dependents

Comparison of pharmaceuticals, which are approved in different countries for relapse prevention of alcohol dependence

Substance	Mechanism	Effect
Acamprosate	NMDA-receptor blockade competitive	Prevention of "conditioned pseudo withdrawal syndrome", approved for anti craving therapy
Naltrexone	Blockade of the n-opioid receptor with indirect inhibition of dopamine release in the striatum	Reduction of ethanol intake, approved for anti-craving therapy
Topiramate	Facilitation of GABA-A-effects, blockade of ionotropic AMPA-receptors	Studies have pointed to a craving reducing effect
Memantine	Non-competitive blockade of the NMDA-receptor	Animal studies have pointed to a craving reducing effect
Baclofen	GABA-B receptor antagonist	Anti-craving effect in placebo controlled studies
Ondansetrone	5-HT3-receptor antagonist	Clinical studies have shown anti-craving effects and a reduction in alcohol intake
Sodium Oxibate	Praesynaptic dopamine agonist	Reduction of Reward craving
Disulfiram	Increase of Acetaldehyde	Aversive reaction

Lenz B, Hillemacher T, Kornhuber J, Bleich S 2007

listed internationally accepted as effective reducing craving and tobacco smoking in tobacco dependent patients, see Fig. 98.

9.6.6 Relapse prevention according to Lesch's typology

Relapse prevention primarily complies with the underlying dysfunctions and the function of alcohol in that particular person. In the beginning, "stabilisation and protection" are most important. After a few weeks of total abstinence, specific psychotherapeutic agreements can be made and individual therapy can begin. This psychotherapeutic therapy is based on personality traits, personality disorders and the patient's coping strategies. Different coping strategies, which can be influenced by e.g. gender, need to be incorporated into the psychotherapeutic setting. Although Lesch's typology offers directions for a correct psychotherapeutic procedure, it still lacks specificity for therapeutic work. The very fact that type IV patients often describe their drinking behaviour as compulsive, or type III patients use the effect of alcohol to improve negative emotions, or type II patients use alcohol to improve their interpersonal skills, might provide information, but is

Fig. 97 Alcohol Typologies and medical relapse prevention treatment

Typologies and medications

- Medication for relapse prevention according to typologies (evidence based)
- Hypothesis: Medication for relapse prevention

Naltrexone	Type A Cloninger II Lesch III &IV	LO-A
Acamprosate	Cloninger II Lesch I & II	Babor B EO-A
Ondansetron	EO-A Babor B	Cloninger II
Setraline	Babor A	Cloninger I LO-A

Leggio L. et al, Neuropsychol Rev. 2009

LO-A: Late onset alcohol dependence EO-A: Early onset alcoholism

Fig. 98 Pharmaceutic relapse prevention in tobacco dependence

Substance	Mechanism	Effect
Nicotine supplements	Occupation of nicotine receptor and dopamine agonist	Reduction of biological craving in Fagerstroem ≥ 5
Vareniclin	Partial Alpha4Beta2 Nicotine receptor antagonist	Reduction of biological craving in Fagerstroem ≥ 5
Bupropion	Anti-depressant with dopamine agonistic effects	Improvement of the basis dysfunction and mood-related craving
Nortriptyline and Doxepin	Anti-depressant with cholinergic and dopaminergic effects	Improvement of the basis dysfunction and mood-related craving
Clonidine	Alpha-adrenergic agonist	Reduction of situation-based craving
Rimonabant	CB1 antagonist and dopamine agonist	Impulse control and reduction of craving in weight problems
Topiramate	Unclear mechanisms	Reduction of compulsive behaviour and improvement of impulse control

not a substitute for a personality diagnostic as provided by axis II of DSM-IV. The severity of a relapse regardless of loss of control is type-specific and therefore this therapy requires different strategies. The choice of anti-craving substances also depends on types and is discussed in depth in the following.

A type-specific choice of an adequate anti-craving substance can double abstinence rates (e.g. acamprosate in type I or II according to Lesch, naltrexone in type III or IV according to Lesch), whereas the wrong medicament for the wrong type can double the occurrence of relapses (e.g. flupentixol in Lesch's type I or III).

9.6.6.1 Relapse prevention in Lesch's type I

From a medical perspective, NMDA-antagonism is the most important relapse-preventive mechanism in type I. Acamprosate matches this profile especially in regards to long-term effects. The aversive substance, disulfiram, is also recommended for type I and can be perfectly combined with acamprosate. It inhibits an oxidative degradation of acetaldehyde into acetate, whereby acetaldehyde accumulates in the blood, simultaneous with alcohol consumption, and symptoms like headache, flush, hyperventilation, hyperhidrosis, high blood pressure and vomiting set in. Disulfiram does not have any known or clinically observed anti-craving-effects. By combining disulfiram and acamprosate, an anti-craving effect is additionally obtained. Besson J et al. (1998) showed that a combination of disulfiram and acamprosate delivers optimal results.

As there are no psychological co-morbidities in type I patients, group psychotherapy is pointless. What is important is that total abstinence is maintained, and that the intake of relapse prophylactic medication is taken for long enough (up to 15 months). Regular check-ups are important and as this group is hyperthymic, they like to have regular check-ups. The abstinence-oriented self-help group is also suitable for type I patients) (e.g. AA-groups, family clubs).

9.6.6.2 Relapse prevention in Lesch's type II

Minor relapses (so-called "slips") don't have any impact on the course of the illness as a whole. Patients in this group don't seek any euphorising effects, but rather suffer from negative craving (desire for anxiolytic and calmative effects) (similar to Cloninger type I patients). Therefore this group requires administration of NMDA-antagonists for at least 12 to 14 months in order to reduce craving. Anxiolytic antidepressants in particular (e.g. buspirone), have been shown to be clinically effective. Kranzler HR (1994) found that patients who were administered buspirone showed more abstinent days, a significant reduction of anxiety and the period of time before onset of the first relapse was longer. Malcolm R's (1992) study did not support these results. Malec et al. have concluded that buspirone is effective as an additional therapy for alcohol dependence with anxiety co-morbidity (Malec E et al. 1996; Malec TS et al. 1996). Sertraline only had positive effects on abstinence rates in type A patients according to Babor (late onset, mild progression) (Pettinati HM et al. 2000). Moclobemide in a dosage between 300 and 600 mg reduces the MAO turnover and therefore can be used as an anticraving substance in this subgroup.

Regular psychotherapy and ego stabilisation is the most important measure in type II patients. Self-help, which is based on the twelve steps used by alcoholic anonymous groups, is often counterproductive in type II patients. This is especially the case for Wikipedia cited steps one (to accept that one is powerless against one's own problems), two (to believe that there is only one power greater than oneself which can rehabilitate the psychological condition), three (to decide to entrust one's will and life to God, however he is perceived/understood), six (to be willing to let God remove "faults in character") and seven (to humbly ask God to remove all personal "faults"). For type II patients, it is crucial that they are in charge of their own life in order to get out of the passive-anxious role and develop more self-esteem.

AA groups are not sufficient. We learned that groups to increase self-esteem or to reduce anxiety, often in a hypnotherapeutic setting, are sufficient.

9.6.6.3 Relapse prevention in Lesch's type III

Similar to type 2 according to Cloninger, patients seek the euphorising effects of alcohol due to their personality disorder (Tellenbach personality, and often also narcissistic tendencies) on the one hand, and depressive co-morbidity on the other. Type III patients are often abstinent for a long time and tend not to have slips. Relapses in the case of these patients, are rather severe. Naltrexone was shown to be effective in relapse prophylaxis (Kiefer F et al. 2005). It has been frequently discussed, whether it is better to administer naltrexone as a daily therapy or intermittently and directed in the case of relapse (Hernandez-Avila CA et al. 2006). Even in longitudinal studies, a depot injection (with 380 mg) once per month resulted in a significant reduction in the number of drinking days compared with a placebo (Garbutt JC et al. 2005; O'Brian CP. 2005); side effects were nausea and headaches. Nevertheless, it should be emphasized that it has been clinically observed in type III patients (individuals with a vulnerability to depression) that the effect of naltrexone decreases after approximately three months. This medication has been observed as having only a mildly depressive effect. The co-morbidity of alcohol dependence and depressive mood always raises the risk of suicide (Cornelius JR et al. 1995; Yates G et al. 1988). Both disorders aggravate each other and influence the neuronal signal system in such a way that established therapies are ineffective or may even have counterproductive effects (Pettinati HM et al. 2000; Johnson BA et al. 2000). Therefore it is vital for this group of patients, in particular, that more work be done to improve and develop pharmacological options. In her overview, Pettinati concludes that SSRIs are effective for maintaining abstinence in uncomplicated alcohol dependents. Yet they are ineffective or even disadvantageous in patients with a depressive co-morbidity (Pettinati HM et al. 2001). Imipramine and desipramine showed positive results in regard to relapse and the reduction of drinking amounts (McGrath PJ et al. 1996; Mason BJ et al. 1996). There is only one study on dual acting antidepressants with milnacipran (Lesch OM et al. 2004). This six month trial has shown that milnacipran is able to reduce relapses. Recently Pettinati et al. published that the combination of sertaline (200 mg daily) with naltrexone (100 mg daily) achieved significantly higher rates in abstinence and that this combination delayed also relapses to heavy drinking. At the end of this trial fewer serious reverse events were reported and the patients tended not to be depressed (Pettinati H. M. et al. 2010).

The 5HT-3 antagonist, ondansetron, seems to be effective against craving and significantly reduces drinking in "early-onset" alcohol dependents

(Johnson BA et al. 2000). A combination of ondansetrone and naltrexone significantly reduced drinking amounts in a placebo comparison study and therefore is more effective than both medications on their own (Johnson BA et al. 2000).

Topiramate antagonises glutamate and promotes GABA functions, which reduces dopamine release in the mesolimbic system. These combined effects also reduce the "reward effect". Topiramate has been found to be successful in both "early onset" and "late onset" types with regards to craving and the reduction of drinking amounts (Johnson BA et al. 2003). 61% of patients with bipolar affective disorders consume increased amounts of alcohol. Topiramate seems to have mood stabilizing and anti-craving effects. Psychotherapy is very important in type III patients. The aim of the therapy is to loosen an overly tight structure so that patients no longer define their self-worth solely in terms of their performance, and increase their ability to cope with narcissistic offences in everyday life, without relapsing.

In regard to self-help approaches, step number twelve of the alcoholic anonymous programme is rather counterproductive ("Pass on the message to others after having been spiritually enlightened ..."), because this is exactly what type III patients should learn not to do (not to always be there for others, not to take the lead, not to be overly smart). In case of narcissistic tendencies, step four can be very helpful however ("to make a thorough and fearless inventory about oneself").

This could form a good basis for further therapy, which should also include narcissistic gain (e.g. imagine oneself being a queen or a king, beautifully dressed, standing on a hill and looking over his/her country and all is peaceful ...)

9.6.6.4 Relapse prevention in Lesch's type IV

Naltrexone, in oral form or as a depot (Garbutt JC et al. 2005) reduces the amount and duration of drinking. Within the group of anticonvulsive medication, valproic acid, carbamazepine and topiramate have been examined. The attempt was to reduce protracted withdrawal symptoms with anti-convulsives and to increase impulse control. Furthermore, it was attempted to use mood-stabilizing effects for affective symptoms. Valproic acid had positive effects in regard to abstinence rates (Longo LP et al. 2002) and irritability (Brady KT et al. 2002). Carbamazepine was able to extend the time until the first relapse, but this effect did not last over the entire period of the study (Mueller TI et al. 1997). Further recommendations are ondansetrone, topiramate, pregabalin, nootropics and if necessary atypical neuroleptics (e.g. quetiapine; Kampman KM et al. 2007). This type shows a high cerebral vulnerability possibly due to frequent withdrawals. Often epilepsy develops independently from the alcohol dependence and anticonvulsive therapy is needed.

Many type IV patients are very difficult to treat within an outpatient setting due to previous cognitive damage (impaired critical faculty often resulting in a high discrepancy between their "wishes" and their "social possibilities"), a lack of socialisation (isolation as a stress factor) or due to their own specific socialisation (an example: a patient's recently transplanted liver is damaged as a result of drinking alcohol with friends). Therefore these patients need long-term inpatient admission with psychotherapy that is specially adapted to this group. In an outpatient setting, sociotherapy can be particularly effective. Likewise, self-help groups that function according to the Synanon model can be helpful (living in a community, own activities, motto: everyone has the ability to live abstinently). However, type IV specific self-help groups need to accept relapses as part of the symptomatology, which often becomes one of the biggest obstacles. These patients tend to display a cyclothymic temperament and changes of mood and activity are often reflected by changing levels of motivation. The most important therapeutic tool is to keep in touch with these patients on a regular basis.

9.6.7 Treatment of relapses according to Lesch's typology

Relapses in type I patients can be treated with Naltrexone for several days. The administration of acamprosate should not be terminated. Benzodiazepines that are administered over a few days should help terminate the relapse and can be administered together with vitamin B1. Therapy sessions should be short, but closely monitored. Admissions lasting one to three days are recommended.

Arguments, agitation, anxiety and stress are typical factors that lead to a relapse in type II patients. A decisive factor is the inability "to say no" to others' expectations. Therapy aims at helping patients to find the courage to make one's own decisions. This new "decisiveness" or learned ability to say "no", might encourage the patient to say "no" to abstinence or to an alleged belief of being in control, no matter what.

Pharmacotherapy and psychotherapy should be ongoing.

If a relapse lasts longer than expected and the patient requests an adjustment of medication, the anti-glutamatergic, caroverine (three times two tablets) should be administered for a couple of days, and for craving, ondansetrone (5-HT-3-blockade) in addition to anxiety relieving medication or alternatively SSRIs can be adjusted to dual action anti-depressants.

Lesch's type III patients usually relapse after a longer period of abstinence and should be advised before the start of therapy that relapses are to be expected, if no significant changes in lifestyle (e. g. the tendency to excessively burden oneself) are made or if phases of depression are still setting in. In case of a relapse, it is important to help the patient to overcome feelings of guilt and to provide objective information on how to combat relapses (e. g. to explain the "buffer" effects of alcohol).

In regards to medical treatment, it is important to continue naltrexone for relapse prevention and to additionally administer gamma-hydroxybutyric acid on a short-term basis in order to stop the relapse. Afterwards, antidepressant medication can be increased or adjusted to a different antidepressant substance. Topiramate, ondansetron or baclofen should be taken into consideration. Antihistamines can have sleep inducing and antidepressant effects (e. g. diphenhydramine).

Type IV patients relapse more frequently than all other types. In the case of a relapse, these types of patients should receive sociotherapeutic treatment additionally to naltrexone. Pharmaceutically, ondansetrone, topiramate, pregabaline and if necessary neuroleptics should be considered (e.g. quetiapine; Kampman KM et al. 2007).

In conclusion, it can be said that relapses in type I progression require medical intervention, whereas type II and III predominantly need psychotherapy and type IV is best treated by using medical and sociotherapeutic competencies. The pharmacological recommendations mentioned above might define the scopes of therapy, but the patient is always the central aspect in the treatment of the relapse. Therefore it is essential to understand the patient's current situation, to reduce stress, to focus away from the patient's failures and concentrate more on things that were successfully done. Furthermore, the patient should be helped to perceive things that are unchangeable (e.g. paralysis after seizure, few psychological and cognitive stress compensation possibilities, unable to do physical exercises and therefore often a dysphoric mood leads to relapse) as a consequence of positive aspects in one's life (e.g. my body had to pay a price for all the things achieved in life) or as part of the current situation (e.g. it is important to concentrate on what I can do for myself today).

9.6.8 Pharmacotherapy of relapse prevention in tobacco dependents

Tobacco dependence is a very heterogenic phenomenon which can be defined by the commonality of nicotine consumption, but the aetiology as well as the craving for tobacco have very different causes (Hesselbrock VM and Hesselbrock MN. 2006; Lesch OM et al. 2004).

Besides the risk of addiction, nicotine has effects that are actively sought by individuals, which is why they continue to smoke. For example, nicotine has been described as having the effects of enhancing concentration, reducing appetite and positively influencing one's psychological state. Often a cigarette is smoked to reduce anxiety in stressful situations and to elevate mood. But also habits and ritualised activities, like e.g. coffee and a cigarette or a cigarette after eating, play an important role. The breaking of these habits is one of the biggest challenges next to the treatment of physical dependence. When medically supporting patients, it is not only important to educate and inform them about the effects of smoking, but also to help them cope with withdrawal. Besides a precise diagnosis of the dependence pattern, a therapy that is precisely adjusted to the patients needs is required because the same kind of therapy is not effective in every patient.

9.6.8.1 Medication for relapse prevention of tobacco dependents

9.6.8.1.1 Nicotine replacement therapy

These products substitute the effects of nicotine at the nicotinic acetylcholine receptor and most likely the effects on the MAO system as well. The "normal" smoker, smoking 20 cigarettes a day, resorbs 20 to 40 mg of nicotine daily and has plasma concentrations of 23 to 35 ng/ml (Benowitz NL et al. 1988). Nicotine supplements often don't reach these concentrations and therefore different forms of administration have been developed. The nicotine patch, which is available in different dosages, is suitable for a basis dosage. During states of craving, during which strong nicotine cravings are triggered, rapid dispersion times, reaching higher concentrations, are required. The sublingual tablet, the nicotine nasal spray as well as the nicotine inhaler seem to be sufficient supplements for these states. Compliance with nicotine patches is usually very positive, but acute forms of nicotine supplementation show a different picture (Shiffman S et al. 1996). The nicotine gum provides a basis medication and can be used in acute situations. Yet it needs to be chewed slowly, which is very difficult for smokers who suffer from strong cravings. All of these products are often under-dosed and therefore have inadequate effects. Today we know that nicotine supplements are especially effective in tobacco dependent patients who have a Fagerstroem score of five or above. These supplements are suitable in withdrawal therapy as well as for cravings in smoke-free episodes and for the reduction of the amounts of cigarettes smoked (Henningfield JE et al. 2005; Sweeney CT et al. 2001; Tonnesen P et al. 1999; Le Foll B et al. 2005; J. Clin Psychiatric Monograph 2003; National Institute for Clinical Excellence 2004).

The most significant side effects of nicotine supplements are nausea, headaches and sometimes states of dizziness and vertigo. Usually these side effects are of low severity and often regress after several days.

9.6.8.1.2 Varenicline

A study that compared varenicline with bupropion and a placebo showed that varenicline increased abstinence rates in smokers more significantly than bupropion and placebo. This effect could still be verified after 52 weeks. In 2007, Cahill et al. published a review on varenicline and summarized data for daily practice:

1. Varenicline is three times better than placebo at improving smoking even in the longitudinal course
2. In smokers, varenicline is superior to bupropion. Studies combining varenicline and other therapeutic measures are still lacking and there is still research needed to better document the role of varenicline in smoking withdrawal.

Further, dose titration studies and studies that investigate symptoms which are a result of terminating medical therapy after long-term administration of varenicline, are needed. However, all in all, side effects seem to be uncommon. Nausea was the most frequently reported side effect.

9.6.8.1.3 Anti-depressants

Mostly dopamine-agonistic and noradrenergic active anti-depressants are discussed in line with nicotine dependence. There is clinical data on bupropion, nortriptyline and doxepin.

Several new dual anti-depressants might also have positive effects.

9.6.8.1.4 Bupropion

Bupropion doubles abstinence rates in both women and men. Studies have used 300 mg of bupropion, which was halved into two daily doses of 150 mg. One study was able to show that a combination of nicotine supplements was able to improve the progression. Further publications reported an improvement of depressive symptoms and in smoking behaviour (Lerman C et al. 2004; Fiore MC et al. 2000; Scharf D and

Shiffman S. 2004; Shiffman S et al. 2000; Jorenby DE et al. 1999).

9.6.8.1.5 Nortriptyline

Also nortriptyline improves depressive symptoms, but it has the biggest effect on smoking behaviour. This applies to both types of tobacco dependents, those who show depression co-morbidity and those without any depressive symptoms (Henningfield JE et al. 1998; Huges J et al. 2004; Ferry LH. 1999; Prochazka AV et al. 1998; Hall SM et al. 1998).

9.6.8.1.6 Doxepine

In older studies, this medication has already been proven to be effective for both nicotine withdrawal syndrome and tobacco craving (Edwards NB et al. 1988; Murphy JK et al. 1990).

All of these anti-depressants have well known side effects. These are elevated heart frequency, dry mouth, changes in blood pressure and increased risk for urinary retention in men. Narrow angle glaucoma is a contraindication for tricyclic anti-depressants.

9.6.8.1.7 Clonidine

Clonidine is an alpha-2-noradrenergic active agonist, which is used in opiate- and alcohol withdrawal. A study included smokers that were not able to stop smoking despite being motivated to quit. Results showed that twice as many smokers taking clonidine were able to quit smoking within four weeks when compared to a placebo group (Glassman AH. et al. 1988). These positive results could still be observed after six months. As side effects of clonidine are quite common, it tends to be a second choice in therapy.

9.6.8.1.8 Rimonabant

Rimonabant is a CB1-antagonist and data suggests a decrease of impulse control in eating, which also applies to alcohol (Soyka M et al. 2007; Despres JP et al. 2005; Pi-Sunyer FX et al. 2006). As impulse control also plays a role in smokers, rimonabant has been tested in studies on smoking reduction. In these studies, 20 mg rimonabant was administered daily and smoking behaviour and weight were monitored. Light smokers and smokers with a Fagerstroem score of five or above were included in the study and results showed that abstinence rates were twice as high and weight was more significantly reduced than in the placebo group (Cohen C et al. 2002; Anthenelli R. 2004; Klesges RC et al. 1997; Klesges RC et al. 1989). Dose titration studies are also lacking for rimonabant. Our study shows that women who smoke are especially suitable for these studies as they smoke significantly more often in order to control their weight than men. The extent to which combinations of anti-depressant medication can be effective should definitely be examined. Women also smoke more frequently because of a prevailing depressive mood (Lesch OM et al. 2004). Nausea is one of the most frequently reported side effects of rimonabant (Soyka M et al. 2007). Rimonabant in daily practice showed an increase in depressive symptoms and we believe that further studies in this mechanism are necessary.

9.6.8.1.9 Topiramate

This anti-epileptic has been examined in alcohol dependents over a period of three months and results showed a significant improvement in alcohol dependents' impulse control. The starting dose of 25 mg/daily was gradually increased to 300 mg of topiramate and was well tolerated by patients. Results also showed significant improvement in smoking behaviour, which was controlled by using cotinine levels. The role of topiramate or similar substances in smoking cessation needs to be further examined (Johnson BA et al. 2003; Johnson BA et al. 2005).

All other substances that are of theoretical interest lack sufficient data to be recommended for smoking cessation (e. g. nicotine vaccine, dual antidepressants, ondansetrone etc.).

In conclusion, it can be stated that the smoker's response to anti-craving substances as well as behaviourally oriented therapy approaches are important factors in withdrawal therapy. Furthermore, patience and the ability to encourage motivation time and again are crucial issues for supporting smokers. The recommended medications have very different mechanisms and clinical data suggests that they are only effective for certain subgroups of tobacco dependents (e. g. improvement of abstinence rates from 20 % to 40 %, but this still leaves 60 % that don't profit from this method). The subgroups described in chapter 6.2 and different forms of craving have different biological mechanisms and therefore future studies need to consider these factors.

9.6.8.2 Therapeutic procedure according to subgroups of nicotine dependent patients

The Institute for Social Medicine and Centre for Public Health with pulmonary specialists qualified in counselling smokers, and the Medical University of Vienna, Department of Psychiatry and Psychotherapy, have developed a diagnostic instrument which has divided nicotine dependence into four different clusters. Different forms of craving (relaxation, coping, stress and depression) are considered. These four clusters with their different craving mechanisms comprise then homogenous groups which are also based on shared biological and psychological aetiologies. (Lesch OM et al. 2004), Fig. 99.

A decision tree is suitable for the definition of particular subgroups. The severity of each dimension is exemplified by simple and weighted categories and thus clear decisions can be derived from this. The score of the Fagerstroem test is very important in withdrawal therapy, but for relapse prophylaxis therapy, consecutive symptoms, like infantile behavioural disorders, seem to be more important than the Fagerstroem score.

9.6.8.2.1 Subgroups according to Kunze and Schoberberger (Lesch OM. 2007)

Moreover, Kunze has introduced three types of smokers, namely level smoker, peak smoker and mixed types, which are defined as follows (Fig. 33):

1. Level smoker: smoking is evenly distributed across the day
2. Peak smoker: consumption in specific situations or notably more at specific times of the day (= peak times), then only little or no smoking for longer periods
3. Mixed types: regularly smoking at steady intervals, but more intensive on certain occasions

9.6.8.2.2 Craving in subgroups of tobacco dependent patients

Data on subgroups needs to be confirmed by further research and there

Fig. 99 Decision tree for the classification of smokers into groups

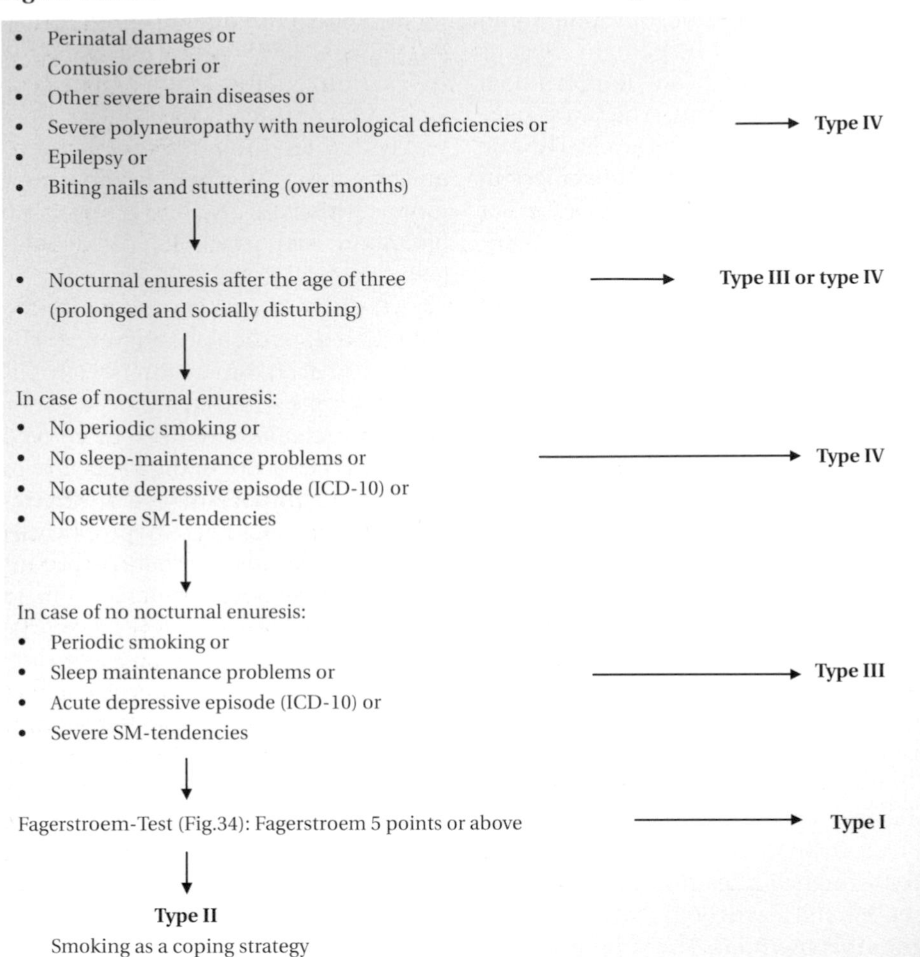
• Perinatal damages or
• Contusio cerebri or
• Other severe brain diseases or
• Severe polyneuropathy with neurological deficiencies or
• Epilepsy or
• Biting nails and stuttering (over months)
Type IV
• Nocturnal enuresis after the age of three
• (prolonged and socially disturbing)
Type III or type IV
In case of nocturnal enuresis:
• No periodic smoking or
• No sleep-maintenance problems or
• No acute depressive episode (ICD-10) or
• No severe SM-tendencies
Type IV
In case of no nocturnal enuresis:
• Periodic smoking or
• Sleep maintenance problems or
• Acute depressive episode (ICD-10) or
• Severe SM-tendencies
Type III
Fagerstroem-Test (Fig.34): Fagerstroem 5 points or above
Type I
Type II
Smoking as a coping strategy

are only few therapy studies on subgroups. Nevertheless, we would like to introduce a therapeutic scheme for subgroups, which should be examined by research in the future. Today we know that there are four dimensions of craving additional to the four clusters of tobacco dependence (Lesch OM et al. 2004).

1. Smoking to increase relaxation and well-being
2. Smoking to cope with situations (smoking as a coping mechanism)
3. Smoking to better cope with stress
4. Smoking to elevate mood

These different types of craving have different biological mechanisms and it is widely known that men tend to smoke for relaxation, due to boredom or to increase well-being, whereas women tend to smoke in order to control weight and to elevate their mood.

9.6.8.3 Pharmacotherapy in relapse prevention in tobacco dependence, according to subgroups

9.6.8.3.1 Relapse prevention of cluster I

This subgroup of tobacco dependents has a Fagerstroem score of ≥ 5 points, but there is no prevalence of psychiatric co-morbidities, premature cerebral damage, behavioural disorders and no other symptoms, which demand a classification to subgroups III or IV.

Pharmaceutical relapse prophylaxis

The effectiveness of nicotine supplements has been proven, but there is no scientific data on duration and dosage in long-term administration. In case of relapse, it is essential to begin a nicotine supplement therapy as in withdrawal therapy (nicotine patches, nicotine gum, inhaler, sublingual tablet). Varenicline could be a useful additional drug for withdrawal therapy, and also for relapse prophylaxis.

To which extent dopamine agonists or MAO-A antagonists play are role in this group has not been investigated yet, but in theory these substances should have a positive influence on smoking behaviour (e.g. moclobemide).

Long-term changes in the glutamate-taurine quotient are expected, which suggests using NMDA antagonists for relapse prophylaxis. Acamprosate and neramexane are being discussed in line with this indication.

Combining these medications could be effective, but has not yet been scientifically investigated.

9.6.8.3.2 Relapse prevention of cluster II

This subgroup of tobacco dependent patients smokes Fagerstroem-negative (Fagerstroem-score ≤ 4 points). There are no signs of psychiatric co-morbidity, no premature cerebral damages, no behavioural disorder and no symptoms that suggest a classification to subgroup III and IV.

Pharmaceutical relapse prevention

To which extent dopamine agonists or MAO-A antagonists play a role in this group has not been documented by research, but in theory these substances should have a positive effect on smoking behaviour.

Long-term changes in the glutamate-taurine quotient are also to be expected, suggesting the use of NMDA antagonists in relapse prevention. Acamprosate and neramexane are being discussed in line with this indication. Anti-depressants (e.g. Bupropion, nortriptyline, doxepine, moclobemide) are likely to be effective in this group.

Combinations of these medicaments might be effective, but this has not yet been supported by research.

9.6.8.3.3 Relapse prevention of cluster III

Symptoms of subgroup IV must be absent. Long-term enuresis nocturna, which significantly influences the development of the adolescent, is no reason for exclusion, if a psychiatric co-morbidity, usually with a major depressive disorder or suicidal tendency has been recorded in the case history. Often an association between the severity of symptoms and smoking behaviour in recurrent psychiatric disorders has been documented (e.g. heavy smoking during severe depressive phases). These patients have often high, but sometimes also low, Fagerstroem scores.

Pharmacological relapse prevention

The dose of psychotropic drugs needs

to be adjusted in the smoke-free phase (anti-depressants, see also group II). Bupropion is the first choice in this group, but nortryptiline is still a possible option in this subgroup.

Nicotine supplements have been shown to be effective in the Fagerstroem group with ≥ 5 points, but there is no data on duration and dosage for long-term administration of these supplements. In case of a relapse a nicotine supplement therapy should be started immediately, as is the case in withdrawal therapy (nicotine patches, nicotine gum, inhaler, sublingual tablet).

As there are usually more women in this group, who tend to smoke for weight control, CB1 antagonists like rimonabant might be suitable, but need clearly a combination with antidepressants.

9.6.8.3.4 Relapse prevention of cluster IV

Infantile cerebral impairments, somatic diseases and/or infantile behavioural disorders lead to considerable developmental disorders. Often, smoking is an additional complicating factor. Critical thinking about one's own health behaviour is reduced in several domains. Smoking is only one of these phenomena. In addition, temporary severe alcohol abuse has often been observed in this group. Primarily, individuals of this group tend to be intellectually impaired and are easily influenced by their peer group. Secondary problems are social difficulties, reactive depressive episodes and more than 70% of these patients have a Fagerstroem score of ≥ 5 points.

Pharmacological relapse prevention

In this group, nicotine supplements need to be administered over a long period of time. Atypical neuroleptics, or topiramate, other antiepileptics and NMDA antagonists are likely to improve impulse control. Scientific data for this group is missing however. Varenicline might be effective in improving the patient's condition, especially if nicotine supplements turn out to be ineffective. If these patients also abuse alcohol a combination with naltrexone is a good option.

9.6.8.4 Medication of tobacco dependent patients in special situations

9.6.8.4.1 Nicotine consumption in combination with other dependences and/or psychiatric disorders

This subgroup of tobacco dependent patients smokes in addition to a secondary dependence or in order to reduce symptoms of other psychiatric disorders.

Tobacco dependence in combination with alcohol dependence

Therapeutic procedure should be in line with the recommendations of Lesch's typology of alcohol dependents. Type I alcohol dependents, who have stopped drinking, but who consume exorbitant amounts of tobacco, still have a shortened life expectancy, just as if they were still drinking. Also the prognosis of alcohol dependence is better if tobacco dependence is treated at the same time. Effective control of nicotine supplement therapy and smoking reduction is done by measuring nicotine and cotinine in urine or by measuring carbon monoxide satiation.

Tobacco dependence in schizophrenia

If a schizophrenic patient is tobacco

dependent, it should be borne in mind that not only do high doses of nicotine reduce the level of neuroleptics in the blood, but also that the schizophrenic patient often experiences the sedating effects of nicotine positively, as it lowers extrapyramidal symptoms (e. g. akatisia). However, direct dopaminergic effects of nicotine aggravate schizophrenic symptoms. In individual cases, we were able to show that a reduction of nicotine consumption leads to an improvement in psychopathological symptoms. Principally, it is suggested that dose adjustments of neuroleptics be considered in this group of patients.

Tobacco dependence in affective disorders

Especially in the case of manic disorders, the same rules as for schizophrenia apply. Yet there is no scientific research on this topic. However, from experience, the onset of a manic and/or depressive episode is often marked by excessive smoking, and sometimes by increased alcohol consumption (as a sign of the incipient increase of energy and unrest). As the first signs of an episode of illness episode set in, some patients have reported a clearly increased craving for nicotine.

9.6.8.4.2 Tobacco dependence and pregnancy

The embryo is extremely sensitive to tobacco abuse during the first three months of pregnancy, but also later on. Impaired circulation of the placenta and a low birth weight of the child are only a few consequences worth mentioning. Changes in tobacco dosage seem to severely damage the growing embryo. It is important to reduce tobacco consumption especially during pregnancy, in which case the use of nicotine supplements at least enables the avoidance of other tobacco ingredients.

This medical-psychiatric presentation of tobacco and alcohol dependence has put particular emphasis on axis I to III to DSM-IV. The following chapter describes the treatment of alcohol dependents from a socio-pedagogical perspective. Mr. Christian Wetschka has delivered excellent scientific data from supporting (homeless projects) and motivating dependents to take an active part in life (theatre projects) and incorporating social institutions into therapy. Every psychiatric diagnosis stands in the context of sociology, psychology and biology and it is our aim to provide sufficient space in this book for a sociological perspective.

10

Sociotherapy of alcohol-and tobacco dependents with regards to Lesch's typology

Written by Christian Wetschka

10.1 Alcohol and Tobacco

Studies have repeatedly supported the assumption of general practitioners that alcohol and tobacco occur together in psychosocial practice.

In "sociotherapy", alcohol dependence is of prior importance, especially because it interferes with re-attaining the ability to regulate oneself and thus complicates any attempts towards stable social integration. Tobacco dependence is often a complicating factor additional to alcohol dependence, with relapses in both forms of dependences being influenced by social stimuli.

As we shall discuss in the section on sociogenesis, there is a correlation between socio-economic status and the development of dependence. Poverty, social stigmatisation (affiliation with a marginal group) and social isolation are important factors that determine the development of somatic and psychological disorders. The concomitant occurrence of alcohol and tobacco dependence increases the risk for sequelae, like dental damage, obesity, malnutrition or cardiovascular diseases.

A factor in tobacco dependence of socially disadvantaged individuals, which should not be underestimated, is that a disproportional amount of income (often up to 50%) is spent onr buying cigarettes, which often leads to further debt. This factor can negatively influence self-preservation and social integration, for example, if the participation in certain leisure activities with others is not possible for financial reasons. Further limitations in socialising activities concern the increasing number of bans on smoking in pubs, agencies, hospitals and public transport, which means that e.g. individuals might chose to miss out on an excursion, or a visit to a theatre, rather than not be able to smoke for two hours in a train/in the theatre.

There are established models and institutions for the support of alcohol dependents in socially precarious conditions (e.g. homeless) which concentrate on alcohol dependence, while nicotine dependence often remains unconsidered. To some extent, there is resignation towards smoking. Models which contribute towards the reduction of tobacco dependence in underprivileged groups, are needed.

10.2 The sociotherapeutic[1] mission

Before we can address dependence-specific interventions with regards to subgroups, the following section will first describe and define the nature of "sociotherapy", in particular because it is distinct from the related disciplines of social work, social pedagogy and psychotherapy. In comparison to these fields, "sociotherapy" puts more emphasis on a mutual and active shaping of the social environment. On the other hand, it is undisputed that all these forms of intervention overlap and represent variations of "networking processes".

As social aspects are of great importance for the development of every dependence, socio therapeutic interventions for people with addictions, especially for those in socio-economically poor conditions, are pivotal.

Herrmann Spaeth, a psychiatric patient, talking about his experiences in the "therapeutic chain":

"To me, aftercare is a gloomy issue ... In a sense the symbol of the topic is the desk. Room numbers, agencies, desks and the particular kind of people who sit behind their desks, control the scenario ... What remains? An act, a sad act unfortunately, a person that is taking notes, who is playing a sad role in this act. The worst of this scenario is this emptiness, this hollowness, this absolute soullessness ... rehabilitation merely means that either you turn into something useful, that is integrated, or you are segregated, which means you become a hopeless case ...

Each one of these "human object gawkers" knows best what he (the affected) is lacking, what he needs, where he belongs etc. and therefore, after a while, you don't really know who you are anymore ... the aftercare consists of a number of activities. Here every affected person asks himeself about the purpose of these institutions and to which extent they are able to genuinely help ...

The affected person feels that no institution or any group is a real community, everything is imposed due to the disease, and this helps lay groups or other groups to exist only because of the disease, you have to be psychologically ill in order to belong to the group. Therefore the disease is the only value the community has, and that's it. The individual history of the affected becomes unimportant due to these conditions, one must adapt to the ill community ... Like in industry, this ill community consists of sub-branches, information centres, workshops for the handicapped (sheltered workshops) and residential care facilities, this industry is then called psychiatric aftercare ...

His despair is the hunger for normality ..."
(Hermann Spaeth, cited by Keupp and Rerrich 1982).

1 The terms sociotherapy and social therapy are used synonymous in relevant literature. In America, the term "multi-systemic therapy" is also used in certain contexts.

This critique by an affected person explains the primary essence of sociotherapy: the overcoming of contexts that are determined by the disease, which, confine patients to their patient role, a role which often continues to define them far beyond their period of psychiatric admission, in the striving towards "normality".

At the same time, for the alcohol and tobacco dependent, the pursuit of "normality" is a social contradiction, because society perceives alcohol and tobacco consumption as "normal" and not as "abnormal/pathological". Children and adolescents adopt the behaviour that their parents and/or peers exhibit as "normal". Growing up continues to be linked with the right to determine for oneself one's contact with psychoactive substances. Therapy must support a dissociation with these patterns of socialisation, or, in other words: the affected needs to redefine "normalisation".

The term sociotherapy has been increasingly differentiated, apart from earlier singular attempts (for example in Elias Salomon, cited by Haag 1976), in the decades since World War II. Like psychotherapy, it can be viewed as a counter strategy against the *objectification* or *alienation of the self*, as well as an attempt, within the context of certain institutions and measures, to safeguard or rather reclaim human subjectivity (self-determination, experimental ability, access to, and utilisation of, resources).

This became more apparent after the two world wars, during which humans were used as "cannon fodder" or/and turned into victims of ideological and political manipulation. In 1947, Viktor von Weizsaecker picked up the term "sociotherapy" again, which he describes as a "method of modern psychotherapy" that seeks to influence and change the "social environment" in order to help the psychologically ill, especially if psychotherapy is not possible. This is a highly problematic definition, above all because it defines sociotherapy as going beyond actual psychotherapy (Schwendter 2000). In the sixties of the 20th century, the psychiatric attribution processes made via diagnostics and psychiatric institutions were subjected to international criticism (Basaglia, Szasz, Laing, Foucault…). At the same time (during late 60s and early 70s), a number of terms in regard to sociotherapy were developed, in which the distinction between sociotherapy and related methods, such as psychotherapy, social work and social pedagogy, was a recurrent theme (Baer 1991/2005). It must be emphasized that sociotherapy is *more* than just the further development of social work and social pedagogy; rather, it is an independent discipline (in theory at least). In the meantime, specific educational curricula for sociotherapists have been introduced, we can now speak of a convergence of concepts which allows for a stable definition. On the other hand, it should be noted, that, in its role as a *mediator*, sociotherapy is (and needs to be) "caught between two stools", those of the disease-oriented realities of psychiatry and "normality". Doerner and Plog state: "Sociotherapy seems to be much too general for it to be defined from the perspective of only one occupation. Arguably, it can be said that the purpose of sociotherapy is to point to the generalized handling of rules and norms, responsibilities and liberties, individuality… and social issues" (Doerner et al. 2002, p. 553).

As an example of this aspiration towards a convergence of concepts, we will cite two definitions. The first one is by Rolf Schwendter, whose "Introduction to Social Therapy" (2000) still belongs to the standards works, and the second by Hilarion Petzold, founder of integrative therapy and an important theorist in sociotherapy. Both strive to highlight the autonomy of sociotherapy in comparison to other phenomena in the psychosocial support continuum, not least because these definitional clarifications pin down specific education curricula (Gesamthochschule Kassel, Fritz-Perls-Institute Duesseldorf).

Rolf Schwendter:

"Social therapy is perceived as an integrating concept of action which connects social, psychological and therapeutic interventions respectively. (...) Socialtherapy can be understood as an interdisciplinary approach which seeks to develop the ability to reflect and act. Social therapy is a special form of perceptual diagnosis, treatment and exploration of the psychosocial distress of the individual, families and groups. The term social therapy implies that the suffering individual is not separate from the social situation which has caused the problems, but that therapeutic approaches (via a double perspective) address both social and psychological conflicts. Social therapy is directed at the misery of socially disadvantaged population groups, who are usually neglected by conventional, predominantly individual therapeutic approaches" (Schwendter 2000, p.8).

Alongside the call for interdisciplinary "diagnoses" and treatments", *an orientation* towards the social field is emphasized, implying that sociotherapy acts in the everyday life of the affected, by integrating those relationships which occur naturally in his life. The final aspect of the definition is of no minor importance: the specific attention given to *disadvantaged* population groups, often marginal groups, who don't have the option of treatment. This points to the sociotherapy's mandate to criticise institutions and society.

Hilarion Petzold:

"Sociotherapy and psychosocial counselling can be described as theory-driven, planned work with people in social systems which maintains an awareness of the influence of such systems and contexts at a micro and meso level, by using methods of intervention that structure these problem situations. The aim of this is to strengthen social competencies and performances of individual groups so that they can better cope with their personal and social life. Sociotherapy also encourages the shaping of one's own life as well as mutually co-operative behaviour and social creativity. In this way, it is possible to change institutions and social domains and to motivate people living and working in these social areas towards an engagement in personal issues, psychosocial health and a humane quality of life. In order to reach these goals, a broad, multi-theoretical model of psychosocial interventions is needed, in which differently tested methodological counselling and

therapeutic approaches are integrated" (Petzold 2003, p. 927).

For Petzold, whose definition is based not least on practical work with marginal groups migrant workers and elderly people, the goal of sociotherapy is to change and shape the social environment by promoting behaviour which expresses solidarity, and by valuing the quality of life. Sociotherapy is not responsible for changing only individuals, but also *institutions*.

Furthermore, *interdisciplinariness* ("multi-theoretically based model of psychosocial intervention") is an essential part of sociotherapy. The equation of psychosocial counselling and sociotherapy is of no lesser importance. Petzold underlines the possibility of sociotherapy for the socially disadvantaged, such as those "difficult" individuals (e. g. psychotic, drug-addicted and borderline patients), who only profit from psychotherapy under specific conditions, provided that they want to engage in such an extensive process and are able to persevere with it over a long period of time – a phenomenon which we will encounter again in the typology of alcoholism and in discussing its consequences for therapy.

The sociotherapist needs to work at psychosocial hotspots (troubled neighbourhoods), where the interventional repertoire of social work and psychotherapy is not able to offer help, not least because of discrimination, and where the social environment needs to be changed to the advantage of those affected. Psychosocial hotspots can however be (total) institutions which are anti-psychotherapy in character and in which psychotherapy comes up against institutional boundaries (prison, compulsory psychiatric treatment, residential homes, approved schools and the like). With the mandate of reestablishing "normality", sociotherapy becomes the manager of the friction which exists between different realities, which obstructs the development of the personal potential of those affected. As a mediator between what are at times extremely different perspectives, sociotherapy is "trans-disciplinary" in essence.

Form a historical and practical perspective, sociotherapy has originated from a "grey area" between social work and psychotherapy. In addition, other required competencies and skills stem from the know-how and experience of pedagogy, art therapy, sociology and social psychiatry.

The *occupational profile* of the socio-therapist has been confined to diverse educational contexts (e. g. as an additional qualification for social workers or psychotherapists), however the professionalization of sociotherapeutic work which has to date taken place, is only a variation of the same thing. In practice, large numbers of sociotherapeutic interventions are carried out by persons who are directly involved in the individual's everyday life. These are of course social workers, psychotherapists and social pedagogues, but in many cases, and presumably to a much greater extent, they also consist of family members, friends, nursing staff, home helps, creative, leisure, and self-help groups, who don't have any sociotherapeutic awareness or self-concept. Clearly this is related to the grass-rootedness of sociotherapy. Its goals are to normalise the organisation of everyday life, where it is most effective, i.e. in the everyday life of the affected. Due to this fact, there is probably no other domain which is as open to individuals working on an honorary basis (or as "volunteers") and who already, by dint of their life circumstances, embody and communicate "normality". In addition, they are rarely completely identified with institutions, as is inevitably the case with professional staff.

> **Example:**
> In a flat-share for type IV alcohol dependents in Vienna, we have deliberately not employed specialised staff and have thereby done without all associated "rituals of social administration" which might provoke a feeling of social difference. It was more important that a network of honorary workers was in regular contact with residents (e.g. at weekly game evenings, helping to clean up the room, in leisure activities etc.).

In this context, Rolf Schwendter highlights the integration of affected individuals who have undergone similar experiences and can assist people with comparable problems, for example the ex-abuser in drug (socio)therapy, the ex-homeless, the ex-alcoholic (the self-help group scene springs to mind, in particular, in this connection) etc. Not integrating the wealth of experiences of "laypersons" who, especially by dint of their non-professionalism, are able to introduce alternative perspectives, would be going against the grain of sociotherapy. Schwendter: "Helping laypersons are able to contribute qualifications, points of views, sociotherapeutic experience, in short, 'educational elements' into sociotherapeutic work, which often seem to be neglected by professionals, who are blinded by routine" (Schwendter 2000, p.280)

> **Example:**
> Peter H., 56 years old, was living in a sociotherapeutic home for alcohol dependents for two years until he was able to move to a council flat. As Peter is a social person, it was a challenge for him to live by himself in a flat. After a relapse, he increasingly sought contact with people from his old home. Then he found out that his former roommate was in hospital with cancer. During the following period, he visited his colleague three to four times a week and was virtually in charge of the patient. The staff of the hospital was very grateful because they did not have enough time and energy resources themselves for these demanding patient visits. As all parties concerned experienced Peter H.'s visits as very positive, the team decided to ask Peter H. to visit patients in the hospital more often.

Fig. 100 Interdisciplinary dimensions of sociotherapy

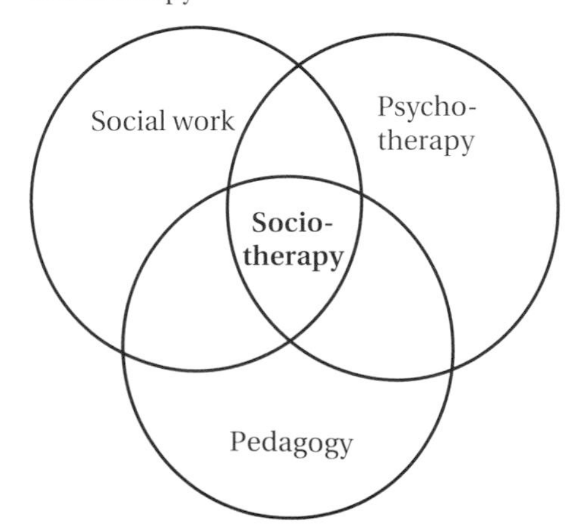

The relationship of sociotherapy and unprofessional support staff needs to be discursive, which means that it works in a complementary and respectful way. Therefore, approaches that link sociotherapeutic action only to certain educational backgrounds, or try to classify it into a hierarchical system (e.g. as being above social work and social pedagogy, but below psychotherapy and psychiatry), need to be viewed critically.

The "hunger for normality" (Spaeth) is probably most intense where the alienation of subjects through institutions is most apparent. As this issue is linked to the need for increased self-determination, sociotherapy continues with its major project of education/ empowerment. Of course, the call for "empowerment" (Stark 1996). has almost become a platitude and, as is always the case with such fundamental dimensions in pedagogical contexts, this call often remains unheard, frequently due to the physical restrictions of the institutions. This is especially the case for "total institutions", in which compulsory therapy always holds a precarious position, but also for relatively "normal institutions", like transitional or permanent homes, which impose different restrictions natures (rules of the house, counselling agreement, obligation to attend group sessions and more). Sociotherapy needs to be aware of tensions and precarious power relationships and needs to counteract them when they obstruct the development of personal potential.

10.3 Classification Psychotherapy-Sociotherapy

In psychosocial practice, such as in psychiatric institutions, it is easy for tensions between psychotherapeutic and sociotherapeutic procedures to arise (e.g. in care or social work), especially if all interactions are interpreted from a "psychotherapeutic" perspective and if there is little room provided for "normality".

Example

"Imagine a situation, in which patients are only perceived from a psychoanalytical, behavioural therapeutic or client centred perspective. In every meeting, the psychotherapist acts according to his therapeutic approach and perceptions: he verbalises the patient's feelings, attends to transference aspects only and hesitates before he acts on the basis that any instantaneous action could reinforce the patient's avoidance behaviour. The therapist is not interested in the rules that the nurses use for regulating cohabitation in the ward, as he is only interested in implementing psychotherapy." (Doerner et al. 2002, p. 555).

In addition Doerner and Plog allegorize in their critical textbook:

"Sociotherapy is the basis! It can't be positioned as just one of many techniques. In fact, it makes the application of other techniques possible. From this perspective, we conclude that the nursing staff (e.g. because of their constant presence) are in charge of sociotherapy more than anyone else." (Doerner et al. 2002, p. 556).

Fig. 101 Differentiation Sociotherapy – Psychotherapy

Sociotherapy	Psychotherapy/Withdrawal
100% dependents	100% dependents
Dependents with severe physical and psychological sequelae (high proportion of co-morbidities)	Dependents without severe physical and psychological sequelae
Organic brain impairment	Neuropsychological deficits of rather subclinical nature
Social disintegration with often disastrous outcomes	To some degree socially integrated

Fig. 102 Classification sociotherapy – psychotherapy

Sociotherapy	Psychotherapy
Low admission threshold, little motivation requirements, "disease acceptance", ability to introspect and verbalise	High threshold, high motivation requirements, "disease acceptance", ability to cooperate and introspect

Sociotherapy supports normal, "non-pathological", healthy aspects of the patient (Doerner et al. 2002, p.556) and, in this respect, complements medical and psychotherapeutic care, from which, however, it fundamentally and/or partially differs. Affected persons are those who become permanently or temporarily limited in organizing everyday life, which in many cases, often goes hand in hand with deficient or instable ego structures. In line with this, there is a difference between sociotherapy and psychotherapy on a methodological level, e.g. in the handling of transference symptoms. Psychotherapy aims at "changing the basic patterns" of personality and in this, the addressing of transference phenomena is standard. Transferences also emerge in sociotherapeutic contexts but they are not actively addressed. That is, transference is recognized and in some circumstances also defined, but never applied by sociotherapists (Walter 2004). In this light, psychotherapy is more biography-oriented, while sociotherapy concentrates on what is at hand, thus being more experience, practice and theme focussed (Baer 1991/2005).

Often characteristics of sociotherapy are influenced by clients' and patients' **personality traits**. Usually patients are considerably impaired in organising and structuring their life. Contrary to psychotherapy patients, **organic brain damages and somatic and psychological sequelae** prevail and patients are often **socially disintegrated**. In some cases, inner structures ("self-regulation") that are needed for leading a self-reliant life have to be established and secured ("formation of structure"). Steingass[2] (2001) compared patients of in-patient psychotherapeutic and sociotherapeutic institutions, a differentiation that needs to be modi-

2 Steingass is the director of a sociotherapeutic home for alcohol dependents in Remscheid.

fied for outpatient services and sheltered housing (for example aftercare, residential homes). This striking dichotomisation of a factual overlapping of both disciplines is rarely observed this clearly in practice, but the divergences are nevertheless apparent when compared.

Clients who receive sociotherapeutic support are often extremely socially disintegrated. There is no contact to family members, relationships are broken and socio-demographic variables suggest low educational background, no school leaving certificates and unemployment. This is also represented by **different admission criteria for various kinds of therapy**. In extreme cases, street work can be interpreted as a sociotherapeutic activity because this is where support is provided or planned.

Bosch (Expert committee in sociotherapy of the AHG scientific council 2000, S. 111–124) defines sociotherapy as inversely related to psychotherapy. While psychotherapy can afford to have its own attitude, which is useful for therapeutic processes but detached from reality, even "escapist", in order to test, experience or discover something that is otherwise unthinkable, sociotherapy works "in touch with reality" and tries to activate healthy aspects of the affected[3].

"Pathological aspects are neither repressed, nor particularly emphasised. While dynamics of relationships are predominant in group psychotherapy, sociotherapeutic group work is generally issue related. Here is where learning and practicing to cope with emotional tensions without using old pathological patterns should take place. If the patient is too reserved or inhibited to express himself or take part in activities, the sociotherapist should not focus on interpreting the patient's behaviour. Instead, the therapist should attempt to motivate the patient towards participation and activity by using available potential and resources. The crucial point is not the elaboration of pathological behaviour, but the encouragement of self-worth, by increasing and stabilising experiences, successfully completing assigned (small) tasks or the mastering of difficulties, and coping with specific moods or situations." (Bosch)

Sociotherapy can support psychotherapeutic work, and in some cases even be substitutive, especially if psychotherapeutic work is not possible or not efficient. Sociotherapeutic approaches emphasize self-awareness in confronting the objective and social environment and the mastering of self-chosen aims and tasks. The scope and specific aims of sociotherapy always depend on the client's abilities and deficits. In regard to clients with severe psychological impairments, this can only be done in gradual steps and within a structured framework. The aim of the sociotherapeutic process is the expansion of autonomy in the client's personality and life with particular emphasis on learning how to cope with everyday life. More important than "personality development" or "self-effectuation", apart from staying abstinent, is that clients are able to find their way around their

3 A finding that has also been documented by Doerner and Plog in their textbook (Doerner and Plog 2002).

Fig. 103 Classification Sociotherapy – Psychotherapy

Sociotherapy	Psychotherapy
Pragmatism and Eclecticisms in the selection of methods	Often purism in the selection of methods (depth psychology, behavioural therapy)
Pedagogical, psycho-educative	Psychotherapeutic method repertoire
Active and directive interventions, "Assisting", participating, sharing	Abstinence, neutrality, professional distance, demanding
Behaviour oriented	Verbal orientation
Focus on problem solving and coping	Focus on the therapy of pathologic, abnormal or deviant aspects
Focus on normal, everyday training of life skills	Creation of artificial "as if" situations
Everyday language	Artificial language ("Feedback"...)
Stable, clear transparent and obligatory daily structure	
Neuropsychological methods, everyday life related brain training	Usually no neuropsychological measures

neighbourhood, e. g. being able to go to the supermarket and to maintain a certain level of hygiene. While psychotherapy seeks "individuation", sociotherapy aims at "socialisation".

Example:
Mr E. has moved to a partially supported living community within the residential care home after the nursing staff has advised him to do so. He lives there together with four other alcohol dependents. Due to his experience in prison (for years), hospitalisation in a home and alcohol-related degradation process, he is overburdened by many everyday tasks. The first issue is self-support; although he used to be a baker, Mr. E. has no clue about cooking. It took a lot for the flatmates to show Mr E. how to open tin cans again and heat them up in the microwave. In doing this, they have to put up with Mr E.'s despondence and resistance towards behavioural change and often have to cheer him up. An honorary employee takes responsibility for accompanying Mr E. to the nearest supermarket and helps him to buy groceries which he can use for preparing a meal. After a few months Mr E. is capable of cooking for his flatmates.

The complementary relationship of sociotherapy and psychotherapy is reflected by sociotherapeutic methods which are based on the everyday needs of the clients/patients. These methods occasionally compensate deficits in a "palpable" fashion:

Sociotherapy is everyday life-oriented and less reflecting than psychotherapy. It's a learning process that takes place through helping, demonstrating, participating, instructing, showing, exemplifying "normal behaviours", but also through control. This usually concerns the skills needed for everyday life, like shopping, cooking, washing, ironing, cleaning, gardening, personal hygiene, handling of money, recreational activities, celebrating etc.

Rolf Schwendter's term, "therapy of the poor" (Schwendter 2000, p. 255), characterises an interesting grey area for sociotherapy, which is underrated, let alone noticed, in the age of professionalization, job-specific classifications and demonstrations of self-esteem.

The "therapy of the poor" represents a therapeutic domain, in which professional resources aren't effective or accepted by clients, despite their need for support. Therapeutic relationships to professional or layman helpers are often formed and this is where helpful therapeutic processes take place. The helper temporarily turns into a "helping-self", strengthens or weakens certain attitudes, projections and transferences in everyday contact are questioned and loosened and new interpretations of the social context are virtually formed "along the way". "Therapy of the poor" implies that psychotherapy can also take place aside from the classic (paid, regulated, professional) context, namely in everyday life and in "normal" relationships, namely, where "psychotherapy" has taken place for hundreds and thousands of years. Psychotherapists are not solely responsible for the application of "therapeutic methods" anymore, but methods have been incorporated with different non-therapeutic forms of interventions (supervision, mediation, life and social counselling, theme-centred interaction, self-help-conversational groups, sociometry, role playing and art therapy etc.), and this is also the case for sociotherapeutic work.

Unfortunately, laymen assistance is repeatedly usurped by professional therapy instead of being seen as something that interconnects with, and supports, it.

Example:
Mrs D. lives in a residential facility for women. In the in-house cafeteria, she meets an honorary member of staff, Mr D., a teacher of religion, who is usually accompanied by his wife, on duty in the cafeteria every Saturday. At times, the women sit together and play "Ludo". Mr D. enjoys playing with them. On a quite night, when the cafeteria was almost empty, Mrs D. uses the opportunity to tell Mr D. her life story. After several unsuccessful and hurtful relationships, Mrs D. has developed a defensive attitude towards all men in general. Some weeks later Mr D. invited Mrs D. to a family trip, an invitation which Mrs D. accepts with mixed feelings. It was a positive experience. Due to the positive contact to Mr D., Mrs D. manages to put her disappointment with men into perspective.

10.4 Sociogenesis and sociotherapeutic chances

10.4.1 Primary, secondary and tertiary sociogenesis

The preferred "subjects for therapeutic treatment" in sociotherapy are those medical conditions that are to a high degree socially determined. Strotzka (1971) differentiates primary, secondary and tertiary sociogenesis. Primary sociogenesis are diseases that are directly caused by social circumstances (which does not imply the absence of other factors); secondary sociogenesis implies the indirect influence of social factors on dependence genesis in the sense that "organic causes in themselves are again causes for the social condition". By tertiary sociogenesis, Strotzka understands the influence of the social environment on the progression and manifestation of psychological disorders. All forms of sociogenesis apply differently to the genesis of dependences. The typology according to Lesch also attempts to focus more precisely on the extent of the impact of social conditions in comparison to other factors. The sociogenesis in type I dependents can be described as secondary and tertiary due to biological/genetic factors (biological vulnerability and high social responsiveness, e. g. social drink catalysts), while socio-genetic conditions in type IV dependents suggest a primary sociogenesis (infantile deprivation/deprivation in early childhood).

With regards to practice, the question concerning the extent to which sociogenesis is significant for diagnostics and therapy, always raises itself. It needs to be borne in mind that, within the current diagnostic paradigm, a primary sociogenesis cannot be diagnosed as the health and/or pension insurance companies only authorizes a restricted code of medical indications, in regards to ICD-10. While "recognized neuroses" like depression, anxiety and obsessive-compulsive disorders are permitted psychotherapeutic treatment, it is very difficult for socially disadvantaged groups, who predominantly suffer from disorders that have social causes (e. g. acute psychosomatic disorders due to stress, psychological problems due to long-term unemployment, broken relationships, poverty etc.), to receive adequate treatment. Diagnostic criteria (Petzold 2003) for some of these "social disorders" don't even exist, implying that there is no prospect of health insurance funds assuming the costs.

Apart from the lack of "social disorder" categories, even existing options, like the axes IV and V of DSM-IV, are rarely used. By considering the dimensions listed on these axes, the aetiology and progression of the disorder can be more comprehensively understood, as social aspects and thus the patient's or client's life environment are included. **Axis IV** assesses **psychosocial and environmental problems** (descriptive) and **axis V** assesses **psychosocial functioning** (global assessment of functioning). A scale is available for the latter (Global Assessment of Functioning, GAF). Additional to the psychiatric and medical diagnosis of axis I, II and III, this scale only assesses psychological, social and occupational functioning.

10.4.2 Sociological factors on a macro-level[4]

The findings that sociological causes are underrepresented by addiction research, as stated by Tasseit (1994) a few years ago, are still valid. On the other hand, "the biopsychosocial structure of condition" of dependence, and therefore the significance of social relationships, has clearly been recognized. However, it is the case that research lit-

4 In sociology, social processes are examined on three levels: macro-, meso- and micro level. The macro level includes phenomena of the entire society (e. g. social stratification), the micro level includes phenomena of smaller groups (e. g. families) and individuals, where sociology often overlaps with sociopsychology.

Fig. 104 Global Assessment of Functioning Scale (DSM-IV)

Global Assessment of Functioning Scale (DSM IV)

The Global Assessment of Functioning (GAF) is a numeric scale (0 through 100) used by mental health clinicians and physicians to subjectively rate the social, occupational and psychological functioning of adults on a hypothetical continuum ranging from psychological health to disease. Impairment in functioning, which has physical or environmental causes should not be included.

Code	(Note: Please use according interim values, e. g. 45, 68, 72)
91–100	Superior functioning in a wide range of activities, life's problems never seem to get out of hand, is sought out by others because of his or her many qualities. No symptoms.
81–90	Absent or minimal symptoms, good functioning in all areas, interested and involved in a wide range of activities, socially effective, generally satisfied with life, no more than everyday problems or concerns.
71–80	If symptoms are present they are transient and expectable reactions to psychosocial stresses; no more than slight impairment in social, occupational, or school functioning.
61–70	Some mild symptoms OR some difficulty in social, occupational, or school functioning, but generally functioning pretty well, has some meaningful interpersonal relationships.
51–60	Moderate symptoms OR any moderate difficulty in social, occupational, or school functioning.
41–50	Serious symptoms OR any serious impairment in social, occupational, or school functioning.
31–40	Some impairment in reality testing or communication OR major impairment in several areas, such as work or school, family relations, judgment, thinking, or mood.
21–30	Behavior is considerably influenced by delusions or hallucinations OR serious impairment in communications or judgment OR inability to function in all areas.
11–20	Some danger of hurting self or others OR occasionally fails to maintain minimal personal hygiene OR gross impairment in communication.
1–10	Persistent danger of severely hurting self or others OR persistent inability to maintain minimum personal hygiene OR serious suicidal act with clear expectation of death.
0	Not enough information available to provide GAF.

erature predominantly examines psychological and biomedical factors, whereas sociological factors are mostly neglected. It is recommended that general health-sociologic factors be considered, which are all significant for the development of an addiction, especially because this is where the border between psychotherapy and pharmacology lies, e. g. in relation to socioeconomic status and health. The imbalance and incoherence of different dependence theories and data emphasise that there is still no "integrative theory of dependence" which examines and systematically correlates all facts on dependence development (Schmidt et al. 1999, Renn 1991), despite frequent calls for such a theory.

In the light of globalisation-related social change, which promotes social inequalities (Razum et al. 2006), an awareness of sociological aspects is needed.

Puls (2003) differentiated three sociological perspectives to explain dependence behaviour:

a) the Stress-Coping Paradigm (alcohol modulates the stress reaction, assists in coping with stress)
b) Theories of Socialisation (long-term socialisation processes, e.g. through family, which influence consumption behaviour)
c) Theory of abnormal behaviour (socio-structural conditions or the environment's reaction towards the consumption behaviour).

The stress-coping paradigm can be used on a macro but also micro social level. Brenner's (1975, in German 1979) established time series analysis has already shown a relationship between economic indicators, like inflation rate, unemployment rate, average income, and diverse health indicators, like psychiatric admissions and alcohol consumption. For example, psychiatric hospitalisations of persons with an alcohol psychosis sharply increased during recessions and decreased again during economic growth. Economic stress clearly seems to be an additional stress factor (an argument that has been strongly criticised).

The sociocultural theory of Bales (1991, 1946), who investigates the social conditions of a dependence development, also belongs to the categories mentioned above. He differentiates between **abstinence cultures** (prohibition of any alcohol consumption), **ambivalence cultures** (conflict between values towards alcohol consumption), **permissive cultures** (allowing alcohol in consideration) and **permissive-dysfunctional cultures** (allowing alcohol excesses). Yet, the relationship between social norms, genesis and the progression of a dependence is continuously put into perspective by research. Therefore we know that social factors are very important for the *acquisition* of specific high-risk patterns of consumption, but that this importance decreases with the progression of dependence development (Schmidt et al. 1999).

Social research has shown "socio-economic status" to be the most important social factor for determining the health behaviour and health status of a population (Hurrelmann 2006). This has also been supported by the WHO[5]. The socioeconomic indicator points to the relative position of persons in social structures of privilege and prosperity. Associations between financial resources, level of education, social acceptance, and physical and psychological disorders have been documented. There is a higher prevalence of disorders among lower classes than among upper classes (see table below). Even rich smokers live longer than poor ones.

Social conditions during childhood, adolescence and adulthood also play a role in the dependence aetiology (of subgroups). As co-morbidities play a large role in the aetiology of most dependences, general information about the patient's health are of interest.

Children

Child mortality and disorders are more frequent among children from lower

5 "Even if medical care improves disease progression and life expectancy in some acute diseases, the social and economic conditions, which make people ill and in need of care, are by far more important for the health of the total population". WHO

socioeconomic classes. For example, the frequency of stillbirths in mothers who went to special school is much higher than in other mothers. Also, infant and child mortality rate is extremely high in low status groups.

Children from lower socioeconomic backgrounds, show relatively poor health behaviour. Their nutrition is worse and they exercise less, compared to children that are better off. Also, children from lower classes take part in fewer medical check-ups.

The standard of dental care, and with it dental health, also continuously decreases with class (from upper to lower classes).

Children with parents of lower socioeconomic status are involved in more accidents than others. Kersting-Duerrwaechter and Mielck (2001) found that children from lower class families have a 24 % higher risk of having an accident than preschool children from higher social classes. This also applies to the severity of accidents (lasting damage), an association that is reflected by the aetiology of type IV dependents.

Adolescents

Trends that were displayed in childhood continue in adolescence: socially disadvantaged adolescents are more often ill than those from higher social classes. Children attending general secondary school are more often ill than children attending grammar school. Nutritional behaviour also decreases with socioeconomic status. Consequently, adolescents from the lower classes are more frequently overweight.

There are clear social differences in consumption of psychoactive substances. Girls' smoking behaviour is also influenced by the family's prosperity and the parent's occupational status. Students from general secondary schools smoke three times more than students from grammar schools.

Adults

The disease and mortality rate is higher in the lower classes than in the higher ones. For example, there are more diseases and higher early mortality rates in working class families than in employed, self-employed or civil servant families. Social differences have an impact on health behaviour, such as the utilization of medical care services. Members of lower status populations smoke significantly more often and more heavily and alcohol consumption is clearly higher in men (women show different results) (Lampert and Burger 2004).

Almost two thirds of men, aged 20 to 59, who are in short- and long-term unemployment, smoke, whereas only 40 % of employed men smoke. Men who are unemployed for up to a year, smoke twice as much as employed men. Men, who have been unemployed for more than a year, smoke three times as much (Dauer 1999).

Differences can also be found in eating behaviour, personal hygiene and physical activity. Lower status groups go to the doctor, particularly the specialist, less frequently.

Higher levels of education and a more favourable economical situation influence all age groups, even age-related dementia is more prevalent in lower social classes.

In, Austria the following data has been published in 2007: the population below the poverty level has three times worse health conditions (11 %) than those with a high income (4 %) and is twice as often ill than those on a medium income (7 %). In regard to educational certificates, graduates from general secondary schools are twice as often (20 %) affected by a chronic disease, than A-level graduates (11 %). 90 % of employees with higher or administrative jobs describe their health as "good", whereas only 76 % of labourers feel this way. The rich live between five and seven years longer than the poor (Statistic Austria 2007).

Furthermore, lonely and socially isolated people are more likely to get ill. They lack a network to help and support them. The elderly especially are affected and migrants and homosexuals also represent risk groups. Cardiovascular diseases and dependences are more frequent in those who are socially isolated.

In conclusion, the following can be suggested: poverty and isolation (lack of resources) promotes disorders. People from lower socioeconomic classes (lower income, lower occupational status, lower educational level, long-term unemployment, single parents, families with many children, migrants, homeless people, prisoners) need a greater degree of health care promotion, to balance their social conditions and state of health. Health costs are highest in this population group.

No less important are the serious socio-political and sociological changes in postmodern society, which are es-

Fig. 105 Nicotine consumption and educational status

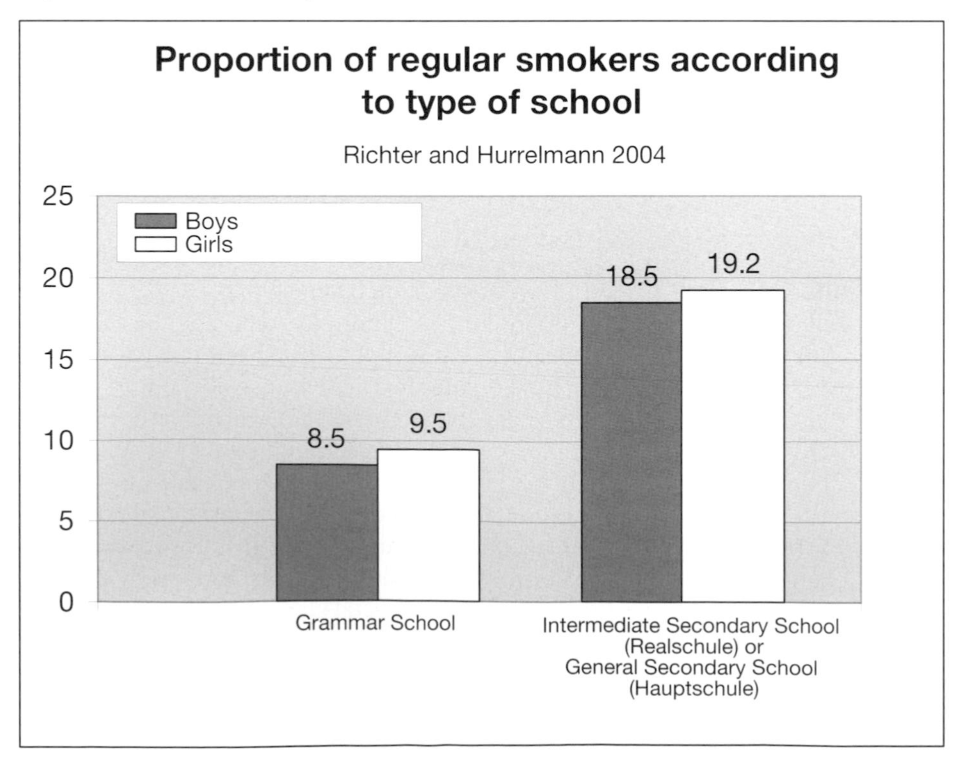

Fig. 106 Health/diseases and socioeconomic diagnoses

Low socioeconomic status	High socioeconomic status
Health behaviour	
– Malnutrition – Poor nutritional rhythm – Lack of exercise – Lack of bodily hygiene – Cigarette consumption – Alcohol abuse in men – Consumption of illegal substances – Violent behaviour – Few medical check-ups – Few early diagnosis check-ups	– Alcohol abuse in women
Diseases	
– Cardiovascular diseases – Diabetes mellitus – Stomach cancer – Bowel cancer – Lung cancer – Kidney-/bladder cancer – Leukemia – Stomach diseases – Teeth diseases – Bronchitis (in adults) – Intervertebral disk degeneration – Overweight/ adipositas – Rheumatism/ gout – Accidents (in children and adolescents) – Mental illness – Multi-morbidity	– Few allergies – Bronchitis (in children) – Few skin diseases, e.g. neurodermitis – Myopia and hypermetropia

Scientific findings in regards to the socioeconomic status, health behaviour and diseases (Hurrelmann 2006

pecially characterised by the dissolving of traditional social networks (Beck 2003), and should be pointed out. The trend towards a single life and the denial of the processes which promote solidarity in society and especially in the cities, make education, the maintenance of a social network and, increasingly, the integration of marginal groups more difficult. The lack of alternative social networks following the termination of withdrawal therapy is one of the biggest problems for the stabilisation of patients with addictions, considering that only a small percentage of patients manage to join artificial social networks (self-help groups, sport clubs, religious communities etc.)

10.4.3 Co-morbidity and marginal group identity

Fichter (2001) carried out an epidemiologic study which examined a homeless population in Munich from a socio-psychiatric perspective by using representative samples (n = 265). Results showed a high degree of co-morbidity (90%) and social deprivation. For example, the extent of social deficits can be illustrated by the predictor "family status".

Fig. 107 Homelessness and marital status

Homeless: marital status: n = 265		Normal population Germany n = 178
53,4 %	single	43,4 %
0,0 %	married	49,7 % (!!!)
6 %	separated	–
3,9 %	widowed	2,5 %
35,1 %	divorced	10,1 %

Fichter 2001

In regard to psychological disorders, substance dependence, especially alcohol dependence, was very prevalent with 72.7 % (vs. 15.2 % in the normal population).

It can't be denied that "social factors" are very significant for the development and progression of a dependence (and other psychological disorders). This pretty much constitutes basic socio-psychiatric knowledge. Within this context, the population group's attitude towards socially accepted norms and values is of importance for sociological discourse. If it is not possible to meet these norms, individual suffers from unbearable pressure, which can only be handled by assuming an anomic attitude, or "apathy" as Merton (Reinhardt 2005) has described it.

The relationship between co-morbidity, alcohol dependence and homelessness is one of the most difficult scenarios to manage when treating groups of multiply and chronically impaired dependents. This can only be handled

Fig. 108 Homelessness and psychiatric diagnoses

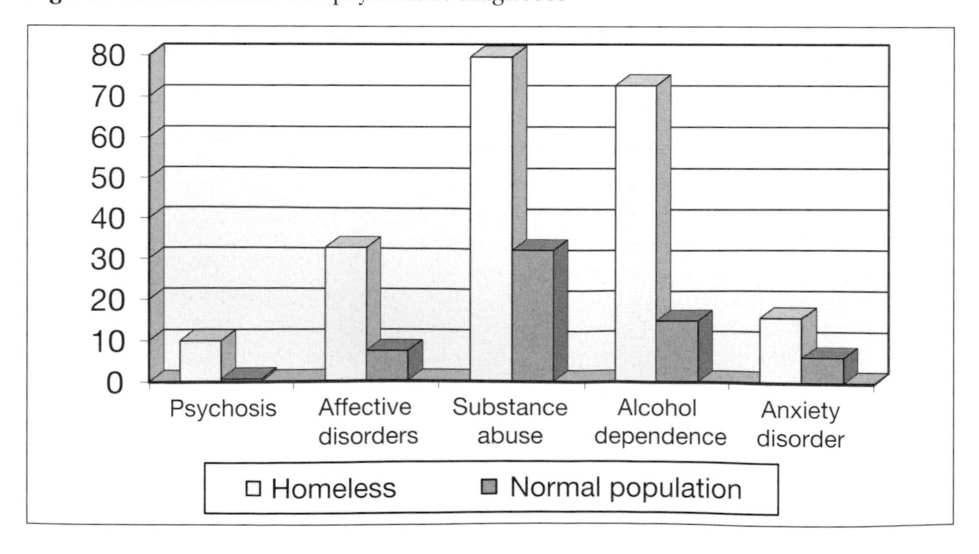

if social work and psychiatry cooperate in an effective way. The threshold of most traditional addiction support institutions, specialised hospitals, counselling centres and self-help groups is too high to provide assistance for homeless clients (Reker and Wehn 2001). In this case, the availability especially of short-term psychiatric help could be very helpful.

10.4.4 The link between social relationships (factors on a social micro level), group coherence and resilience

In line with Coleman (2006), we can indeed speak of a "new science", if one looks at the multitude of data and hypothesis from fifteen years of neuroscientific research. Imaging techniques for exploring brain functioning have been introduced and relationships between social and a number of organic and psychological functions can be demonstrated. These range from the regulation of stress hormones via childhood influences to the regulation of the immune system through the quality of social relationships. Psychosomatic medicine and various psychotherapeutic schools of thought have been making use of this knowledge for some time. Social causes have always been considered in cases of dependence (e. g. examination of family background of alcohol dependents), although they are still undervalued in biologically based models. There is no doubt that the formation of neuronal networks depends on the quality of interpersonal relationships, even to a greater extent than has been supposed. This applies for both children and adolescents, who have high brain plasticity (social control patterns are

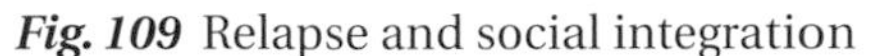
Fig. 109 Relapse and social integration

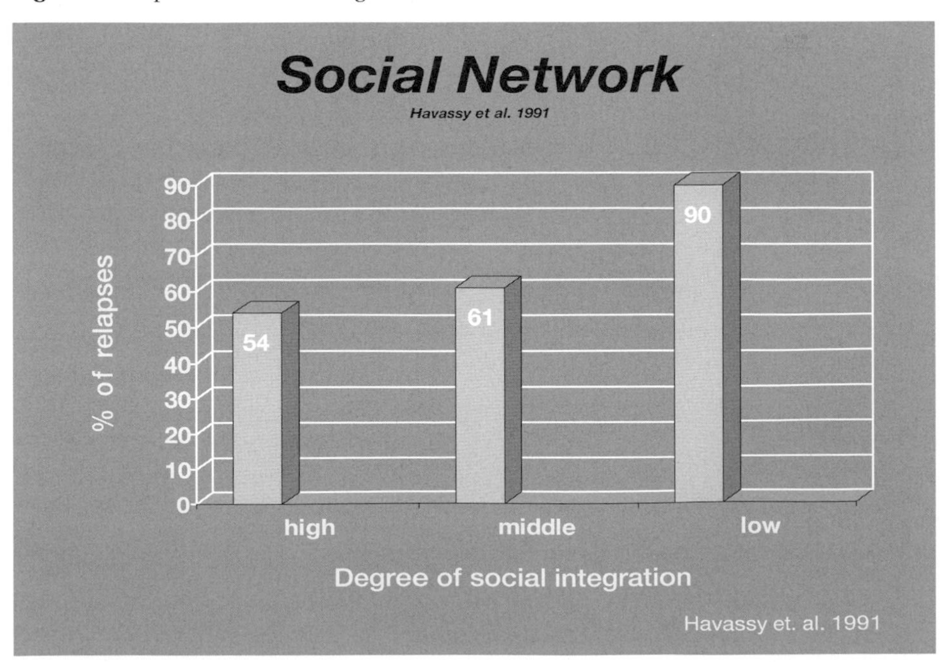

formed up until age 25), but also for all persons beyond the age of 25, in whom neuronal networks are still formed, yet to a lesser extent and at a slower rate.

The importance of social relationships is represented by the therapeutic effectiveness of group experiences. The integration into a stable group is undoubtedly a highly effective therapeutic factor and the goal of group therapy. In his textbook, Yalom (1999) rates "group cohesion" as one of the most important healing factors.

Another eminent finding is the relationship between social integration, utilization of therapy and therapy success. Further, it is uncontested that broken social networks increase the risk for a relapse in dependents (Havassy et al. 1991). Havassy (1991) found that those dependents who relapsed after twelve weeks of therapy, were badly or not at all socially integrated (e. g. living alone, no or few close friend or relatives, no association to groups etc.).

The quality of social relationships, the number of important attachment figures and the extent of social contacts, especially to people that are not linked to institutions, and friends are crucial for the stability of a successful therapy (Roehrle et al. 1998).

Result from neurobiological research supports this by showing that motivation primarily depends on social impulses (see according paragraph in this text) (Bauer 2006, 2007) and that psychological and physical health to a great extent depends on social integration or disintegration. Social interactions and physical activity, for example group activities, have a stress-reducing effect and therefore have a positive effect on psychological and physiological disorders (Unger et al. 1997).

Further support for the healing potential of social relationships and integration comes from resilience research that examined which social and individual factors contribute towards a positive coping with crises (Welter-Enderlin and Hildenbrand 2006). These are:

- growing up in one's own family and a relationship to at least one stable attachment figure (who does not necessarily have to belong to the family),
- the ability and opportunity to express one's feelings
- the integration into a stable, active community (youth group, church community, self-help group, sport club etc)
- a completed professional or school education
- a stable marriage or partnership

The above factors above are, next to individual personality traits like intelligence, interests, positive philosophy of life, flexibility etc., fundamental **long-term factors for protection**[6].

6 Emmy E. Werner's long-term study counts to the fundamental works of resilience research. On the Hawaiian island Kaunai, she observed 698 children, born in 1955, for 40 years. Around 30 % (210 children) grew up in poor conditions: birth complications, stress in the family, parental psychopathologies, divorce. Two thirds of these 210 children developed learning and behaviour problems, turned delinquent or/and mentally ill. Yet, despite these adverse conditions, one third of the children turned into competent, confident and caring adults who successfully completed school and coped well with societal norms. By age 40, none of these persons was unemployed or had problems with the law. Divorce rate, mortality and the number of chronic health problems were average when compared with the normal population. Certain personality traits that were already present in childhood turned out to be resilience factors. These were e. g. certain active behavioural patterns already apparent during babyhood, later, a relationship to at least one stable attachment figure, mostly from within the family, the children's ability to recruit a substitution for parents, integration in groups (e. g.

"Social support" also determines whether resiliencies are being activated or whether new resiliencies can be formed (Mueller and Petzold 2004)[7]. In summary, this implies that a human being is another human being's best medicine. The establishment and cultivation of stable relationships, especially the integration into a collective, has a very high protective and healing potential. This is especially interesting as results from resilience research have suggested that psychotherapy only assists the stabilisation process to a subordinate extent[8].

In his theory of salutogenesis, the Israeli stress researcher, Antonovsky, has outlined a similar perspective: not only pathogenetic factors determine the development and the progression of diseases, but the availability or lack of **resistance resources** in the person. Whether resources are used or not depends on the manifestation of a sense of coherence ("SOC"= sense of coherence).

"The SOC (sense of coherence) is a global orientation that demonstrates to what extent one experiences a pervasive, enduring, but yet dynamic feeling of confidence, that

(1) the stimuli that arise from the internal and external environment throughout life, are predictable and explainable;
(2) resources, to cope with the demands that these stimuli request, are available;
(3) these demands are challenges, which are worth the effort and engagement" (Antonovsky 1997, p. 36).

This sense of coherence is formed by specific life experiences, which allow the person to be largely in control and which don't over or under challenge the person. A precondition of this is the availability of general resistance resources like physical factors, intelligence, coping strategies, social support, cultural stability etc., are available.

If the sense of coherence and, as a result, the effect of the resistance resources, are too weak, a state of stress sets in, which affects existing vulnerabilities (e.g. tendency for substance abuse)[9].

In regard to the resource-oriented approach of salutogenesis, the pathogenic diagnosis, which assesses deficits and impairments, is opposed to a salutogenic diagnosis, which assesses different resistance resources. For this, data from resilience research can directly be transferred.

10.4.5 Analogy to Gerontology: an atrophy of the "social atom"

The atrophy of the "social atom" (Jakob Moreno) represents an undeniable analogy with chronic alcoholism at ad-

church). A crucial result was also that adult subjects experienced a fundamental improvement in their ability to succeed in life between age 32 and 40. This often manifested in "turning points", especially where chances came up that they could better take advantage of at this age. Of eminent importance for the effective use of turning points was the successful coping with crises (e.g. recovery from a life-threatening disease or accident). Werner 2006

7 The questionnaire developed by Petzold and Mueller (PMFR) to assess resilience and protective factors, can be recommended for social work.

8 In the case of the Kaunai-study cited, only 5% of the group, which showed the strongest resilience, were in psychotherapeutic treatment. They were better educated and rather introverted (Werner 2006)

9 For information about the application of the salutogenesis approach in addiction research, see Franke et al. 1998.

Fig. 110 Pathogenesis vs. salutogenesis

Pathogenic diagnosis:	Salutogenic diagnosis:
– alcohol and medication abuse – major depression disorder and sleep disorder – dependant personality disorder	– social skills (ability to communicate with all kinds of different people, dependable, sensitive) – ability to carry out certain organisational tasks – stamina, discipline – used to doing different sports (and still interested) – humour (sometimes cynicism) – several long-term relationships – likes to read (e. g. newspapers) – acceptance of disease – fond of animals (used to have dogs before)

vanced stage, which is always accompanied by chronic tobacco abuse and geriatric problems. Moreno, the founder of psychodrama, was one of the first to suggest that social relationships are part of one's identity (Petzold 1985, 2004[10])[11]. The collapse of the social system is caused by the loss of important attachment persons. These can't be replaced due to individual or social circumstances (disease, restricted mobility due to dependence on (home) care, stigmatisation due to long-term unemployment, admissions to psychiatric hospitals, homelessness, old age, social deficits etc.), and this consequently leads to a permanently destabilised identity. It has been shown that the deterioration of the social network is linked to suffering, diseases, accelerated aging processes and even higher rates of mortality (Petzold and Bubolz 1979, Bauer 2006/2007).

With regards to aging, "social death", with the decay of the "social atom", takes place prior to physical death. This applies for alcohol dependents, especially the type IV group, according to Lesch, whose social integration is very precarious and shows deficits. Apart from the instability of the "social atom", the alcohol dependent, who usually lives among other alcohol dependents, is often confronted by the early death of attachment persons. The mortality rate in alcohol dependents is extremely high, with 12 to 23 years lesser life expectancy in com-

10 "The role of the group in therapy with the elderly – concepts for an "integrative intervention"

11 "The consistency of the social atoms changes when we get older, especially the possibility of replacing lost family members or friends. The social atom changes intermittently when we are young and full of resources. When a single member is gone, another individual can take his place by playing a similar role. A friend is lost and quickly replaced by someone else. This social repair seems to take place almost automatically ... When we get older it is more difficult to replace people we have lost, just like it becomes more difficult for our body to repair itself with increasing age. This describes precisely the phenomena of the "social" death: not in terms of the mind and how we are dying internally, but how we are dying externally ... When we live longer than those we love or hate, a small part of us dies with them, by seeing how the shadow of death strides from one person to the next in our social atom." (Moreno 1960 [1947], S. 63 f.)

parison to the normal population. This often depends on aetiology, progression (type) and treatment history (Lesch et al. 1990). Without treatment, type IV patients don't live longer than 60 years, implying that they don't reach senior age. It is not exaggerated to assume that alcohol dependents who have actively consumed alcohol for years, especially those without any prolonged periods of abstinence which allow the organism to recover, are affected by premature aging. In particular, cerebral degeneration (cerebellar atrophy, frontal lobe syndrome, organic psycho-syndrome), which has been sufficiently described in the literature, stimulates or accelerates the development of a dementia similar to old age dementia. This also applies for social conditions, where isolation and alienation, related to a reduction or loss of an intact social environment, can lead to enormous deprivation.

In regard to premature aging, gerontological, geragogical and even thanatological therapeutic aspects may be suitable for the support of alcohol dependents in confronting behavioural restrictions and the presence of the topic, "death". Clearly, this needs to be considered in academic training, self-awareness and supervision (Petzold 1985). As affected patients or clients are normally older than the carer and develop deep attachments and a need for attention, child-parents dynamics often result via transferences and countertransferences. Here, the personnel might set harsh boundaries and behave in a patronizing way.

Topics like the death of someone close (especially one's parents), dealing with the need for closeness (e.g. with regressive defiance and protest), dealing with one's own age and death need to be emphasised in the training and supervision of care workers.

Example:
Mr W. has been living in a community flat for three years, to which he moved by the help of political friends from his "old" life after being evicted from his house. After insolvency, he lost his petrol station, the cafe and the house in which his family was living. He and his wife became virtually homeless. The reason for this was his sustained alcoholism and the repression of threatening reality. Since the eviction from his house and the separation from his wife and family, he has no contact to his family or friends. His "social atom" has collapsed from one day to the next.
At present Mr W. is living off social welfare. After falling down the stairs in an intoxicated state, he became handicapped and suffers from permanent pain. He is episodically depressed and thinks that he will die soon anyway. After his 60th birthday, the depressive thoughts increased. Despite repeated recommendations, he has rejected medical treatment. Furthermore, he needs to undergo a cataract operation, but he constantly makes up excuses because he is too afraid. He rejects all offers of support. Neither has withdrawal therapy been successful in the long-term. Brain atrophies that have been detected by a computer tomography, cause loss of energy and forgetfulness and the therapy centre advises a custodianship. Yet, this has not been approved by

the Court, as Mr W. is categorized as a "borderline case".
What kind of reorientation is possible in this context?
How can Mr W. establish a new social environment?
As Mr W. is in contact with a political group, he has tried to build new, stable and non alcohol-related contacts with the help of this group and has managed to do this to a certain extent. Furthermore, he has managed to get in touch with his children again. The contact with his family and his "political party" improve his affective state episodically but not permanently. Two to three times a week, he visits the political party's office in order to get some things done (ironing, running errands, copying ...), tasks in which his OPS-related forgetfulness plays a considerable role. He has learned to write down all his appointments and is not alone anymore during festivities.

10.5 Sociotherapy in the context of therapeutic phases

10.5.1 Socio therapy location(s)

(Schwendter 2000)

In contrast to psychotherapeutic contexts, sociotherapy is determined by the location, function and aim of the sociotherapeutic intervention. Sociotherapy is often about genuinely participating and "exploring" character and assisting the affected in their life environment. Sociotherapy can take place in:

- Open outpatient institutions: marriage and family counselling centres, parenting, pregnancy and motherhood advisory services, school psychological services, probation and judicial support services, psychosocial support societies, organisations for community-based work, extramural initiatives.
- Semi-public in-patient institutions:
  Day and night hospitals, transitional institutions, sociotherapeutic residential homes, open prisons, probation homes, special daycare facilities for children ...
  As a result of decades of experience, Petzold suggests "collective living facilities" as alternatives to residential homes or single apartments for certain groups. Assisted residential homes have become common for both old and handicapped persons. For alcohol dependents and certain subgroups, permanent or temporary housing in collective living facilities seem to be a sensible option. These have emerged from the atrophy of the "social atom" as mentioned above. All forms of collective living mentioned by Petzold can be found in sociotherapeutic practice: residential homes, housing groups, therapeutic communities, therapeutic residential homes and therapeutic housing groups (Petzold 1985). Some are limited in time and context by withdrawal therapy, while others are long term and represent rather less restricted forms of collective living.
- Closed institutions like approved schools, mental institutions, closed prisons etc. However, these institutions usually inhibit develop-

Fig. 111 Motivational stages

Motivational stages according to Prochaska & DiClemente	
I.	**No intentions**
II.	**Development of intentions**
III.	**Preparation stage**
IV.	**Action Stage**
V.	**Maintenance**
VI.	**Relapse**

ment and are therefore anti-therapeutic.

10.5.2 Therapeutic phases and settings

In line with international standards, the treatment of alcohol dependents can be divided into four groups. A "closed therapeutic chain" is only effective if adequate tenders for healthcare services for all four phases are provided. The requirements for treatment setting and sociotherapy depend on whether treatment is carried out on an outpatient, semi-inpatient, or in-patient level. The structural approaches of the setting are influenced by the patient's **phases of motivation**. The model of Prochaska and DiClemente (1992) has established itself in practices and also applies for the therapy of nicotine dependents. There are six phases of motivation and actual therapy is not realized until phase four. Insight into the disease and a readiness to deal with the dependence, increase with every phase.

Therapeutic phases

1. Phase: initial contact, initiation of therapy

In sociotherapeutic settings like day centres for the elderly or homeless, or assisted living institutions, the initiation of therapy is an everyday requirement, which often becomes the responsibility of sociotherapeutic workers. People, who are chronically impaired, often face precarious housing provision, homelessness and co-morbidities. The situation requires the close cooperation of social work and psychiatry, which actually makes therapy possible. High threshold settings with high normative requirements often prevent integration into a support system. Besides in-patient and outpatient options for healthcare services, explorative concepts are needed for subgroups with multi-morbidity and high social vulnerabilities/pressure.

Generally, the initiation of therapy takes place in an outpatient setting. If the patient has no insight into his disease, the first aim is to establish a trusting relationship, so that the patient can be made aware of his substance dependence. These conversations should take place in a quite atmosphere (no disturbance, no telephone calls), also sufficient time should be granted (at least 35 minutes for the initial meeting). The method used in Millner´s and Rollnick's[12] *motivational interviewing*

12 Miller ER, S.Rollnik Miller WR and Rollnick S (2002). A sound description of this method for practical use has been offered by Koerkel, Kruse 1997, chapter 15

serves as a standard and can be used as a guideline for this context. A premature confrontation with a "diagnosis" should be avoided. By asking open questions, the patient should gradually become ready to confront his alcohol dependence.

Open questions:

"You are saying that alcohol helps you to switch off? How should I picture this?"

"You are saying that you couldn't endure stressful situations without any cigarettes – what would happen if you do not smoke?"

"You have mentioned that alcohol has helped you to cope with difficult situations? What kind of situations were these? And what were the effects of alcohol?"

In the first phase, objective information, similar to that sought in medical examinations (e.g. elevated liver tests, blackouts, lung functioning tests etc) should be gathered. "Suggestions" for changing drinking habits that are formulated too early, can be counterproductive. The highlighting of discrepancies (contrasting advantages with disadvantages) in phases of indecisiveness is recommended. Therapy can only be initiated with the patient's agreement. The therapy setting or the outpatient counselling centre then arranges an initial or admission meeting. Here it needs to be decided whether **inpatient admission or outpatient treatment**[13] is more suitable.

13 There is almost no available therapeutic provision for tobacco withdrawal therapy in regard to inpatient withdrawal or cessation.

An outpatient treatment is viable if the patient is socially integrated (family, occupation, friends, daily structure a high GAF score) and if his health condition is good. The institution in charge needs to assure the **continuity of treatment.** It is crucial that the therapist and patient have a **positive relationship** (transference), because otherwise the relationship is likely to be terminated in times of crisis.

In the case of poor health, severe withdrawal symptoms, **co-morbidity** (typology) and an **unsupportive social environment,** an inpatient admission is indicated. In this case, the principle of **low threshold** should be demanded, that is, the patients should not be promised a later admission in order to allow them time to "clarify their motivation", but should *immediately* be admitted. Once more it must be emphasised that a dependence is a **life threatening disease**, which requires very prompt intervention.

Further, it should be advised that the **cooperation** between sociotherapeutic institutions and the withdrawal setting should be optimally coordinated so that necessary in-patient admissions can be carried out quickly and smoothly.

2. Phase: withdrawal treatment (around 14 days)

In this phase, sociotherapy is usually secondary, while the treatment of withdrawal syndromes is predominant. (The nicotine withdrawal syndrome lasts longer, around 1 month, with most symptoms manifesting in the second week [Lesch 2007].)

Many therapy institutions tend to confine or control the dependent's curfew. Occupational therapy is limited in its possibilities, as patients tend to be psycho-motorically impaired, as a result of high doses of medications. Sociotherapy raises the question about how to maintain a minimum daily routine for clients.

3. Phase: withdrawal treatment (around 1–2 months)

On the one hand, the dependent's confrontation with his own dependence now becomes the focal point, whilst on the other hand, his physical and psychological well-being (e.g. capacity to experience, recovery, sleep etc) should be supported by health-promoting measures. Motivational crises and protracted withdrawal symptoms might set in (according to Scholz, motivational crises become more frequent in weeks 7–9 of therapy).

The **ambulant therapy setting** is limited to one to two contacts per week at the maximum. The correlation between therapy success and frequency of contacts has been documented by research.

The in-patient setting usually combines a variety of therapeutic approaches, with medical, sociotherapeutic, psycho-educative and psychotherapeutic approaches overlapping. Parallel to these, the social worker assists in clarifying occupational and financial issues and organising subsequent housing arrangements.

4. Phase: aftercare, crisis intervention (1–2 years)

From a sociotherapeutic perspective, this phase is the most important one in combating dependence because in this phase the patient starts to properly confront reality. All catamnesis studies have shown that aftercare, subsequent to an in-patient therapy, acts as a stabilising factor (Koerkel 1992). This also applies for self-help groups. Therapy options that are offered by institutions are often insufficient which confirms the impression that aftercare is seen as little more than an appendage to in-patient therapy.

It is certain that the vulnerability to dependence, e.g. spontaneous recurrences of withdrawal symptoms, cravings etc., is heightened during the first two years and, with this, the risk of a relapse (Scholz 1996). During this period of time, stable contact with the therapy institution, preferably with the therapist-in-charge, and the availability of instant crisis interventions, should be provided.

A night hospital is a valid alternative for transferring the patient from the therapeutic environment to his "old" world: patients are able to work during the day, are in touch with their social environment, but stay in the hospital overnight during the week. This option can be offered for up to two months.

Interval therapy, another concept that seeks to counteract the increased relapse rates of certain subgroups, permits patients several short-term stays (lasting two to four weeks) which are spaced over a year. Patients are allowed to come by, regardless of whether or not they are suffering a relapse. In this way, the therapy institution protects patients during particular relapse-vulnerable phases, like birthdays or Christmas. This form of provision practically anticipates crises interventions and helps to maintain the patient's contact with the therapy institution.

The sociotherapeutic contribution towards aftercare within this therapy setting, is distinguished by **networking efforts.** These assist the patient in making and maintaining contact with the institution responsible for aftercare. In this, sociotherapeutic counsellors are often restricted by institutional borders, e.g. when the amount of therapy hours are cut down due to economic measures, when "crisis intervention" is misinterpreted as being mere breathalyzer tests or if "aftercare" is no more than a series of short 3-minute meetings stretched out over 14 days.

Often sociotherapeutic helpers are personally affected by the defence mechanisms of an overstrained psychiatric system. Suddenly the institutions in charge (admission pavilions, detoxification clinics, counselling centres) demand rituals designed to prop up motivation from the severely censured, relapse patients ("Attend the breathalyzer check-up twice a day, then we will proceed") or appointments can only be arranged in far in advance, not to speak of waiting lists. At the "other end" of the "closed therapy chain", the psychiatric world shows a very different picture, which has nothing to do with "motivational talks", "empathy" and "understanding". The "verification of motivation" argument is often used in this context. Indeed, with these separate mechanisms, the psychiatric system's precarious role in the medical system becomes visible: shortness of resources, permanent confrontation with mentally ill patients, difficult patients, a lack of acceptance and other critical factors create a system, in which many employees are at risk of "burn-out" (Heltzel 2000, Fengler 2004).

An example from practice should illustrate this:
Mr B., 52 years old, looks back on a long history of counselling. After his mother's suicide, the tragic death of his brother and sister and the loss of two fingers due to a workplace accident, he is suffering from acute, recurring depression. Over the years, he has developed an alcohol dependence. Extreme drinking phases are always linked to depression. Whether his delinquency in early adulthood and subsequent imprisonments are related to the depression, has never been examined. Several long-term withdrawal therapies in Germany and Austria have not improved the relapse rate. After several months of abstinence, he usually relapses, which lasts for weeks and during which suicidal ideations are dominant. Two previous suicide attempts have been documented. He barely eats when he is in a depressive phase.
In the meantime, Mr B. has moved to a council flat in Vienna and receives social welfare. He finds it more and more difficult to endure the loneliness in the flat and considers abandoning his flat to move out to live on the street.
During the last crisis, Mr B. again decides to "really end it all". He hasn't eaten for three weeks and bloody sputum indicates a stomach inflammation. A visiting carer finds him in a weak condition and immediately calls emergency, but Mr B. resists and, as a consequence, he is not being picked up. He insists: "I want to die now".

The next day he changes his mind and calls his helper asking for help. At one o'clock the next day the carer meets with Mr B. at the local hospital pavilion. Mr B. has dark circles around the eyes, is just skin and bones and can hardly stand upright.
When the psychiatrist in charge appears, she passes the waiting clients without saying a word and avoids eye contact as she disappears into her office. A little later, Mr B. enters her office. It is decided that he will not be admitted. He should come back four days later for an admission interview at 9 o'clock sharp. Mr B. says that he won't be able to manage this. The psychiatrist replies, "Then you have to make an effort!"
The carer points out Mr B.'s suicidal tendency and problematic health condition, but he is ignored. Four days later, still not having eaten anything, Mr B. drags himself to the hospital pavilion, but he is half an hour late. He is told to wait four more days because he was late.
Following this, Mr B. seeks out his former therapy unit in the same hospital, but even after having spoken to his former doctor, he still has to wait four days for an appointment with the psychiatrist.
On the advice of his carer, Mr B. drags himself to another hospital with a psychiatric unit. In the meantime, he has developed acute withdrawal symptoms. The outpatient department immediately sends him away due to his condition. Mr B. breaks down in the hospital foyer.
Only after the carer, who has to come to the hospital, intervenes, does the psychiatrist offer to see Mr B. Mr B. is admitted the next day.

Apart from the occasional task of networking, sociotherapy is responsible for structuring the patient's daily life as part of aftercare. This means, supporting the maintenance of a daily, monthly, or yearly structure and the development of a (mentally) stabilising environment. Methods available depend on the setting, the available facilities and the options open to sociotherapists but are usually determined by the individual's situation. Some examples of this are as follows:

- crisis intervention, relapse support
- supporting job-seeking, cooperating with employment centres
- searching for suitable work or projects that structure daily life, e. g. day centres for seniors etc.
- recreational activities in groups (swimming, bowling, playing cards, ...)
- organizing festivities
- arranging furniture in a new room
- cleaning up the flat together
- regulating debt
- stabilising health (establishing adequate contact with doctors, nutritional advice ...)

10.6 State of the Art: overlapping perspectives for sociotherapeutic housing and support projects for alcohol dependents

Analyses of the experiences of different care facilities in Austria and Germany over many years, have provided very helpful structures and approaches to improving the course of the disease of chronic alcohol dependents[14]. They reflect the institutions' therapeutic and pedagogic orientations. The "concept" reflects the accumulation of practical and reflected experience and usually documents a lengthy learning process. It allows assumptions to be made about the current position of care facilities or how concepts develop. The tension between the ideal and the reality, that is, between the concept and daily life itself, is always present and may serve as a yardstick for improvement. An essential characteristic of social facilities is that they adapt to changing situations (trends, political climate, situations, changes in clients etc.) and that they connect marginal groups with society. Furthermore, local solutions, that is, procedures that conform to local conditions, are more efficient than general concepts (e.g. procedures in rural areas are different to the ones in cities).

The following formulates overlapping perspectives which are based on different concepts of aftercare facilities and the practical implementation of their work. These are "standards" which are largely valid today and can be found in various forms in most aftercare institutions for alcohol dependents.

10.6.1 Standard categories

1. The differentiation of (a) patient group(s)

The most established differentiation criteria are

- gender (e.g. male and female houses)
- age (minimum and maximum age, e.g. houses for the seniors or for adolescents)
- nature of substance (separating alcohol dependents from drug dependents)

The terms "high-threshold" and "low-threshold" are further ways of differentiating certain aspects. The institution's differentiation and specialisation may promote a "high threshold", which means that clients have to meet certain criteria[15]. Care facilities tend to select according to **"motivation"** and **"competency"**. These factors are generally difficult to assess as they always depend on the phase in which an alcohol dependence is diagnosed (it must be borne in mind that the regeneration process takes several months). Therapy places are expensive and scarce and this is why the system supports those in whom an investment "pays off". This is how the terms "motivation" and "competence" become criteria for the allocation of financial and personal resources.

There is a danger of losing "low-threshold" as a value, especially in terms of therapy and the support of alcohol dependents. If alcohol dependence is considered a disease, a low-threshold approach which serves the clients' needs, should be employed.

Apart from these general assessment criteria (age, gender, lifetime history of drug consumption, motivation

14 The Vinzenz House of the Caritas in Vienna, ALOA and GOA in Upper Austria, Aloisianum in Graz, the alcoholics housing community in Feldkirch, SOALP in Salzburg, the residential home in Schillerstrasse, Berlin, Hans-Scherer House in Munich, Type IV housing community in Vienna.

15 In most cases, the care institutions for alcohol dependents have developed from housing projects for the homeless, in which the specialisation on the group of alcohol dependents has resulted in higher-threshold therapy offers.

and competence), any further differentiations, and their realisation in practice, become more difficult. Requirements are:

- Clear conceptions, which have been theoretically and practically considered, about which patient group will, and can, be treated in the respective care facility. As a rule, the facilities' written concept plan will already contain the core of this differentiation as long as it has been developed in tandem with the learning and adjustment processes, which is generally the case, if one considers the history of the institution and its relationship to the concept plan.
- The differentiation does not imply that only one group (types) should be allocated to one institution, but special emphasis should certainly be given to one particular target group. An example of such a differentiation is the therapeutic programme according to Lesch's typology at the Humboldt University of Berlin, which does not permit type IV patients into the normal programme. Admission criteria like "autonomy" and "social competencies" are often used in differentiations.
- Differentiations are made in structured and focused admission interviews or procedures, which are mostly conducted by specially trained and experienced workers.
- Differentiations also lead to non-admissions and rejections. The team is likely to develop the attitude "that they can't help all alcohol dependents" and that the respective institution has strengths and weaknesses, which may or may not stabilise or help certain subgroups.
- Differentiations promote the transparent handling of house rules, concept-based rules and especially the management of "exceptions" to these rules, which are made in practice at times; for example, in relapse assessment, a differentiation is made between "hidden and visible relapses" or different levels of motivation (= cooperation, "compliance") (e. g. sanctions for extending admission).

2. The written concept plan as a sign of an institutional learning and maturation process

- The concept plan grows along with the institution and is representative of the institution's different maturation and learning phases because it is regularly adapted in line with any institutional changes.
- The concept plan is usually available in written form and serves as a basis for orientation for employees in training.
- The concept plan is important for decision processes in the team. That is, it is more than a "dead paper", which is never referred to, but rather a description of the team's values and reasoning.

3. House rules/user agreement

- The house rules (or user agreement) show the client who has moved in, which care strategies and therapeutic mindset are being used. It reflects the facilities' concept plan.
- The house rules can be seen as a therapeutic instrument in them-

selves as, when adhered to, they regulate daily procedures for living together.
- The house rules are signed at the time of admission.
- House rules may need to be revised, in accordance with changes in daily life, as required.

4. Practice
Practice is not only implemented "intuitively", but is based on specific theoretic/scientific systems of thought which distinguish between different levels of reflection (a continuum ranging from very general to very specific levels) (tree of science).

- Principally, any action is, or can be, linked to professional discourse. This is manifested in the ways in which field-related topics are examined.
- Knowledge about the following kinds of therapy is integral to meeting general practical standards:
  - **Psychoanalysis** (e.g. knowledge about certain *defence mechanisms* like repression, projections and about constellations like *transference* and *countertransference*)
  - **Person-centred conversational therapy** (showing empathy and respect)
  - **Behavioural therapy** (reward and punishment; employing praise, critique and strategies that promote self-enhancement)
  - **Psychiatry** (Psychoses, affective disorders, personality disorders, prescribed medication etc.)
- More or less explicit **knowledge about alcohol**, that is, more knowledge about disease-specific processes and symptoms, e.g.
  - Knowledge about the dangers of withdrawal symptoms, withdrawal epilepsies and delirium tremens
  - Knowledge about organic sequelae (fatty liver, liver cirrhosis, gastrointestinal diseases etc)
  - Knowledge about the relationship between depression/anxiety and alcohol consumption as an attempt to treat oneself etc.
- More **specific practical standards** are:
  - Legal foundations for occupational activity (social welfare law, immigrant laws etc)
  - Enforcement regulations in regard to payment of unemployment benefit, emergency support or social welfare (benefit system); but also
  - Knowledge about developments in related institutions
  - Specific knowledge about housing and work projects and their admissions' criteria etc.

5. Teamwork
Teams are usually *multi-professional* and *mixed gender.*

Team communication is structured by the use of several tools and media (log book, team meeting minutes, records, shared calendar etc).

The most important tool, however, is the team meeting and special meetings (workgroup, specialist division group etc.)

Team meetings usually take place *weekly* and have a pre-assigned structure (agenda, presentation). In either case, the team meeting is an established *form*, in which all problems are discussed and concerns expressed by all team members. It is a sign of severe structural damage and relationship problems, if topics are not tackled or if colleagues are not "heard".

The team meeting is the central forum in which cases are discussed and decisions are made, for which everyone is responsible. Topics that are discussed by the team usually concern disciplinary measures, crisis interventions or the transition of the patient from one therapy phase to the next. In these team meetings, a common "language" and pedagogical approach towards certain situations is developed.

Requirements for team members are: social competence, ability to give and receive criticism, learning aptitude, empathy, autonomy, organisational skills, flexibility, and the ability to follow the institution's rules.

6. Further training/supervision

There are certain standards for supervision (SV). It is important to determine the setting at the beginning.

- The determining of who needs SV. (Directors? Compulsory community service workers? Volunteers?)
- The SV is paid for by the institution and organized by trained supervisors (there are lists with the national supervisory association, e.g. Austrian Association for Supervision).
- Sometimes team supervision and case supervision are separated (which has been criticised by specialists).
- The directors of institutions or those in charge are responsible for the continuous training of their staff (once or twice a year).

7. Definition of aims

The definition of therapy aims is standard procedure especially in the case of transitional care facilities, where residents are prepared for independent living and where the length of stay is prearranged and time limited. The aims are set as a result of agreement between the therapist and the client and checked from time to time, e.g. the client receives feedback about his developmental process. The goals that have been attained serve as positive reinforcement. Progress and failure in regard to these aims are reflected on at regular intervals (e.g. every three or six months), both alone with the client and together in the team.

8. Documentation

In many cases, supervisors demand the documentation of the course of therapy, possibly in digital form, which is regularly monitored (through samples at least). Annual reports are usually documented in written form.

Although evaluation seems to be becoming more and more important, valid instruments for evaluation (questionnaires, quality circle) are still needed.

Apart from monitoring what takes place, this systematic documentation serves other functions too, such as facilitating the transfer of a case from one therapist/institution to another (therapy substitution) and facilitating case reflection for therapists or the team (e.g. in case supervision).

9. The phases of support

Principle: Maximal orientation at the beginning, followed by increased autonomy and a reduction of control from the outside.

1. Admission procedure (house inspection, housing trial, admission interview, introducing the client to flatmates, reading the house rules etc.)
2. Trial period
3. "Fixed-term care" usually divided into several phases of reflection (e.g. every six months) – case conference, possibly changing to a different type of housing (e.g. from a shared room to a single room, from a residential facility to a flat-share or assisted living etc.)
4. Detachment phase (through external changes: e.g. obtaining the house key, less frequent breathalyzer tests).
5. Aftercare

10. Relapse regulation

As relapse is a fundamental part of dependence, regulations determining the handling of relapses can be found in all rehabilitation care facilities. These regulations set sanctions and boundaries that determine at which point, according to the degree or frequency of relapse, the client will be obliged to leave.

This regulation is usually divided into three phases, e.g.

1. Relapse: verbal warning
2. Relapse: written warning
3. Relapse: moving out

The stricter the rule, the more likely it is that exceptions are made in practice. However, making exceptions and not insisting on a specific rule is a sign of professionalism because it shows that factors relating to personality and life events are being taken into consideration. This is in line with scientific findings that suggest a relapse has many types and causes.

In flat-shares or living communities, it is common practice to discuss the relapse of a flatmate in the presence of the affected.

A common perception is that every relapse reflected on in the group, is an opportunity for learning for the individual affected and the whole group.

11. Abstinence regulation

In aftercare institutions, abstinence regulations for dependents in withdrawal are essential.

That is, **no alcohol is to be consumed in the institution (flat, home).** If this rule is broken, in most cases the dependent will be asked to move out immediately.

A more difficult question however is the **intoxication level** of clients coming to the institution. Often the institution orders an intoxicated client to stay away from the institution, but some institutions have a "drying-out room" (in the sense of "learning from the relapse"), in which the affected can sober up/cope with withdrawal. Contrary to critics labelling this procedure as relapse promoting "co-alcoholism", it should be seen rather as an **interruption of relapse** (if carried out appropriately). However these institutions sometimes don't have enough space for a drying-out room.

12. Violence regulation

Violence is not accepted and there are no exceptions to this rule. Violent assaults generally lead to the offending individual having to move out immediately. The possession of guns is prohibited. This is also stated in the house rules.

13. Regulations for returning
If the client has moved out early, usually due to several relapses, there are concept plans that stipulate the conditions under which he may be allowed to move in again, and the timeframe.

14. The group as a medium for learning (mandatory conversations)
In most institutions, the "peer-group", that is, a group of like-minded people, is seen as an important medium for promoting self-awareness.

Normally, several group meetings take place per week/per month. Having to undergo such group processes and long hours of conversation can, for some alcoholic dependents, become a reason leaving the therapeutic programme.

The (sociotherapeutic) community has three functions:

- to provide protection (protective structure)
- to provide orientation (orientation structure)
- to stabilise (stabilising structure).

15. Using daily life for the creation of pedagogical interventions or incentives
The most important field in sociotherapy/social pedagogy is the daily life and the collective coping with, and structuring of, daily life. For all alcohol dependents, it can be assumed that the addictive substance has come to dominate and structure their daily life. The acquisition and consumption of alcohol in certain environments has gradually pushed out all other interests (**absorption of interests**). The buried interests have to be taken up again during abstinence or alternative ways of structuring the addicted's life need to be developed.

Therefore it makes sense that both **recreational activities** and **occupational therapy** (creative work) are undisputed in their importance for withdrawal therapy and the aftercare of alcohol dependents. In both areas, alcohol-free forms of social contact are established and practiced.

- Cooking and eating together
- Cleaning together/cleaning for the group
- Coping with financial shortage
- Festivities
- Recreational activities
- Watching TV
- Common projects (e.g. excursions, travelling)

Often a fundamental value related reorientation of personality, a discovery of meaning, results from social integration and more stable relationships (e.g. resuming contact with one's family, friends, partner).

16. Concept of aftercare
Scientific research has shown that aftercare subsequent to withdrawal therapy improves the success rate of therapy.

As the first two years of abstinence are known to be times of recurring crises of adjustment (organic-social), it is important that aftercare should cover this two-year period at least.

Further, it is important that transitional care facilities continue to stay in touch with the clients, provided that institutions aren't responsible for the assisted living themselves.

Some treatment facilities encourage contact to alcohol-specific, self-help groups (International Blue Cross, Alcoholics Anonymous, AHA etc), however only a minority of alcohol dependents profits from these groups and takes part for a longer period of time. It is probable that exclusive focus on the topic of "alcohol", with all its negative connotations, leads to boredom over time. Also these groups may fail to address issues that are more fundamental to the life of an abstinent alcohol dependent.

The integration into non-alcoholic groups that structure social contact by using certain mediums (sport, games, handcrafts etc.), are more helpful and easier to endure. These can be sport clubs, theatre groups, game groups (playing cards), cooperating in social projects (e.g. in mobile homeless support, doorman service in homeless shelters, kitchen service ...), integration into a church community and the like.

The integration into such projects is difficult and requires the affected to be brave and willing and the therapist to be patient and ready to cope with failure.

Yet from practical and theoretical experience, it is uncontested that the integration into social networks is one of the most important pillars to abstinence, not least because it supersedes the often tightly structured phase of inpatient therapy and assisted living.

17. Framework of attachment figures

The aim is to build supporting and helpful relationships. Relationships are essential impulses for motivation. One of the most important preconditions of relationship building is the conscious creation of interpersonal closeness and distance, which is continuously reflected upon. Examples of relationship building are:

- **Role reflection** and **clarity in therapy**, that is, the adherence to professional standards (e.g. not taking clients to one's home, no friendships or partnerships).
- Awareness of **transference** and **countertransference phenomena.**
- **Detachment.**
- The therapy relationship is usually **temporary** (the separation from this stabilising relationship is taken up as a theme and takes place within a gradual process of detachment).

18. Expense contributions

Clients pay a contribution towards the total fee, which serves as preparation for paying rent later on. Fee contributions (which don't apply in some places, e.g. in rehabilitation facilities) are a pedagogical concept which represents the principle of reality and, as a result, makes possible an engagement with rights and responsibilities.

19. Networking

Networking with other institutions is an important resource. All topics significant for therapy work are discussed within this network (concept formation, detachment, detection of system deficits, development of alternatives, initiatives etc.). Networking can also foster political awareness.

The adjustment and optimisation of measures and offers of provision for clients are crucial and include:

- regular network meetings with cooperating institutions
- participating in work groups
- visiting other institutions
- development of collective essays, campaigns, projects
- preparation of meetings, seminars, etc.

The connection to medical-psychiatric support systems is especially vital for subgroups with repeatedly impaired alcohol dependents, especially if crisis interventions are needed. Often *short-term, reliable* external medical help is unavailable, which leads to even further damage to the dependent's health (and related, additional costs, especially if the affected does not receive support from the health system). Furthermore, this situation overly stresses therapy personnel who are often left "alone" with relapsing clients. Although the networking standard is often not attained, its functionality can't be doubted (Reker and When 2001).

20. Autonomy and control

On principle, the goal is the client's attainment of the maximum autonomy possible. This entails the systematic reduction of initial control.

The extent and nature of this control depend on the institution's style on the one hand, and on the needs of the clients on the other hand (and therefore also on the typological focus of the alcohol dependents life in the institution).

Measures include **breathalyzer tests** (ranging from occasional to strict and regular checks e.g. when entering the house); **unannounced spot checks on rooms** (mostly "on suspicion"); **attendance lists** (in one case, even surveillance by camera of persons entering the house); **notice of departure,** following long absences; curfew regulations (including exceptions to these regulations); and of course checking the therapy goals set by social workers (progress in debt regulation, savings, visits to doctors and agencies, job search, attendance of aftercare sessions and the like).

If the aim of the initial phase is the establishment of a stable relationship between therapist and client and integration into the community, then this progress must be reversed in the **detachment phase** (fewer therapy sessions, more activities/social contacts outside of the home, less frequent or no breathalyzer tests etc.)

10.6.2 Excursus: supported housing projects – worlds of their own

Many characteristics described above are predominantly valid for transitional care homes (e.g. definitions of aims, structuring of phases, relapse regulation etc). Homes have a different dynamic than supported housing projects. Further, whether care facilities are denoted as transitional or permanent is a constitutive factor which determines different attitudes towards care and different objectives. The following outlines some observations from practice:

Transitional or permanent habitation: different group dynamics

In transitional institutions, the bridge towards permanent residential facilities, only provisory relationships are established between the carers and residents because from the start everyone knows that the relationship is only transitional. This "temporary arrangement" often leads to poor compliance, on the part of members of the household and carers, with the house rules. In additional, the need to defend and demarcate one's private sphere, which is made difficult by the lack of space, is very intense in transitional homes. Many years of experience in different transitional homes have shown that the relationships formed between co-habitants are less stable, despite similarities in residents' backgrounds. This partial isolation in transitional homes often leads then to total isolation in the permanent housing arrangement. Apart from the motive of defence, which is pronounced in larger institutions, the permanent change in residents, due to people moving in and out, also plays a role. A further factor in the dynamic of transitional residential homes for alcohol dependents, are personal experiences from previous residential home stays during childhood, adolescence or imprisonment respectively, which reinforce ambivalence towards the transitional care facility and its residents.

Some of these tendencies are even stronger in transitional housing projects. Reports from carers that the common rooms are always empty or that they are only used for arranged group meetings, are not rare. In this context, sociotherapeutic/social pedagogical approaches require a high level of commitment and personal resources, which are often not available for the support of alcohol dependents. Permanent supported housing projects exist primarily for the handicapped, secondarily for older people, and quite rarely for the addicted. The only sociotherapeutic permanent housing project for chronic alcohol dependents in Austria is the type IV supported housing project of the organisation, "VEREIN STRUKTUR", in Vienna.

The social dynamic of permanent supported housing projects is different to that of transitional care facilities. The dynamic is also very important for the course of the disease, albeit not solely. After residents have stayed aloof for a while, behaviour which is often linked to heightened social anxiety, a "substitute family" emerges. What is important here, is which kinds of crises arise, and how the group copes with them. A stable and flexible social organism also develops in permanent supported housing projects against a background of social deprivation which is nearly always present, to the point of traumatic experiences in their own families, foster families, in care homes and prisons. Most residents have never had a "normal" socialisation, but have often had to confront very difficult social experiences. Social insecurities, to the point of social dysfunctions (e.g. social phobia), are certainly a normal part of living together. The path to a "substitute family" is marked by ambivalences and conflicts. While intensive processes don't take place in transitional institutions, they are always present in permanent housing projects. The community offers an intensive, long-term setting for this learning process.

It is likely that the initial insecurities of such housing projects promote stability seeking group dynamics. Miles mentioned the "phase of insecure scanning" and the "phase of depressive stagnation", which might be followed by a phase of "euphoria". According to Bion (Antons 2000), "basic assumptions" and their corresponding behavioural patterns, dominate at the beginning. These serve as orientation in the initial, insecure phases:

1. Dependence (fixation on the leader), followed by counter dependence (turning against the leader),
2. Fight (members face conflicts among each other),
3. Escape (occasionally through relapsing) and lastly,
4. Pairing

In regard to the shared life of people with psychological disorders, especially social traumas, the fact that traumas can be reactivated whilst living together should be expected. This can lead to a temporary deterioration of the psychological condition.

If people who have experienced isolation, aggression and rejection whilst living in a big city, join a community, they are likely to find the warmth and love that they need in life. They let go of masks and barriers and become vulnerable. They experience a time of solidarity and profound joy. However, precisely because they let go of their masks and allow themselves to become vulnerable, they discover that the community can be intimidating. This is because the community is a place of relationships which expose our hurt feelings and show us how difficult it can be to live with others, especially with certain people. It is much easier to live only with books and objects, with the television, and with dogs and cats! It is much easier to live alone and do something for others only when you feel like it.

Jean Vanier[16]

16 Jean Vanier has founded the international project "Arche", where handicapped individuals live with non-handicapped individuals in a community.

Trust, determination, responsibility

Trust is one of the most important factors when living together, especially for dependents who have had negative experiences with other dependents. The question is: "How much can I trust you?" At the beginning, it is common for residents to spend time observing each other and testing each other out. Often, the collective concealment of relapses from carers is a sign of trust amongst dependents and needs to be continuously addressed in the group.

All residents have to be genuinely *determined* to live together with other people, in order for a housing *community* to develop. This is a process that can take any length of time. If one or more persons are not committed to living together in this way, any further processes or development are contaminated. Alliances, exclusions and conflicts, which are linked to an increased relapse rate, are likely to take place. Only when this phase has been mastered, can the phase of *encounters* and *responsibility* be reached, in which a mutual interest in each other's lives becomes possible.

Many or few rules

Once the decision has been reached to live together and the group is ready to assume responsibility, the rules have to be changed, regardless of whether they are explicit (mutually determined) or implicit (determined by everyday practice). The need for regulations is different in each housing community. Some seek their "salvation" in "regulations" of all sorts, while others want as few rules as possible. Often, regulatory authorities (strict parents, schools, homes, prison etc) are associated with negative experiences, and are therefore avoided.

The following must be clear: too many rules interfere with one's life and the ability to find flexible solutions, yet a minimum of rules is helpful, especially for residents, who need direction. In other words, it depends on the quality of the community and how it wishes and needs certain areas to be regulated. This needs to be found out first. The institution needs to provide a minimum number of rules (e.g. prohibiting alcohol consumption in the housing space).

Example:
When setting up a new community housing project with dependents, the carer addresses the cleaning up of the flat and kitchen. "Which rules should be implemented?" The tenor of the residents' replies comes as a surprise: "No rules at all!" The carer finds this hard to believe, because the topic of cleaning, in particular, has always been one of the bigger problems in community housing projects. When asked how this should work in a housing community, the residents suggest "Everyone cleans up their own mess" – The carer has doubts about this "method". But after only a few weeks, he needs to revise his attitude. Even after several months, the cleaning of the flat and kitchen has never arisen as an issue at group meetings and the flat is clean. Thus, even here, "self-organising systems" exist. This system only collapsed in the second year because of an accumulation of relapses.

Relapses:
If a relationship system emerges from the processes described above, in which everyone finds their place and has their own responsibilities, psychological stability is positively influenced and the frequency of relapses is reduced. Although relapses which are jointly experienced, are always a strain on the community, if discussed openly and with trust, they also serve as an important learning experience for everyone. Although the sanction of having to move out is common way of handling frequent and continual relapses in transitional institutions, it needs to be questioned in permanent housing communities, especially when stable relationships have been built.

This especially applies in the case of chronically dependent individuals who don't have any housing alternatives, and can only expect a drastic radical deterioration when having to move out (e.g. relocation to a nursing home). When mutual sympathy is present (phase of responsibility), the community won't want to take the step of evicting someone until all other options have been exhausted (crisis intervention, therapy etc.). It goes without saying that in well-functioning housing communities, it is first and foremost the group who should make the decisions and generate solutions at times of acute crises. Sociotherapeutic interventions should focus on structuring the process of conflict and spurring things on, but should not take away from the group its responsibility for making decisions. This applies for as long as the community is capable of acting. Psychological crises however, like relapses, can weaken the social organism and cause a "collective regression", which impedes a sense of responsibility. In this case, the community becomes incapable of making far-reaching decisions , and carers have to intervene.

> **Example:**
> Flatmate X. has relapsed several times over the past weeks. Numerous stays in hospitals failed to improve his condition and after returning home, he started drinking again. His general condition deteriorates rapidly. Neither do attempts at persuasion and confrontations during group meetings within the living community have a stabilising effect. Nevertheless, none of the flatmates dare to demand that X. move out. Two other flatmates start drinking again due to the ongoing situation. As a consequence, the "community" is not able to make decisions anymore. The fourth flatmate seems terrified and distressed and virtually "escapes" into a pseudodepressive state. The fifth flatmate reacts with a sleep disorder and increased panic attacks. This marks the start of the "collective regression" and the group's incapacity to make decisions. Only after the carer in charge decides that X. has to move out, does the situation start to calm down. The community was not (yet) strong and articulate enough to consciously and explicitly make such a decision itself (although the decision was made at a defensive level, to be sure). In such cases, specialists speak of "systemic relapses".

Thus, the coping with relapses is the primary task of the residential community's social system, which also includes external attachment figures (carers, volunteers, therapists etc.). From the start, the mutual handling of relapses needs to be a priority in the community. If one member of the community relapses, every flatmate's reaction must be heard. The expression of one's opinion is an important impulse for the relapsing individual, but also for non-relapsing individuals because it prevents repression. This is important because alcohol dependents have become accustomed to denial and looking away. Often, nonrelapsing persons are cautious in confronting the relapsing flatmate because they are often personally affected as well ("I have relapsed before and it could always happen again"). This inhibition is not entirely negative as it suggests a careful approach to others' weaknesses, which is very important when living in a community.

The ability to repress something harmful, the Freudian "defence mechanism", is an important life competency. Its stress relieving function is often not realized until it is no longer sufficiently present and the affected is overwhelmed with negative thoughts and flashbacks which cause anxiety and depression.

Mutually determined sanctions can also be helpful in certain groups (e.g. certain additional joint services). If this path is chosen, it is pedagogically advisable to make sure that sanctions are voluntarily accepted and don't humiliate the individual. Therapeutic "sanctioning" should not be employed as it has nothing to do with co-habituation in everyday life.

Especially "fascinating" are the rather rare "collective relapses" of two or three residents. This can in some cases be described by Bion's mechanisms of "pairing", a strategy which serves to compensate insecurity in a group.

Any clarification of the motives and the, for the community, very distressing course of events, is difficult for the community because of different needs and underlying pathogenic mechanisms. Yet, an attempt should at least be made to understand the underlying mechanisms. In the long run, collective knowledge about personal backgrounds and dependence causing mechanisms should be developed In this respect, it is important to let resistance towards reprocessing (coming to terms with the past) "dissolve", whereas tough confrontations are rarely productive or necessary. Timing plays a big role: one must be able to wait until "it is ok". Therapeutic processes, e. g. positive development cannot be forced.

Example:
In a residential community for five people, two residents are "co-relapsing". A. buys the alcohol which is consumed by A. and B. in A.'s room. The relapse lasts several days. B. suffers from epileptic seizures and needs to be admitted to an in-patient hospital. A. is drinking so heavily that he also requires outpatient support.
The analysis shows very different motives for the relapse. B. has been relapsing for a longer time. His physical condition has deteriorated in the past months due to compensated liver cirrhosis and cardiac problems. He tries to "endure" his organic disorders (digestive disorders, shortness of breath, oedema in the arms and legs) as well as his anxiety and depression by drinking alcohol, which further worsens his condition. It is in fact like a vicious circle which he can't escape.
A. has very different motives. Since he moved to the residential community several months ago, A. has been very withdrawn. Most of the time he stays in his room, only goes to the common room to eat and never takes part in mutual activities (playing cards, excursions, visits to the theatre etc.). A few weeks ago, he started to go to the common room more often and soon after also started to play cards. Everyone was very happy about this openness. With this step, A. became aware of his general social anxiety. Just as he had delayed taking a step towards the community, so he is now delaying the move from the residential community flat back into "life". In order to go outside and meet people, he needs alcohol, just like before when he used to live on the street. The opening up to other people caused him to come face to face with his social phobia.
The clarification of the motives behind the relapse is a relief for all the other residents.
While B. is in hospital, A. imposes a sanction upon himself of cleaning up B.'s room that was messed up during the relapse.

As already mentioned and as the example above has shown, the connection of medical-psychiatric care facilities is essential for crises intervention and the support of multiply affected alcohol dependents with severe organic impairments. Cooperation between the care

facilities and the hospital should guarantee that essential interventions, like temporary in-patient admission, take place quickly and reliably. For this to happen, a basis of trust needs to be first established between the psychiatric clinic and the care facility in order to neutralise the institution-based boundaries and misjudgements. This shortens the duration of relapses and limits organic damage.
The carers of the residential community are responsible for crisis intervention, but the support from flatmates is also desired and helpful.

Violence
On principle, in all social institutions, violence (and sometimes the mere threat of violence) means that the individual concerned has to move out. This is usually written down in the tenancy agreement. Of course, this rule is subject to modification if the resident has had a longer period of occupancy and is deeply rooted in the community (attachment), especially if the majority of residents want the affected to stay. If this is the case, it is important to collectively and objectively confront (including by visualizing) the dangers and the possible preventative strategies. (What can be learned from this episode? Were there identifiable triggers? How can protective mechanisms be integrated? Were there any danger signals? Would an alternative course of behaviour have prevented the violent incident?). Further, it is important that other residents admit their share of the blame, although without doubt, the institution itself has ultimate responsibility for violent incidents, and by the same token, for the protection of its employees.

Example:
A resident goes "overboard" in the residential care community. Although he is only slightly intoxicated, he threatens one resident with a knife. The latter escapes to his room and calls the police. The police bring the offender to a psychiatric unit which discharges him the same evening. The psychiatrist points out that, due to brain degradation, only a small amount of alcohol is needed to cause a psychotic reaction.
The offender is repentant and apologizes to the "victim". All residents advocate the offender's staying in the community, although they know that such reactions could happen again during a relapse. They hope that the readjustment of the medication will improve the situation. The housing carers accept the experiment after having discussed it with the institution. The offender receives a warning.

Role and function of the carer
The past paragraphs have shown that personal and pedagogical requirements and tensions in permanent residential care facilities are very different to those in transitional settings. Certainly the community's learning and development process also serves as a learning process for the carer(s), a process which should be constantly reflected upon (supervision). In a setting without temporal restrictions, carers and residents form stronger attachments which can also lead to deeper emotional involvement. This implies that classic transferences and countertransferences are more frequent, e. g. disappointments (anger, ag-

gravation), deeper involvement in private matters (worry, grief), reduced ability to set personal boundaries in cases of relapse and disease (not being able to switch off) etc. The carer's involvement in such a community is an intensive and rewarding experience, which should not be overlooked. A natural give and take of attention, care and help etc. is "normal" and its attainment a constant aim. Yet, it is also important to continuously explore the boundaries in regard to what is "healthy" and "viable" for the community and the carers.

On principle, the classic divergence of social work which takes up positions between the poles of *personal responsibility* (the community's) and *external responsibility* (the carer, the institution), applies likewise to the running of a residential care community. In a supported housing project for psychologically and physiologically impaired people who live in a communal environment that is vulnerable to conflict, the institution is, unquestionably, in charge of financial, legal and safety related issues. Within this framework, personal responsibility should be striven for as far as possible.

The fundamental decision to live as a community, which needs first to be made by the group, implies permitting each other sufficient living space, facing crises together, not running away or marginalizing someone (mobbing). This creates a highly effective learning situation, for carers as well: not being able to (nor wanting to) kick someone out so quickly, but instead finding solutions, together with the community, even in the most difficult situations and phases of tension and conflict, is an enormous pedagogical challenge which can only be met if the carer is willing to learn, which also perhaps implies, critically appraise previous experiences and knowledge, not stick too hard and fast to the rules, or resort to institutional violence as a solution because these interfere with motivation (positive relationships) and co-creative processes. The biggest challenge is to trust the self-organising processes of the community and to remain reticent despite irritating or chaotic phases. This includes accepting helplessness, disorientation and disappointments and being able to wait for developments and not always pretending to have answers for every question that arises, and an intervention to fit every critical situation. Working with a community of psychologically impaired dependents in a family-like situation is surely a job which can tax carers to their limits. Those who haven't developed an awareness of their personal limits and haven't learned how to take care of themselves, might be at risk of burn-out. The unavoidable requirement for handling these processes is honesty with oneself and this is also what we expect from our patients and clients.

Countertransference

One of the most important dimensions of self-awareness in sociotherapeutic practice is the detection of transferences and countertransferences in relationships, which are activations of early, often infantile, relationship patterns. The blending and reactivation of different relationship types and needs is a reality, which is a general part of human communication, but should be sensibly handled in psychosocial practice. The following will list some recommendations which can help to identify one's own tendency towards countertransference (Baumgartner 2003):

- If I am experiencing strong feelings of uneasiness, sadness, despair or the opposite, adoration, enthusiasm, excitement in the presence of a client with whom I am in conversation.
- If I am suddenly experiencing sudden surges of interest or feelings of rejection, and vigorous and long discussions with the client
- If the client's criticisms and reproaches hurt me.
- If I am experiencing vivid and conscious gratification as a result of his open praise, signs of contentment, attention and acceptance of me.
- If I am not in a position to refuse to give what the client demands of me (e.g. reassurance, encouragement, praise, an assertion of authory).
- If I constantly encourage dependence in my relationship with clients through continually reassuring them.
- If I feel obligated to help him by interfering with the client's social life, taking initiatives in his stead (e.g. calling the doctor), or using my personal influence to smooth out difficulties.
- If I am encouraging the client to aggressively free himself from a relationship he no longer wants (family, boss, spouse).
- If I am indifferent to the therapy situation at hand (delay, choice of the room, appointment of a date), or the opposite, if I handle material details with special accuracy and punctuality.
- If I like telling my friends and acquaintances about the client by emphasising his importance and character traits, or by talking ironically or cynically about him.
- If I am constantly wanting to find out whether things turn out all right for him, or whether he is following my advice, or if I am trying to maintain contact with him for as long as possible.
- If I am dreaming about my clients.

Each of these behaviours or experiences *can* be a sign of an insufficient boundary but on the other hand, it should be made clear that each of these signs only becomes significant within a specific context. Furthermore, reflection about one's own style of communication and support is required in order to understand the meaning of these patterns. This list consists of suggestions not principles.

10.7 Motivation – a challenge for whom?

10.7.1 Ambivalent functions of motivation

Unfortunately, the expectation that psychiatrists, doctors and other specialists are unbiased, neutral and non-judgemental morally with regard to alcohol and other substance dependents, is often unjustified. Projections, the consequences of which are mostly borne by patients and, because of which, the whole system of dependence support suffers, are very common. On the one hand, this is linked to the practitioners' poor self-awareness and the demanding working conditions which prevail in psychiatric settings, but also to society's unchanging attitude towards alcohol dependents. Society's high expectations of alcohol dependents, namely complete abstinence, crassly contradict its negative valuation of alcohol dependence.

Every practitioner can cite instances where the diagnostically defined, pathological significance of alcohol dependence has not been sufficiently, or only half-heartedly, brought to bear on the case. For example, in some places it is common practice to charge alcohol dependents for rescue operations, or to support, in case conferences, the mythical argument that suffering, especially a high degree of it, has therapeutic value. ("The patient has not yet reached the decisive low point of his alcoholic career. The level of suffering is not high enough."). Although stated a century ago, it is probable that Ziegler was right in suggesting:

> "Dependents are still seen in a negative way, despite all the education and information, so that it takes a long time until the patient accepts the diagnosis of "addiction" and makes uses of the treatment on offer. To wait for motivation which has been induced by the pressure of acute suffering, is unethical, produces irreversible damage, worsens the prospects for treatment and increases the mortality rate in dependents.
>
> *(Ziegler 1992)"*

This still (in our society) widely accepted moral concept of alcohol dependence has led to its definition as a degenerative disease for which the individual himself is largely responsible. One of the historically tragic consequences of this type of thinking is to be found in National Socialism where alcohol dependence was defined as being an "unworthy life" and thereby used to legitimate the killing of people.

Why then is the motivation paradigm still being used in practice today? Probably because it is in line with modern society's performance orientation: "If alcohol dependents are able to booze", then they can make an effort if they want to receive therapy. Such demands towards cancer patients or people with diabetes would be rejected with outrage. Alcohol dependents are more like "us" because they do what we do: consume alcohol, reward themselves with alcohol, celebrate … this is why they have to meet the same performance criteria as we do. This attitude probably entails the widespread opinion in society that dependences are a result of a lack of willpower and weakness of character, which only supports the unrealistic demand for performance[17] [18]. And in all this, they demonstrate to normal citizens quite plainly the collapse of their own performance ideology.

The use of the term "motivation" is often used to select certain "subgroups" of alcoholics who are appar-

---

17 In a survey, carried out in 2006, asking 1,000 Austrian citizens about the causes and target groups to which they donate money, it was shown that most sums went to children (40%), catastrophies (27%) and the handicapped (17%). Only 1% of donations went to drug and alcohol dependents who therefore represented the end of the "popularity scale". Source: APA-market research.

18 The sociological arguments for this thesis can be found in the anomy theories ranging from Durkheim to Merton, see Reinhardt 2005. Here, civilisation's request for the individual to demonstrate self-control is explored as a theme (Norbert Elias). The failure to demonstrate the required self-control leads to sanctions or compensations, like stigmatising the ill, which relives both the individual and society.

ently more likely to profit from withdrawal therapy. Grosso modo this is one of many selection processes within medical and psychiatric selections. No state or society can afford to pay for psychiatric and sociotherapeutic care for all those who are psychologically ill. Only a certain percentage of the psychologically ill receives specialist treatment and a specific selection programme then decides which treatment is offered. The assessment of "motivation" is one of these selection methods. What is really assessed in this selection can only be assumed because there are only a few valid investigations. Unfortunately, it is probable that the aim of these processes is the selection of those patients who can be best taken care of by the respective therapy system. It is not the clinical condition, nor the degree of suffering, that is considered, but the suitability of the individual for a particular therapy system. Conversely, this has an effect on the system's success rate: if I am only treating patients who are still able to self-regulate themselves (e.g. type II dependents), I shall obtain better results as a therapist/therapy system. In this way, it is not the quality of therapy that determines the success of therapy, but the selection of patients. If these hypotheses are valid, it seems logical that type III and type IV patients, who have a poor prognosis, are less frequently admitted to therapy programmes than other subgroups[19].

In regard to the therapist-client relationship, Schwoon has discerned a further function of the concept of motivation: "Although we don't have much scientific knowledge about motivation, the investigation of this concept fulfils a very important function. It leads all practitioners involved in treatment to distant themselves from disappointing experiences. The reason why therapy failed, e.g. due to a relapse, is ascribed to the patient's non-existing or weak motivation. Like this, deficiencies in theoretical and therapeutic concepts don't have to be critically examined (Schwoon 1992).

A doctor's, counsellor's or social worker's criticism of the patient's inadequate motivation towards therapy is often a projection or, at least, a reduction of the underlying complexity of the disorder[20]. In any case, the concept of motivation is usually seen as an attribute of the patient, without considering the therapeutic environment. Yet it is obvious that motivation depends on interaction, which requires successful and satisfactory interaction between counsellor/doctor and patient. Also, many other "contextual factors" play a role: conversational situation, patient's condition, acknowledgement of the disease, transference and countertransference, the patient's case history in the institution, the doctor's ability to show empathy, mutuall sympathy or antipathy etc. (Ziegler 1997).

19 The number of type IV patients receiving continuing treatment is below average. "It seems that therapists are still trying to make work easier by motivating patients, who already show certain amounts of self-motivation, in both motivational and withdrawal therapy". Oberlaender, Platz, Mengering 1998

20 Also Rauchfleisch, who argues from a psychoanalytical perspective, has stated that a unilateral motivation concept could be debilitative. He thinks it possible that the patient experiences the therapist's rejection as a narcissistic insult: "If we want to offer efficient and professional help, then we have to critically analyze the traditional concept of motivation and examine whether the so-called "lack of motivation" really is a characteristic of the client or whether it might represent a problem belonging to the therapist." (Rauchfleisch 2002)

When aetiopathology claims the existence of several subgroups of dependents, then it makes sense to assume that different "motivation types" exist as well. But this typology is probably psychologically questionable because dependence type and motivation are not necessarily linked. Nevertheless, the typology leads one to expect that there is more than just one right kind of "motivation" and that it is more appropriate to speak of a "motivational process". This process is always determined by a number of people who can change over time and during treatment.

10.7.2 The relationship between dependence and motivation systems

Abstinence is the most common measure of motivation. This urgently needs to be questioned, as we know that dependents are psychologically and neurobiologically different. This is especially important when abstinence is already the aim at the beginning of withdrawal treatment and when psychoorganic brain disorders (e. g. symptomatic transitory psychotic syndrome) are causing increased psychological and physiological instability. It should be noted that even after "somatic withdrawal symptoms" have diminished after five to ten days, relapses must be anticipated for weeks and even months[21]. The assessment of motivation during this withdrawal crisis which gets more and more acute, is rather absurd.

From a neurological perspective, "motivation", namely the ability to follow a certain goal, takes place in the same system in which the biological correlate for dependence is located.

These are the *reward* systems in the striatum and ventral tegmentum (Rommelspacher 1992), and in particular in the nucleus accumbens. Here, the "motivation aggregates for survival" are located which stimulate the motivation process by releasing dopamine, endorphins and oxytocin (the hormone which produces emotional attachments). At the same time, all neurological processes that lead to the development of a dependence, take place in the so-called "mesolimbic and mesocortical dependence axis".

Motivation and dependence therefore are rooted in the same neuronal mechanisms, suggesting that dependences are in a way also "disorders" of the motivation system. The impairment of these systems makes it even more difficult to judge dependents in regard to their motivation.

Knowledge about the brain's *reward* centres and results from neurobiological brain research, show that the motivation systems operates "socially", implying that its aims are sustainable relationships.

"The natural aim of the motivation systems is a social community and positive relationships with other individuals. This does not only concern personal relationships that encompass love and affection, but all forms of social interaction.

For the individual, this implies that the essence of motivation is to find and to give interpersonal acceptance, appreciation, attention

21 In the literature, these phenomena are described as "protracting withdrawal syndrome" (Feuerlein, Schuckit) or as phases of degradation (Scholz). (Schuckit et al. 1994)

or affection. From a neurobiological perspective, human beings are designed for social resonance and cooperation."

(Bauer 2006, p. 34)

The notion that the motivation system (Bauer 2006b) is stimulated by social factors can be understood by examining the loss of social integration. Isolation (mobbing, exclusion from the community) can lead to a psychogenic death. Social isolation or exclusion, if protracted, can lead to apathy and the collapse of all types of motivation. Stress systems are activated, blood pressure and the risk of a heart attack increases, the nucleus accumbens decreases in substance and is less active and pain centres in the brain are activated. On the other hand, an intact social integration has positive effects on health and socially integrated people live longer. Unintentional loneliness is a life-threatening factor.

These results are of great importance for all human sciences and their applications (school, education, social work, psychotherapy etc.), because the basis of every motivation is primarily the formation of sustainable relationships and not just the expression of competitiveness or the sexual drive.

Joachim Bauer (2006a), who hypothesizes that the "social brain" is the centre of motivation, distinguishes between five elements of motivation and relationship respectively:

1. **To see and to be seen (attention)**
   Motivation, which means that sustainable relationships start by noticing the other and vice versa, and with the willingness to show oneself to others

2. **Mutual attention**
   Mutual interest in something and interest in the other's concerns promotes the formation of a relationship. To be mutually interested in, or to stick up for something, conveys the feeling: *I care about you!*
   It is important to me to understand the way you see the world.

3. **Emotional resonance**
   This is the ability to adapt to the emotions of the counterpart or to get one's emotions across so that the other is able to adapt to them. People who are emphatic are perceived as likeable.

4. **Cooperation**
   Doing something together, planning and realizing it, enhances the relationship. This is "motivation" in the strictest sense, namely to "mutually set something in motion for the sake of something/someone" (Latin: movere). This factor is used by sociotherapy in the shared organisation of daily life.

5. **The reciprocal understanding of motives and intentions**
   A relationship requires the ability to intuitively and analytically understand the other's motivation. In doing so, often opinions (diagnosis) from third parties and from one's own life history, which could be projected onto others, need to be checked and in some cases corrected. This demands good observation skills during conversations.

Thus, motivation is not just "present" or "not present" or "not sufficiently present", but is established in the formation of a mutual relationship. It might be that it is difficult to establish a relationship with certain people and it might be that institutional circumstances (e.g. lack of time, strict observance of privacy rules etc.) complicate the establishment of a relationship. Yet, in regard to motivation for treatment, the question as to how a relationship with the patient/client can directly or indirectly be established should always be explored. If this does not work out or is not even attempted, the motivation concept should not be used.

In regard to motivational work in dependence support, it is important to meet the dependent at the level "where he is at" currently. Distance is usually counterproductive. Kuntz emphasises that it is more efficient to approach the patient than to wait for him to make the first move as it establishes a positive "transference". A high-threshold attitude, which waits for the patient to act, only embraces patients that are already sufficiently motivated to come to the institution (Kuntz 2000)[22].

This is in line with epidemiologic analyses that have found that dependence support institutions are very competent and successful in high-threshold domains (counselling centres, hospitals), but only reach a small target group of dependents that are better structured (type I and type II dependents). In regard to therapy policy, traditional dependence support meets all criteria of the "Inverse Care Law": The individuals who are doing relatively well, receive the most, and the best quality, help – and vice versa (Poerksen 2001).

Should the dependents' motivation be confronted with the high-threshold approach of most therapy options?

10.8 Sociotherapy as network promoter

The number of differentiations and specialisations in both health and social occupations, and institutions (with their scarce resources), leads to unclear boundaries and competitiveness as well as alienation towards those depending on these systems (see Hermann Spaeth's statement at the beginning of this chapter). Social therapy is also responsible for the identification of any "negative consequences resulting from these differentiations, specialisations and hierarchies and, following an examination of this area, for generating solutions." (Schwendter 2000, p. 13) In this context, micro-and meso levels of sociotherapy cover these aspects:

- **optimising flow of information**
  (Who needs which information in order to act? Who works together? Who communicates the information to the clients?)
- **clarity of client contracts**
  (Who is in charge of the case? Where are the boundaries of the contract?)

22 In line with this, the renowned expert for personality disorders, Peter Fiedler, has summed up: "It is quite terrifying how we have adapted to specific schools of therapy and methodological therapy and profession stereotypes. In reality, the attempt to generate solutions and perspectives with individuals who have reached the limit of their possibilities is often hopeless. Dialogue-based psychotherapy, which only takes place in the therapy room, is mere nonsense in many of these extreme cases. The antiquated and possibly completely absurd 45-minute rhythm of a private practice with a "come attitude", binds the psychotherapist to his armchair in his role as a helper. Especially this approach needs change gradually, when dealing with people, who have come to grief in life!" (Fiedler 1998, S. 399).

- **informing the affected person**
  (Is the institution still acting on behalf of the client or is it already detached from the client's level of knowledge?)
- **integrating family and other attachment figures**
  To this end, the interconnection of all persons involved, and thereby the creation of *multiple perspectives* and *transdisciplinarity*, is indispensable for *casework*.

On a macro level it is essential to:

- **Create cooperation between all domains involved.** It is important to understand how an institution functions and "thinks" (e.g. separation and selection mechanisms) so that clients who are particularly difficult to handle, are not pushed from one institution to the next. This applies especially to psychiatry and the homeless sector. These domains often lack political solutions.
- **Gather and provide resources and regulate them** (admission criteria, enforcement acts), e.g. subsidies, government aid and project support programmes etc.
- **Develop, discuss and implement standards for care, pedagogical support, housing etc.** (guidelines, handbooks, expert meetings ...)
- **Do public relations, lobbying and political work.**

10.8.1 Micro and meso levels of networking

In regard to its "networking" aspects, sociotherapy is similar to "network therapy", where systemic and behavioural therapeutic principles are often predominant within community psychology (Roehrle et al. 1998). Florian Straus and Renate Hoefer (1998) have highlighted the sociotherapeutic orientation towards community, integration and empowerment and list seven important characteristics of networking:

- **Network analysis** is needed before networking can take place.
  The psychodramatic perspective of the "social atom" can be used in this case. The social atom in-cooperates all attachment figures and their respective relationship to the affected person. Closeness and distance, conflict and empathy are described as follows: "A social atom with a good consistency is marked by a high number of positive and a low number of negative relationships between close individuals and by numerous relationships between individuals (...), a balanced distribution of closeness and distance in all relationships as well as connections to other social atoms." (Petzold)

  Example:
  Mr B. got divorced four months ago and had to leave the marital flat. At the moment, he lives in a double room in a transitional residential home. He has completely lost touch with his family. As he doesn't have his own flat anymore, his children can't visit him at the weekends. As he has no reason to visit his wife anymore, he loses all contact to the mutual friends. His only contact is with his sister, who he meets once or twice a month, but she is suffering from cancer – a

further stress factor for Mr B. Network analysis shows that he has enormous social deficits, which need to be compensated for. Together with his social worker, Mr B. looks for people he knew before he got married. He decides to contact friends from school and further considers visiting a single club. Despite his reluctance, he decides to buy a mobile phone so that people can get in touch with him more easily.

- Often networking functions as **replacement work**.
  Networking **disintegrates problematic networks.**
  If the network consists of negative members who fail to change and negatively affect one's sense of self-worth, it is important to separate oneself from this network. This is the case when, for instance, alcohol dependents stop going to pubs with "old friends" as they know that these contacts might promote a relapse. If the affected manages to give up the old "pub contacts", he becomes socially isolated. Thus, abstinence comes at a high price. The depravation of the social atom causes stress and is destabilising. In order to prevent relapses, these defective relationships need to be replaced with stable, alcohol abstinent contacts. However, individuals with social deficits often find it very difficult to handle this.

Fig. 112 Deficient social atoms

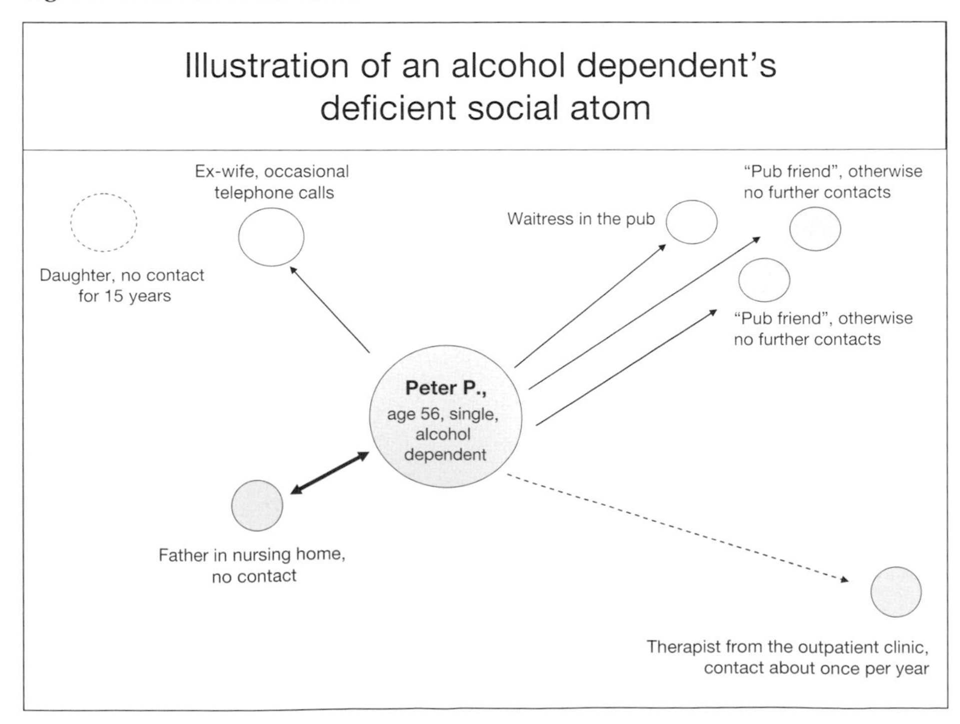

One aim of networking is to detect social resources:
Are there any possible contacts in the client's family?
Are there any possible contacts in the occupational environment?
Are there any possible contacts in recreational activities? Etc.

The following example tackles whether a client could (and would like) to contact his daughter or whether the contact to his ex-wife could be intensified. In addition, further resources need to be sought in the client's biography.

The disintegration of networks might also entail a separation from one's own family. When evaluating networks, it is important to consider the quality of the relationships: are they strengthening or weakening? Do they create or protect from crises?

Example:
After Mr B. got divorced, he started visiting his parents more frequently. His father constantly criticises him because, after having completed withdrawal treatment, he moved to a transitional home ("living with the homeless"). His mother is worried that "now he won't get back on his feet at all". Mr B. experiences these meetings as very strenuous and constantly has a bad conscience, even many days after visiting. Mr B. doesn't dare to even think about visiting his parents less often. He feels indebted towards his parents and puts up with their attacks.
It is important that Mr B. re-evaluates his relationship with his parents. Their expectations and the dynamics of interaction need to be questioned. Systemic or transaction-analytical interpretations of this relationship could show Mr. B. that his parents try to confine him to a dependent child ego role. His "bad conscience" is a crucial factor in this. How could a parent-son relationship be formed which does not cause a "bad conscience"? What are the parent's fears? What are the son's fears? What is being defended against? What kind of function has the "bad conscience"?

- Networking also promotes **social identity.**
Integration into a social system provides resources, security and identity. The peer group is the matrix of identity. It pretty much describes which "role" the individual plays in regard to others and the world. Individuals who live on "the edge of society", often suffer from extreme fluctuations in self-confidence. Sociotherapeutic interventions can stabilise identity. In doing so, the sociotherapists' feedback is an important input into the system. Also the network (family, living community…) can learn how to provide feedback by receiving extrinsic positive feedback and frequent up-dates about what the affected has "achieved" so far. In this process, "diagnoses" and other stigmatising attributions are disregarded, while the individual becomes the centre of focus.

Example:
Every year the theatre project "Kreativ am Werk" stages a new production. Mostly alcohol de-

pendents and individuals with other diagnoses take part in the play. After the opening night, participants receive feedback. This includes watching a video recording followed by discussion and also intensive feedback. Especially compelling were feedback sessions that took place in an educational institution, where every participant sat down in a "hot seat" and listened to what the others appreciated about his/her "input" into the project. This kind of long-term collaboration paired with open feedback has significant effects on the development of identity. Everyone who was part of this project experienced a feeling of belonging, despite competitiveness and crises. Furthermore, this ritual encourages people to provide feedback to others as well. After this ritual, one participant said: "Now I finally know, that I am actually good for something".

- Networking monitors and develops **helper networks.**
  Many clients have a long history of helper experience. As a result of having stayed at several institutions and after countless withdrawal treatments, clients may have 'collected' a number of helpers who are "more or less" active. Often diffuse and even confused helper-client relationships are encountered which need to be resolved. It must be made clear which relationships are helpful and stabilising and which are destabilising (e.g. due to a strong dependence, or manipulative behaviour etc.). It is possible that a *helper conference* needs to be organised. In this conference, the person who will be responsible for the case and the supporting measures which still need to be taken, should be determined.

  Example:
  Thomas L., 38, has been suffering from diabetes since childhood. He drinks to cope with his disease-related depression, which has lead to fluctuations in his sugar level resulting in several hospital stays. Motivated by his fear of social isolation, he has accumulated an entire "network of helpers": once a month he visits a diabetes self-help group, every week he goes to a "fun group", he takes part in a theatre group in the neighbourhood support centre and he attends regular therapy meetings with a psychologist and social worker who are located at two psychosocial institutions. Furthermore, his debt counsellor arranges private insolvency and once a month he goes to dependence aftercare at the outpatient clinic for alcohol dependents. Lastly, he found a mentor at a church group (where he sings in the choir) who helps him improve his housing situation by arranging a change of residence.
  In the meantime, Thomas L. starts to feel very exhausted due to all of these appointments. To this day, no one has attempted to initiate a case conference to enable all helpers to meet.

- Networking **creates new networks**.

Radical life events (retirement, chronic disease, divorce etc.) can cause a collapse of the "social atom" which means that important attachment figures and resources are lost. The compensation of missing persons in the network becomes more and more difficult with increasing age or/and psychosocial problems. Sociotherapy needs to focus on creating "prosthetic social atoms" (e.g. recreational groups, visits, day care…). The organisation of telephone chains, e.g. when working with the elderly, has proven to be an effective strategy. Other possibilities could be postcard chains, rotating venues when visiting people (e.g. playing cards at different hosts' places), meeting at certain events, organising a "jour fixe", taking part in group, recreational and cultural activities etc. Groups that are too homogenous become boring and instable over time. This also applies to self-help groups in which clients only define themselves by their "problems". An effective approach for organising and stabilising a social network is **collaboration**. Active contributions make social situations more interesting and strengthen self-efficacy by shaping social conditions. Additionally, having a certain place within a social environment (through being given responsibility for a certain task) reduces anxiety. If one wants to integrate individuals who suffer from anxiety into a social network, assigning them a specific task has been shown to be the most effective method.

Example:
For many years, Mr V. lived in several assisted housing institutions and five years ago he moved to a retirement home for the formerly homeless. He is an alcoholic and regularly faces crises. Usually he relapses due to anxiety or "when he can't switch off his thoughts". His live-in partner died one year ago. As both spent most of their time together, Mr V.'s entire daily structure collapsed all at once. Through contacts in his church community, he joins a theatre group, where he takes a small part. Due to frequent rehearsals, he meets many other members of the group. Furthermore, he starts going to mass every Sunday. He also gets in touch with an occupational therapy centre again. An adjustment of medication helps him to control his panic attacks and sleeping disorders. Once a month, he takes part in a sociotherapeutic group. The diversity of these measures helps Mr V. to stabilise his social atom.

- Networking **strengthens existing networks.**
  Network analysis has shown that clients often lose contact to any former social groups. Often clients feel very ashamed about any dependence-related events (divorce, loss of flat, receiving social welfare) and fear social stigmatisation, so they escape into isolation. Sociotherapeutic intervention can support clients in getting back in touch with their social contacts. For example, the support person in charge can join the

client in going to a football pitch, if that is where the client regularly used to go.

Example:
Mr C. has told his social worker that he used to go to a football pitch with his friends every Saturday and Sunday when he was younger. Due to the divorce, the loss of his job and his flat, he has isolated himself more and more and has lost almost all of his contacts. Recently he met one of his friends coincidentally and they exchanged numbers in order to organise a get-together at the football pitch. Mr C. is not sure whether he wants to get in touch again because he is afraid his friend will find out about his social comedown and reject him. The social worker encourages him not to be ashamed of his "different life experiences" and to contact his friend. In a spontaneous role play, they practice the "confession".

It needs to be pointed out again that sociotherapy uses the potential of **non-professionals** (volunteers, laymen helpers etc.). This is a fundamental sociotherapeutic networking strategy, not least because laymen helpers, who aren't paid and or appointed by institutions, can more easily connect the client with "normality".

Furthermore, networking considers "changes in daily life" on a political level. It uses **PR and lobbying** (Schwendter 2000), which for example leads to the founding of **self-help groups** or **citizens' initiatives**. Also, alternative facilities (places where affected individuals from institutions meet with "normal" people e.g. inpatient cafes, tearooms, mixed theatre groups, recreational groups, neighbourhood help projects, housing projects where old and young live together) are interventions that support the community.

Medication-oriented health systems which work with diagnoses and specific rules, often have debilitating effects on the client (see hypothesis on motivation in this chapter).

Generally it is important that networks are not **homogenous** (e.g. consisting of only old or alcohol dependent individuals). A homogenous group promotes stigmatisation and separation and due to a lack of human and spiritual vitality they become instable and unsustainable. Heterogenic networks have more resources, offer more diversity, stimulation and activities. Also, heterogenic groups have a tendency to grow, as new people are consistently brought along and new connections to other networks are made (Hass and Petzold 1999).

A concluding example illustrates the "radicalness" and, at the same time, efficiency of sociotherapeutic networking. In America, "multi-systemic" therapy has established itself in social work with recently released prisoners. This form of intervention is an explorative method which accompanies the client in his respective life environments, e.g. to school, flats, homes, on the street – pretty much everywhere where released prisoners spend their time. This method does not use diagnoses. The aim is that the sociotherapist gets to know the client's social network and discovers its weaknesses. The main focus is on the network's available resources, thus on the availability of persons who could stabilise (mentor) the adolescent delinquent. This could be a former schoolmate, a relative, someone from the church community etc. In the second phase, the sociotherapist assists the client in spending lots of time with his mentor and breaking ties with people who could lead him into prison again. This therapeutic intervention can take up to 4 months. Several studies have shown that 25–70 % of clients managed to stay relapse-free three years after having been released (Boruin et al. 1995.

10.8.2 Macro levels of networking

Social conditions (see chapter 10.4.2) are mirrored on all levels and thus also on the institutional and political level. Political conditions not only promote or impede certain interpretations of cases, but also determine the methodologies and standards for institutions to use (e.g. closing of drug counselling institutions or homes for the mentally ill). Thus on a macro level external communication is very important for institutions that rely on political and financial support. On the other hand reasonable legislation would not be possible without the inclusion of institutions that work "at the basis".

The reformation of psychiatry (1975 in Germany, 1979 in Italy, around 1980 in Austria, in the US much earlier [Szasz 1980, 1994]) has lead to an increase in outpatient and extramural care of mentally ill patients. Yet, it has failed to consider the selection process of patients, which has led to a reduction of in-patient therapy places. The fact is that there are not enough places for all patients who require in-patient treatment. Psychotic patients, who are at risk of self-harm or harming others, are preferred over alcohol dependents. In short, general psychiatric hospitals use the "motivation argument" (see section on motivation) to "de-select" alcohol dependents regardless of their acute somatic and psychological co-morbidities. Therefore, more and more mentally ill live in homeless institutions because they don't receive adequate psychiatric care. Homeless institutions are pressured and need solutions, which however can't be implemented without political assistance. Therefore the aim of networking should be to bring together representatives from homeless care and psychiatry and initiate an exchange between them. Yet these attempts often fail because of the different "terminology" used in these sectors, a terminology which in turn is based on different interpretations of reality. The aim of the networking process should be that both partners realize that available resources can only be used optimally by working together and that unilateral separation strategies are counterproductive.

Another essential function of networking on a macro level is the creation or optimisation of legal contexts, e.g. for the "hospital" – "residential home" connection.

Example:
A cooperative network has formed between retirement home A and hospital ward B as a result of years of contact. Clients and patients are directly transferred from the hospital to the residential home, whilst at the same time relapsing patients can be admitted to the ward for stabilisation or assessment. After finding out about this "flow of patients", the hospital su-

pervision intervenes and notices that these cooperative networks are illegal, despite having been shown to benefit patients. In this case, there is no legal protection for such networks.

Although psychosocial care institutions clearly need more networking, the drawbacks of networking processes need to be considered as well. Over time, the cooperation between institutions leads to mutual standards, which cause a uniformity of rules, methods and criteria. Thus, niches for certain clients might disappear.

10.9 Sociotherapy with alcohol dependents in the context of Lesch's typology

10.9.1 The critical relationship between psychiatry and sociotherapy

Although sociotherapy strives to focus on "normal" and "every day matters", in order to counteract the way in which the "ill" are treated by the medical system, and so as to refrain from superficial diagnoses, diagnostic attributions can't be avoided[23]. This is especially the case when working with target groups (e.g. admissions to type IV housing communities).

Psychiatry has become an institutional part of the judiciary and it returns verdicts of enormous diagnostic, social and judicial relevance, covering such issues as preventative detention, forensics, custodianship and compulsory committal.

Lesch's typology is a psychiatric classification system with a biological focus. It is used by practitioners "within the system" and is therefore located, from the outset, within this tense constellation. Although the typology considers social aspects, they are subordinate to biological factors.

This critical relationship should not be severed because it is basically productive and useful, as long as the dualism between psychiatry on the one hand, and the daily e living environment on the other, can be bridged. In this respect, psychiatry has an obligation to deliver, above all in view of the hierarchical gap between the medical and caring professions which exists in practice, whereby social work is often only seen as "unskilled work" and not as a discipline with equal value (Staub-Bernasconi 2007). In many areas, a systemic "non-cooperation" and alienation between psychiatry and social work exists, which has lead to pre-assigned roles, ignorance about working conditions and the other's perspectives, and political myopia. In regard to the current situation, which goes beyond German-speaking countries, the aims of psychiatric reform ("outpatient prior to in-patient-settings") are still poorly implemented in the health system even after two centuries. Many mentally ill individuals who need therapy still have to live in unsuitable housing facilities, which worsens their condition and overstrains the often poorly trained personnel. For this reason, social psychiatry is needed.

Only a mutual effort to accept alternative perspectives can lead to desired results. The nature of sociotherapy is "interdisciplinary" or "transdisciplinary" respectively and aims at discourse

23 As we have seen, the admission to, and payment of, sociotherapy is linked to assessment, thus to the diagnosis of a medical specialist

and networking, as described in previous sections; it seeks to initiate and encourage the "polylogue" (Petzold), which is the dialogue between all affected parties. Psychiatry needs to acknowledge that, apart from the patient's individual abilities, interventions are never effective on their own but always in combination with different interventions and resources ("polylogue"). In order to maximise effectiveness, factors should be assessed as follows:

The potency of sociotherapy lies in its complementary relationship with a variety of disciplines and standpoints. Ultimately, the aim of psychotherapy, psychiatry and sociotherapy is to become dispensable. The "client" or "patient" should disappear so that the "person" can emerge.

10.9.2 Application of the typology in sociotherapeutic contexts

Due to its transdisciplinary approach which brings together biological, psychological and sociotherapeutic aspects and allows conclusions to be drawn accordingly, the typology according to Lesch has also proven itself to be effective in sociotherapeutic practice. It is a valuable contribution to the differentiation process, especially in regard to the differentiation of aetiologies, which is the basis of sociotherapeutic intervention and planning. In Berlin, Lesch's typology was used for the development of the "residence at Schillerpark", and, in particular, in relation to the admission of patients from psychiatric facilities (Humboldt Hospital), where Lesch's typology has been used to categorize patients according to typology for over 15 years (type IV patients receive different care to patients in groups type I, II and III), an emphasis which has led to significant changes in the patient population (Oberlaender et al. 1999). In Austria, Lesch's typology is applied in several hospitals. Ginner (2006)carried out a study in which he used Lesch's typology in a homeless facility in Upper Austria to develop criteria for successful therapy.

Fig. 113 Therapeutic impact factors (Lesch)

Therapeutic impact factors:	
Medication	1/10
Psychotherapy	1/10
Social support	3/10
Patient's decision	5/10

For years, Lesch's typology has been incorporated into the training programmes of different institutions (for example, the newly created Caritas curriculum for social carers, training courses for social and health care managers etc). The Caritas' Vinzenz House in Vienna has been using the typology for years and has provided important data on typology. An analysis of residents confirmed that only few type I and type II alcohol dependents are found in homeless institutions, whereas types with acute personality disorders, previous cerebral damage or poor progressions (types III and IV) are in the majority (72%).

On the basis of two decades of experience in the field of social care in Vinzenz House, in the context of which it has been shown that certain alcohol dependents often manage to stay abstinent over many years as a result of the "dry environment" and their integration into the housing community (usually through becoming responsible for precise household duties, e.g. regular kitchen or porter duties) – and it should be added that these cases are almost always type IV alcohol dependents – an association named "STRUCTURE" was developed which established a permanent housing community for type IV alcohol dependents) in April 2006.

Five type IV alcohol dependents with a long history of therapy and whose goal is abstinence live together in a semi-assisted sociotherapeutic housing community. In order to support group culture, individual therapy is intentionally reduced to a minimum and is increased in cases of crises, while group work, which is adapted to the group's capabilities and needs, takes place regularly. The following two topics are the main focus of group work: living together on a daily basis and coping with relapses, whereby the factor "living together" is far more important, as it, in itself, prevents relapses. The aim of sociotherapeutic approaches is to develop "normality" in the context of living together i. e. in the daily life of the community (renovation work, setting up cable television, visits to the doctor's, cooking, organising recreational activities etc.). It could be shown already within the first year that disease progressions had dramatically improved. According to Lesch's (1985) Catchment Area Study, the average duration of abstinence (CAD) per year in type IV patients was *below 10%* (and was even less over a period of four years). In the type IV housing community, the duration of abstinence was very much above this trend (Annual report of the „STRUKTUR" society 2006/2007).

It can be concluded from this that the development of stable networks has a positive effect on patients and that the stability of the primary group, i.e. the residential community itself, is also an important factor, whereby the open-ended nature of the housing is

Fig. 114 Lesch types in homeless institutions

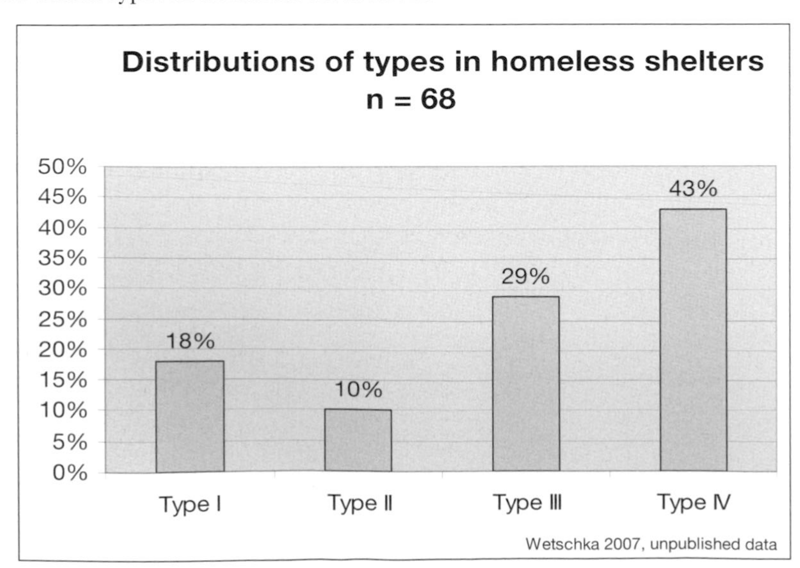

Fig. 115 Abstinence rates of type IV community residents

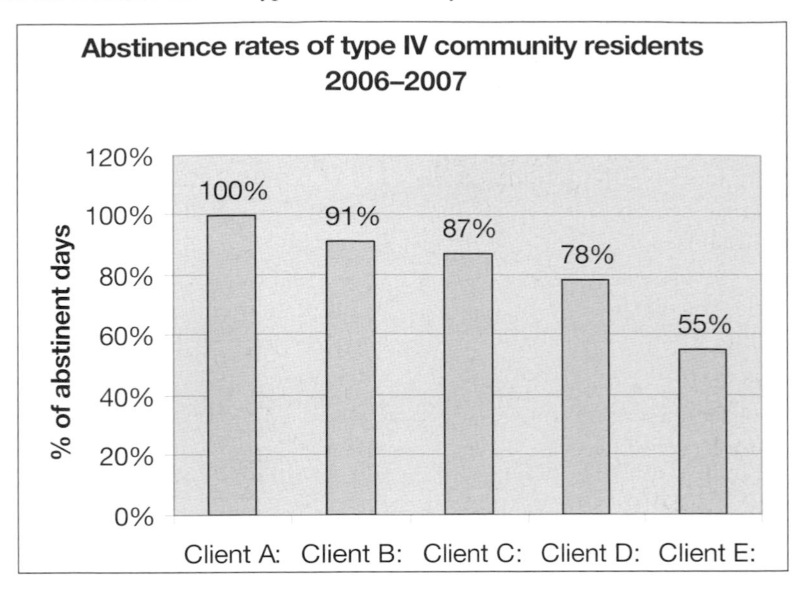

also likely to be significant, and this has proven itself to be relevant to group dynamics.

Transitional communities are clearly less stabilising housing forms.

Considering the fact that some clients in this community have severe traumata, the success of the concept is remarkable. There are four principles which seem to be efficient (Jahresbericht Verein Struktur 2008):

I.	principle: efficient treatment of the basic disorder
II.	principle: availability of immediate support
III.	principle: being productive on behalf of others/safe position in the social network
IV.	principle: connection to the outside – growth of the „Social Atom"[24]

24 The embedment of the individual in a social network is described by Jakob Moreno as the „social atom".

10.9.3 The relationship between type and self-regulation

Recommendations for all stages of treatment and care can be derived for every type, based on typology which suggests an association between aetiology and long-term progression. Strictly speaking, these four types are four different forms of alcohol/tobacco dependence, which consequently also need different therapeutic interventions and aims (see chapter 6.3).

Neurobiological conditions are represented on a behavioural and personality level. Every type correlates with different personality traits. In regard to the therapy of these different types, a leading criterion is the client's level of **self-regulation.** The ability to organise one's own life is a basic dimension of personality. It requires the interaction of cognitive and emotional aspects. Within the context of behavioural therapy, the term "self-efficacy" is often cited. The psychoanalytical perspective has described this notion as "ego strength", which is the apparatus that mediates the libidinal drive (id), the demands of the super-ego and the environment (social adaptability). The ability to regulate oneself implies that the individual is oriented around reality, but is "nevertheless" able to live a fulfilled life. The ego has several control mechanisms which affect the internal world (for example by blocking inappropriate momentary impulses) and act on the environment (e.g. a conflict is noticed and actively dealt with). Thus, ego strength is the systematic interaction of cognitive, emotional and social abilities which are located in the brain and which are linked to brain development and damage (including genetic dispositions). Sociotherapeutic and psychotherapeutic approaches should consider specific neuropsychological impairments in alcohol dependents. Although such impairments have been investigated and supported by research worldwide since the 60s-and 70s, they are rarely considered.

This low level of interest in, and often insufficient level of knowledge about, neuropsychological issues leads to misjudgement and mistreatment in the therapy of alcohol dependents and to an over- and under challenging of patients. Cognitive effects of impaired brain functions are often interpreted in a psychodynamic light. We only see what we know, and if we don't know enough about the causes of certain behaviours, we use our extensive depth psychological terminology and describe the things we see as resistance, defence mechanisms, repression, denial, belittlement, avoidance or unwillingness to change, in any case something neurotic (...). "In order for therapy to be successful, the therapist should know which of the patient's cortical structures and its related functions are impaired". (Steingass 1998)

Cognitive make-up (intelligence, noopsychological functions), level of education, the repertoire of social and emotional experiences and skills are the result of an interaction between genetic and biological structures (abilities, psychosexual orientation, cerebral deficits etc.) and socialisation (background). The personality which emerges from this complex dynamic, is *more or less able to be self-reflective,* plan his own behaviour and to be responsible for consequences, thus signalling a readiness or an ability to "adapt" to his social environment or positively arrange it ("high intelligence"). Linguistic and other levels of expressions are a further requirement for organizing one's life. These structures, which form the neuropsychological basis for dependence development, are located in the frontal cortex and need to be further discussed.

As each of the subgroups has different drinking and relapse patterns, it can be assumed that each has a different kind of *self-regulation ability:*

Type I (Allergy Type, biological causes):

Self-regulation usually breaks down in combination with alcohol (and nicotine). Generally, the ego is intact and there is enough ego-strength for coping with daily life.

Example:

Mr S., 36 years old, married, computer expert, was admitted to a detoxification centre. At the time of

Fig. 116 Lesch's typology in key words

Type I:	"Allergy"	The cause of the problem lies in the alcohol-metabolism
Type II:	"Anxiety"	Alcohol/nicotine as a solution to the conflict
Type III:	"Depression"	Alcohol/nicotine as an antidepressant
Type IV:	"Habituation"	Cerebral dysfunctions, impulse control disorder

admission, his blood alcohol level was at 3.5‰. Mr S. needed large amounts of alcohol every morning in order to control his withdrawal symptoms. He had to drink out of the bottle, as his tremor kept him from drinking from the glass. Further symptoms were acute sweating all over the body, rapid pulse and episodic anxiety. Three weeks ago, Mr S. collapsed while skiing on a slope. The emergency doctor suggested a circulatory collapse, while the doctor at admission suggested an epileptic seizure.
The anamnesis showed that Mr. S. is socially well integrated. At work, Mr S. experienced some alcohol-related problems for which he was able to compensate however.
Two weeks after withdrawal treatment, Mr S. is able to work at the computer again. In his spare time, he starts to train at the institution-owned fitness studio.
As Mr S. enjoys taking part in psychotherapeutic group meetings, he considers doing group therapy after he has finished with withdrawal therapy.

Type II (Conflict drinker, psychological causes):
Self-regulating ability breaks down in situations of tension, stress, conflict, anxiety etc. The ego is weakened in certain stressful situations; coping strategies have not been acquired or have been lost. A lack of self-esteem and a heightened emotional sensitivity further promote psychosocial instability.

Example:
Mrs P. has been living in homeless shelters on and off for the past several years. Whenever she needs to make a decision, she asks someone else to decide for her. She permanently needs affirmation and recognition in other areas of her life too and is unable to say "no" in most contexts. In the past, Mrs P. used to have partners on whom she was emotionally and financially dependent. At times, Mrs P. feels down and depressed and anxious during alcohol withdrawal. She is not able to live on her own. The severity of withdrawal symptoms is limited (two-dimensional tremor) and she has never had an epileptic seizure. There are no signs of polyneuropathy. Occasionally however, Mrs P. suffers from sleep-onset insomnia. The doctor found no organic brain damage. In the past, Mrs P. has always had abstinent phases, but just recently she has been drinking so much

that her blood alcohol level rose above 2 ‰.
Through talking to her counsellor, Mrs P. realised that she drinks alcohol in order to help her cope with stressful situations and emotions, e.g. when quarrelling with her boyfriend or a member of staff at the home. The medical specialist recommends psychotherapy as a way for Mrs P. to learn how to cope with stressful situations without drinking alcohol

Type III (affective disorder, mood swings, depression):
Self-regulation breaks down in phases of affective instability (depression, mania, hypomania). In some phases, ego strength decreases. Alcohol is used as a substitute for this loss of self-regulation. In stable phases, however, self-regulation can be maintained.

Example:
After several attempts, Mrs M. manages to go to a psychiatrist. She shows up blind drunk at the psychiatrist and drops onto a chair. She has been feeling exhausted for weeks. For months, she hasn't been able to sleep for more than three hours a night. Only when she has drunk a certain amount of alcohol is she able to sleep for four of five hours. Her psychiatrist knows that Mrs M. has previously undergone four withdrawal therapies. She had to give up her job as an accountant three years ago and she now lives off welfare. Her suicidal fantasies have become more frequent in the last months but she doesn't speak to anyone about them. Mrs M. knows very well that the sweating in the morning and slight hand tremor are withdrawal symptoms, but feels totally controlled by alcohol. She has lost a great deal of weight over the past months and in the last two weeks she has repeatedly collapsed due to vertigo. She takes the medication prescribed by her medical specialist only occasionally and the medication has no effect when combined with alcohol. Further in-patient therapy is inevitable. The course of the disease shows that acute depression has developed at least once a year over the last ten years. The medical specialist suggests Mrs M. undergo an "interval therapy", with shorter but more frequent in-patient stays.

Type IV (previous cerebral damage, reduction in performance, social deprivation):
Self-regulation is limited from the outset. The reduction in performance is constitutive and irreversible. Usually, not all areas of the personality are affected. The deficit is more visible in some aspects of personality than in others (inability to handle money, speech disorders, partial impairment of performance, sexual disinhibition, homelessness, negligence etc.). External mechanisms are needed to replace the missing self-regulation (structure formation).

Example:
Mr W. was diagnosed as a type IV patient. His father was alcohol dependent as well and Mr W.'s childhood and adolescence were affected accordingly. Furthermore, a birth defect was diagnosed. This

defect caused a partial impairment of performance. As it wasn't detected and treated, Mr W., although he had a wide range of interests, had to go to a special school. Even today, he is still substantially linguistically impaired. He still has reading and spelling difficulties. In later years, Mr W. developed an alcohol dependence. At the age of 28, he lost his flat and subsequently lived with relatives or in residential homes. A variety of alcohol therapies failed to have any positive effects. An analysis of his problems indicated that he has a sex, money and alcohol related regulation disorder. In order to fulfil his sexual desires, he needs to drink alcohol, which he needs to overcome his social phobia. Drinking alcohol in turn consequently leads to massive financial expenditures. Numerous withdrawal treatments, which only focused on Mr W.'s alcohol problem, were ineffective. A therapy that tackles his sexual issues is not possible and also questionable. The current carer of Mr W. takes care of his finances and tries to organise satisfying activities (a daily structure) for Mr W. His "alcohol" problem becomes seen as secondary.

10.9.4 Types and aims of therapy

When considering the different aetiologies of alcohol dependence, it can be assumed that alcohol consumption has different functions in each deregulated self-system. For different reasons, the ego loses its self-regulatory ability and alcohol is used to cope with any unpleasant and distressful aspects of a stressful situation. This is especially the case when interpersonal relationships are missing or instable. The progression of type I and type II patients differ from the poorer progression of type III and type IV patients in terms of social skills and resources (competencies and performances). Type I and type II patients tend to possess more social skills and resources than type III and type IV dependents. The absence of relationships and previous experiences of loss influence the psychodynamics of type III and type IV dependents. The treatment and compensation of dysfunctional relationships is very difficult and sometimes nearly impossible, due to a lack of therapeutic resources. Stabilising environments (therapy centres, homes, living communities etc.), which have a "holding function" (Winnicott), need to be temporarily activated.

Different deregulations of ego functions require different therapy goals. This is part of general therapeutic knowledge which suggests that in order to pin down any therapy goals for the phase after withdrawal, the patient's aetiology and personality need to be understood. Yet there is still a counterproductive monism in the treatment of alcohol dependents, whereby "psychotherapization" and total abstinence are the only therapy goals. The typology suggests that a number of treatment options should be chosen from. Furthermore, results from studies on long-term progression remind us to be humble in regard to therapy objectives: even a reduction from acute relapses to slight relapses should be seen as a success, while total abstinence is rather inadequate as a therapy goal[25].

Before we can answer the question as to which kinds of goals should be defined on the basis of the typology, it should be noted that any answer will again be a "typological answer", which needs to be adapted to the client's individual personality traits in practice. So what should therapeutic goals look like from a typological perspective?

Any relapse should also be interpreted according to type. Whilst type II dependents can, if need be, handle phases with low intakes of alcohol/ nicotine ("slips") reasonably well, types III and IV generally can't do this (and "relapse" with loss of control).

Then, which kinds of therapy and forms of care are in line with the aims of the particular psychosocial condition?

Type I patients have a biological dysfunction and therefore don't require any intensive psychotherapy. This is not the case for type II and III patients. Often analytic (exposing) psychotherapeutic procedures are effective. In contrast, self-help groups, which only focus on the topic of alcohol or nicotine, are not suitable for these groups as the constant preoccupation with this "problem" weakens the ego.

Chronically affected type III and IV patients are a challenge for every care system. Due to a reduction in performance and an impairment of self-regulatory skills in social life, any support offered needs to be aimed at these issues. While type III patients profit from medicamentous and psychotherapeutic support, type IV benefits more from sociotherapeutic measures (the organising of a daily structure, occupational therapy, stimulating recreational activities, the relief of pressure, sociotherapeutic residential homes etc) than from any other measures. Due to the rigid personality of depressive alcoholics ("type melancholicus" according to Tellenbach), whose orientation towards achievement coincides with a tendency towards self-devaluation and a latent compulsivity, the willingness to have therapy, and thus the willingness to change one's personality), is often not sufficiently present. The "loosening of the ego", a therapeutic requirement, which aims at increasing the ability to enjoy and experience things, at the same time activates the fear of change. Many small steps are needed and long-term perspectives (over many years) are required. Last but not least, it is important to change the patient's "social world", e.g. improving instable and conflict-laden relationships in type III dependents.

Many type IV patients are not able to live alone when they get older. Often they have to move to **sociotherapeutic residential or nursing homes**. Yet, these housing projects are usually oblivious to residents' alcohol dependence (that is alcoholisation and alcohol consumption are accepted in such homes). The common opinion that older chronically alcohol dependent individuals who suffer from sequelae are not able to stop drinking and "just need the alcohol", is unacceptable as both practical experience and results from research have shown the contrary. Instead, a consideration should be made of *which approaches* are suitable for this group of dependents. However, it is still the case that traditional systems of dependence support don't suf-

25 For example the „Ambulant group programme for controlled drinking", which has been taking place in Nuremberg since 1999. (Koerkel et al. 2001).

Fig. 117 Typology based aims

- Type I: Absolute abstinence (necessary due to biological factors and realistic due to psychological and social conditions)
- Type II: Long intervals with absolute abstinence, infrequent small relapses ("slips") without loss of control (sometimes also "controlled drinking" or "controlled smoking", that is a reduction of the number of cigarettes smoked.)
- Type III: reducing the occurrence of acute relapses (also smaller and shorter relapses should be rated as a success).
- Type IV: Acute relapses are to be expected despite of therapy; minimizing the severity of a relapse. Social dependence is of prior importance, that is abstinence is possible if sociotherapy is administered adequately! Whether aims are reached depends on the setting. In some cases the securing of survival will have to be the most important aim.

ficiently incorporate the existence of different subgroups of alcohol dependents. Due to the high threshold of most outpatient clinics and hospitals, the group of poorly structured dependents can't be adequately reached, so most cases don't receive adequate treatment. Dependence support systems prefer dependents who are still able to independently come to the institution,

Fig. 118 Typology based aims and methods

- Type I: stabilising psychotherapy, self-help groups (e.g. anonymous alcoholics), focus on alcohol-and nicotine problematic
- Type II: Ego-strengthening is predominant; therefore all psychotherapeutic options need to be considered, no groups that focus on alcohol
- Type III: Ego-loosening is predominant; therefore psychotherapy is preferred over alcohol-centred groups. The first stage of psychotherapy needs to focus on motivation (relationship formation), before solutions can be formulated.
- Type IV: Stabilising conversations, no "explorative" therapeutic procedures. Sociotherapeutic stabilisation and practice of relapse strategies is more relevant. Self-help groups are successful. Assistance can be carried out by e.g. a practitioner in cooperation with a sociotherapeutic setting (social worker, home, occupational therapy, custodianship etc).

which is wrongly equated with motivation (see section on motivation). This finding also applies to self-help groups which have established themselves as part of the traditional dependence support-triad (outpatient departments, clinics, self-help groups) and haven't developed any treatment options for type IV dependents, nor provide any benefit for marginal groups (Arenz-Greiving 2001, Wienberg 2001).

10.9.5 Sociotherapeutic aspects of therapy with alcohol dependents who are fundamentally impaired in their performance

Type IV focus in social institutions

10.9.5.1 Type IV characteristics

In most cases, type IV dependents show a combination of infant deprivation (early loss of mother, residence in homes and care institutions, violent environment or the presence of other factors which damage brain development) and later sequelae (acute polyneuropathy, craniocerebral injuries etc.). Sometimes performance impairment is linked to direct organic causes like epilepsy, meningitis or perinatal damage. Often infant behavioural disorders (enuresis, stuttering, biting nails) point to stressors in childhood. Often there is an indication of learning disabilities and difficulties at school. Type IV dependents show a higher frequency of stays in prisons, homes and hospitals and experience more withdrawal treatments than other types. The mortality rate is rather high due to alcohol sequelae (in combination with tobacco abuse). In Germany, the term "chronically multiply affected dependents" (CMA)[26], (Hilge 1997) has been developed to describe this group.

The use of alcohol and tobacco starts before age 20 and is usually associated with a certain kind of social environment and forms part of the daily structure of the dependent. Sociogenesis is very common and thus, in many cases, the stabilisation of social conditions improves the dependence progression.

The mortality rate in alcohol dependents is many times higher than in the general population, that is alcohol dependents die 14 to 23 years earlier than individuals with no alcohol dependence. Life expectancy in type IV patients is shorter than in other types. If the disease is untreated, it is unusual for type IV patients to reach their 60s due to previous damage.

Type IV patients who don't receive proper treatment and regularly relapse for longer periods of time, need more hospital admissions and care. This is supported by Lesch's long-term study which showed that type III and IV patients had the highest number of hospital admissions (more than half of type IV patients were admitted three times or more to hospital during the period of time under study: 51.6 %, see fig. 38). The offering of adequate support for these groups would significantly reduce costs.

---

26 A dependent is chronically affected if his chronic consumption of alcohol or other substances has led to acute or gradual physiological and psychological damage (incl. co-morbidity) and above normal or gradual social disintegration, so that he can't activate any vital resources by himself and doesn't have enough support from family or other people, which makes him dependent on institutional support … CMA (almost always, H.H.) have an impaired or no ability at all to structure their day." (Boettger, quoted by Hesse 2004.)

10.9.5.2 Cerebral damages as a result of chronic alcohol abuse, frontal lobe syndrome

Alcohol, as well as tobacco[27], directly, (through contact with alcohol and its aldehydes), and indirectly, (e.g. through vitamin deficiency, especially thiamine), damage the central and peripheral nerve structures. Numerous studies have shown which brain areas are especially damaged (Mann et al. 1988, Mann 1992, Steingass 1994, Happe 2000, Heinz and Mann 2001) and distinguish between diffuse and specific damage. Examples of diffuse neuropathological changes are enlargements of ventricles (brain chambers), enlargement of the sulci (brain furrows) and a reduction of brain weight and/or volume.

Damage is mostly caused by lesions and degeneration in the following areas:

1. The **limbic system**, which leads to memory problems, especially in episodic and autobiographic memory;
2. The **frontal cortex**, which causes very complex changes in behaviour;
3. The **right brain hemisphere,** which influences spatial stimuli processing (decreased performance in visual-motor tasks, spatial and visual organisation of perception as e.g. in face detection, face-name-combination etc.) (Steingass 2004).

27 Nitrosamines, which are released during smoking, are synthesised into formaldehyde and thus have toxic effects additionally to aldehydes, which are synthesised from alcohol.

The symptoms of frontal lesions are multi-facetted and appear contradictory. This is mainly due to information from deeper brain regions being interconnected and classified into higher schemata ("scripts", "pattern") in the frontal lobes. Therefore not all non-frontal brain functions are affected. The frontal cortex servers as a controller and regulator that is responsible for the planning, executing and controlling of behaviour. This includes the processing of environmental stimuli when planning behaviour (sensomotoric functions). The frontal lobe syndrome can be divided into two parts: changes in personality and cognitive changes. Schneider, in fact, has suggested three forms of the frontal lobe syndrome (Schneider 1927, 1929).

Changes in personality which are due to damage to the frontal lobes, lead to pseudopsychopathic (positive symptoms) and/or to pseudodepressive syndromes (negative symptoms) (Blumer and Benson).

The former is similar to an acute personality disorder with neuropsychological causes: Hyperactivity, motoric unrest, euphoria, impulsiveness, silly, immature behaviour and "Witzelsucht" (or joking mania). The social behaviour is socially inappropriate and social norms are not followed with the result that affected individuals appear indiscreet and lack personal boundaries. The disorder is also characterised by sexual deviant behaviour (e.g. exhibitionistic behaviour, public masturbation ...). Some cases match the symptoms of a dissocial personality disorder. Many established alcoholism typologies consider this characteristic (Cloninger, Zucker etc.)

The pseudodepressive form of the frontal lobe syndrome is characterized by a lack of motivation and initiative, an ineffective and careless attitude to work, affective indifference, slow cognition and reduced psychomotoric activity. It can be well compared to depressive symptoms.

One of the most serious cognitive deficits caused by frontal lobe lesions is the inability to learn from direct experiences in the social environment, e.g. integrating incoming information when planning behaviour and, if necessary, changing the strategy. Affected individuals with frontal lobe lesions have a tendency towards perseveration, they obstinately "stick" to a topic or to a chosen strategy, even if it is clear that the topic is of no interest to others, or that the strategy is inefficient.

The learning ability also seems to be limited when the affected have to combine two classes of different categories of stimuli (e.g. name and face).

Short-term memory is severely impaired in terms of the chronological order of information.

The generation of problem solving strategies is slowed down, deficient or not present at all.

Individuals show reduced performance in divergent thinking (many different answers to one question), however show no deficits in the field of convergent thinking.

Linguistic impairment (incomplete, simple sentences, confabulations) are quite frequent, although the speech faculty of alcohol dependents is in fact less affected.

By analysing the results of neuropsychological tests, Cramon (1988) has summarized typical cognitive weaknesses of affected dependents with frontal lobe lesions (which does not apply to conventional intelligence tests):

For sociotherapeutic practice, the degradation or damage of brain structures is also important in regard to the changes in the sensitivity to toxic influences. The combination of brain damage and alcohol and medication abuse can cause psychosis-like states.

10.9.5.3 Executive Cognitive Functioning (Giancola and Moss 1998, Frank 2002)

Research studies of alcohol dependents have examined the relationship between self-regulatory skills and dependence in regard to changes in EEG values. The reference point used in these studies was the "Executive Cognitive Function". ECF is defined as "self-monitoring of goal oriented behaviour" and is responsible for a number of performances, which are located in the cerebral cortex (particularly the frontal cortex):

- Attention
- Planning
- Organizing
- Conceptual thinking
- Abstract thinking
- Cognitive flexibility
- Self-control and monitoring
- Motor behaviour in planning and execution

Psychiatric disorders are often associated with ECF deficits. ECF deficits have been found in

- Antisocial personality disorder
- Psychopathy
- Substance abuse
- Social behavioural disorder
- Attention deficit disorder and hyperactivity
- Aggressive behaviour

Fig. 119 Frontal lobe damage: symptoms

- impulsive, hastily behaviour
- impaired generation of (sub-) solutions
- no goal oriented behaviour
- insufficient extraction of relevant information
- extraction of relevant features/subplans without following consequences for behaviour
- "sticking" to (irrelevant) details
- poor adjustment ability-/preservation of preceding action sequence
- rationalisation of difficulties occurring at tests
- poor learning from mistakes
- poor development of alternative plans
- breaking of rules
- poor coordination of (sub-) plans
- increasing inaccuracy in planning (during testing)
- usage of routine behaviour that is irrelevant to the plan

As the performance of type IV dependents is very reduced due to cerebral factors, it seems viable to employ the concept of reduced ECF and frontal lobe damage when treating this group. Low values in the ECF are represented in low P300 amplitude levels in the EEG. Children of substance abusers with a high risk for addiction also showed lower behaviour control and lower ECF values. At the same time, it has been shown that children of substance abusers have a lower P300 amplitude in frontal cortex EEGs (Frank 2002). An association between low aggression thresholds and low ECF seems very likely. Yet this also suggests that this personality dimension plays a role in psychiatric conditions of type III dependents which are linked to outward and inward aggression. This "antisocial" personality is emphasised by Cloninger, Babor and Zucker. In other typologies, alcohol dependents with dissocial personality traits form a separate subgroup (Windle and Scheidt, NETER typology).

Limited self-regulation is also represented in respective disease progressions. While type I and II patients usually have optimal (abstinent for over three and a half out of four years) or good progressions (abstinent for at least three and a half years out of four), type III and IV patients have significantly poorer progressions (type III: abstinent for only three months of four years, type IV: abstinent for less than three months of four years). It can be assumed that the small group of alcohol dependents who manage to drink controllably over a longer period of time predominantly consists of type II patients. It is impossible for type III and IV patients to drink controllably. In general, it is suggested that realistic and moderate aims be set.

From practice we know that when the patient has managed to stay abstinent, cognitive and social functions improve (Mann et al. 1988, Mandl 2002). Yet in case of frontal lobe damage, regeneration is limited, because there is no restructuring occurring in this brain region, although physiological changes (increase in brain weight and substance) can take place. In some brain areas, however, specific training does lead to improvements. However these improved performances are not global but "domain-specific" as they are limited to trained skills and abilities, so transfers to comparable behaviour patterns can't be made (Steingass 1998).

Therefore training needs to focus on skills that are life-relevant for the affected. "Thus it is surely more important for the residents of our institutions to learn how to independently find their way to the supermarket and shop without the help of others (which is self-esteem and autonomy enhancing), than to be able to solve labyrinth tasks or reproduce long, memorized word lists by heart." (Steingass et al. 1998).

10.9.5.4 Coping with violence

> The wise man uses his mind like a mirror, – he does not run after things, nor does he go to meet them. Whatever heads his way, he picks up in his mirror but he doesn't try to hold on to it. Just that, however, is what enables him to win out over things without ever getting hurt himself.
>
> *Dschuang Dsi*

Although violent acts are frequent in dependents' biographies, they only play a secondary role in everyday social and therapeutic work. Yet the practitioner has to expect aggressive comments and acts. Despite growing literature about causes of violence and aggression, descriptions of ways of behaving and interventions which could be useful for practice, are still rare. Therefore we would like here to make a few recommendations for practice. These recommendations are in the context of psychiatric interventions made during manifestations of violence and aggression (Anke et al. 2003, Ketelsen et al. 2004).

Violence is not a personality trait and thus can't be classified according to a specific subgroup of alcohol dependents. However, it will be discussed here in connection with the set of problems associated with type IV patients, including the previously mentioned correlations, (frontal lobe syndrome) and their reduced ability to regulate themselves and their affects.

Violence in alcohol dependents is often linked to continuous and protracted alcohol intoxication or loss of frontal control, caused by certain noxa (schnapps, psychotropic drugs). Biographies often show criminal convictions for "alcohol offences", e. g. assaults during intoxication. The role of permanent stress in the loss of self-control should not be underestimated. It has noxa-like effects on the brain and can weaken control mechanisms. This points to the frequently neglected analysis of *situational factors* which contribute towards aggressive outbursts, like housing conditions, inappropriate implementation of in-house rules, general stress during hospital and home admissions, crises among staff – shortfalls in numbers of important carers, divergent or unclear behaviour of staff, conflict between staff and the management etc.

One can generally assume that everyone would prefer to have control over their own behaviour and emotions. Thus, violent acts in social contexts are generally a result of an unwelcome fragmentation of the self, which the individual doesn't seek out. The aim of sociotherapeutic interventions is to support the individual in avoiding conflict situations which induce, and are caused by, stress (prevent escalation), regaining self-control, as well as being a means of protecting him from the consequences of his uncontrolled behaviour. In many cases, not always, but very often, the violent individual is the psychologically weaker party.

The *attitude* even more than the actual *behaviour* of the intervener is one of the most important variables in handling outward aggression. The following have been show to be of help in situations of aggression:

a) The absence of anxiety

Both opponents and the social environment are sensitive to the intervener's body language. Facial expressions, gestures, posture, and tone of voice – all of these signals are used by individuals' in-born protective mechanisms as a means of orientation. Ideally, the intervener *should not be anxious*. This allows him to serve as a means of orientation for those involved in the aggressive attack. At the very least, he should try to control his own *arousal* and/or insecurity.

Self-confidence can be increased by deliberately using the following body language, which has been summarized by Anke at al. as **anti-victim signals**:

- One's gaze should be directed at the aggressor. To look away and pretend that nothing has happened, only makes the aggressor feel more sure of himself.-**"Ready to fight" posture**: walking uprightly, keeping the head up, shoulders straight, expanded chest.
- **Confident, determined behaviour,** with a steady, unhesitant stride.
- Not hiding one's **hands in one's pockets**, rather, if appropriate, clenching one's fists and bending one's arms as if ready to punch somebody. (The clenched fists can enhance one's own feeling of self-esteem.) Generally any **gestures of insecurity** (any fight or flight behaviour) should be **avoided** (standing too far away, looking at the ceiling during the conversation, biting one's lips, looking down at one's feet, scratching one's ear etc.).
- When communicating in aggressive situations, **sentences** and instructions should be **short**, clearly pronounced and repeated, when needed.
- As one easily gets out of breath in these extreme emotional situations, it is important to **consciously breathe in and out**.
- **Positive self-talk** which can be visualised or quietly said during the crisis situation is supportive as well ("I will get through this!" "I can do this!" "This can be sorted!"...).

b) Boundaries – recognizing countertransference

Sometimes violent situations evoke memories of violent experiences in the past (traumata) in both patients and staff. It is recommended that staff who work in psychiatry or do social work with marginal groups, develop an awareness (via self-exploration) of their tendency towards transference in violent situations and their ability to act responsibly in violent situations. In aggressive situations, it is sometimes better to delegate the responsibility to somebody else and withdraw from the situation.

In this context, one's *current mental state* needs to be considered:

- What is the threshold of my stress level?
- At which point do I lose control?
- Do I have enough power, calmness and assertiveness at the moment to manage such situations?
- Is it (currently) better to call the police instead?

The manager of the institution is always responsible for the mental state and protection of their staff. Previous traumata in members of staff should be known and taken into consideration. If a member of staff is immediately at risk, client/patient care becomes secondary and the reestablishment of security the main focus.

c) De-escalating behaviour

Furthermore, it is important for the intervener to know which of his interventions promote or de-escalate aggression. Aggression promoting behaviours are, e.g.:

- loud, hectic and insulting comments (e.g. swear words, shouting)
- insecurity in voice
- unexpected intervention without any previous contact with the aggressor
- (unexpected) physical contact
- arrogant behaviour (e.g. to raise one's head and eye brow, contemptuous expression, staring at the patient, shrugging one's shoulder, laughing at the patient, schoolmasterly tone etc.)
- authoritarian behaviour (threatening, demonstrating distance and power, e.g. jingling keys, interrupting the patient, using jargon ...)

In contrast, **de-escalating interventions** are:

- rying to **speak quietly and calmly** (yet assertive and firm in voice and conviction)
- S**hort sentences** relating to the situation at hand (avoiding complexity)
- Keeping in touch with/trying to make contact with the aggressor
- Distraction in "stuck" situations, e.g. offering a glass of water or cigarette, changing the topic etc.
- **"LIMO"[28] – Conversational technique**
  Praising: "I appreciate your ability to call things by their name."
  Interest: "I would like to learn more about this."
  Admitting **f**aults: "Of course we all make mistakes!"
  Openness towards further conversation: "I would like to talk more about this topic with you."
- **I-statements** ("I am really upset that you are intimidating the other patients.")
- **Stop-sentences** (Exclamations, which might disrupt escalating

28 LIMO means in German: LOBEN, INTERESSE ZEIGEN, MÄNGEL ZUGEBEN, OFFENHEIT, it is translated here as PRAISING; INTEREST; ADMITTING FAULTS AND OPENNESS and could be taken as „PIFO"-Technique

situations): "Stop!" "Hold on!" "Enough of that!" "Get out of my way!" "Please let it be!" etc.

d) Clarity, coherence and explicitness in words and behaviour

Context variables of conflict situations are a further central category in managing aggression:

a) ***Consulting others*** (a third person)
It is likely that other qualified **helpers** who are more experienced and feel more confident in such situations need to be brought on board. Maybe a member of staff is around who has a **better relationship** with the person or persons affected than oneself. The presence and/or intervention of a higher ranked person (Medicus 1994) can also have de-escalating effects (ward management, senior physician, (home-) director etc.). Practitioners point out that older, professionally experienced women (e.g. nurses, social workers...) have a better influence on people who are upset.

b) ***Resolution of the conflict***
The immediate focus is to protect and **separate** the victim from the aggressor. The same applies for the opponent. The resolution of the conflict situation is one of the most important interventions. For example, changing the location can be an effective measure.

c) **Sending bystanders away (or creating distance from the bystanders)**
Send away the "audience" (helpers, "initiators"), or leave the location with the aggressor. Public aggression often attracts "public interest". Bystanders increase the stress level, especially if they interfere with the conflict. The principle has to be stimulus reduction.

"Debriefing" (Ketelsen and Pieters 2004) **the incident**

In social and therapeutic environments, every conflict needs to be debriefed. This is done with both the client/patient and the staff involved. This can take place in the form of a meeting between the aggressor and the victim, the aggressor and aggressor, or the aggressor and the staff. Debriefing, that is, an exact and collective analysis of the incident, can be done in a single one-to-one meeting, but also in the course of several conversations, in which everyone's opinion can be heard. In case of very vulnerable situations, more detailed debriefing is needed (e.g. individual supervision for staff). In regard to conversations with patients/clients, a person to whom the affected is closely attached, could be asked to join. In debriefing, it is important to analyse any triggering factors, but also to analyse the behaviour displayed in light of the client's life/care situation. In regard to the client, the following needs to be reflected upon:

- Which factors have triggered the destructive behaviour? (Which need has been frustrated?)
- Has the client encountered any similar situations? What has happened? Do his aggressive outbursts follow a certain course?
- How is the client affected by his own aggressive behaviour?
- How does the client's aggressive behaviour contradict his (therapy) goals?

- What could the client do to remain calm in similar situations? (e.g. retreating, breathing/relaxation techniques, calling someone to reduce aggression by talking etc.)

In regard to any similar future situations, it is therapeutically sound to write down, together with the patient, the form of intervention that is desired and thus accepted by him.

A recurring demand in regard to aggressive behaviour is the call for **psychotherapy**. In the process, the fact that there are fewer psychotherapy options for individuals from lower social classes, with lower levels of education and financial possibilities is frequently overlooked. And even if the therapist is suitably qualified and willing to therapeutically assist a dependent individual with an acute aggression problem, it is questionable whether the patient will actually be able to stay the course of an often intense, long and expensive therapy process.

For further treatment of aggressive behaviour in alcohol dependents, existing therapeutic contact could be activated or intensified in aftercare.

10.9.5.5 Sociotherapeutic structures instead of psychotherapy

The course of the disease in untreated type IV alcohol dependents is rather poor, which is shown by reduced life expectancy. Data shows that even in type IV patients who have received withdrawal treatment, the disease progression is unfavourable. On the other hand, findings from sociotherapeutic practice indicate that there is a group of type IV patients who are able to reduce their drinking and stay permanently abstinent. Studies in Vienna (The Caritas Vinzenz House, type IV housing community, the Caritas community) and Berlin (Schillerpark housing community) have supported this finding. We will outline a number of significant type IV case studies. Successful long-term stabilisation of type IV individuals is predominantly associated with the "creation of structure" and the integration into a positive social environment ("stabilisation via social stimulation") and not necessarily with (psycho-) therapeutic intervention. These sociotherapeutic processes reduce ego deficits which are responsible for drops in performance and weak self-regulatory skills. The deficient ego is replaced by external mechanisms/a system of social, cognitive and emotional substitutes, ranging from stable friendships to custodianship. If ego deficits are successfully compensated, many cases manage to reach and obtain total abstinence, despite a negative anamnesis and acute organic alcohol sequelae.

With some limitations, these observations are transferrable to tobacco dependence as well. Often type IV dependents smoke heavily because it is a norm in their social environment, to combat boredom or due to a lack of motivation, which again is caused by a lack of a daily structure. An active and structured daily routine with rewarding relationships can have positive effects on nicotine consumption.

The disparity between sociotherapy and psychotherapy is blatant. While therapy activates ego-potentials through self-reflection, the creation of structure compensates ego-deficits through external resources. Psychotherapeutic "activation" of ego-resources in type IV patients is generally ineffective as either the required resources have never been available or they can't be activated due to life-long degenerative processes. It's the responsibility of psychotherapy to decide whether the patient can be stabilised by external or internal resources. In psychosocial practice, it is sometimes not possible to distinguished whether institutional or clinical measures are needed. This is the consequence of insufficient differentials and inadequate knowledge.

On occasion, changes in personality are expected by psychotherapy which do not materialise, or not to the required degree. This criticism can also be levelled at social work, which sometimes waits two, three or four years for the development of "autonomy", the "ability to work" "ability to live independently" (especially the case in cost-intensive settings) to set in. Yet this expected adjustment is rather unlikely to materialise since the psycho-organic pre-conditions are not present. The reasons for such erroneous judgements about clients'/patients' resources are rooted in a lack of cooperation/networking between psychiatry and social work. Clearly all parties involved in such processes would benefit from personal abilities and boundaries being realistically appraised. To this end, knowledge about neuropsychological conditions is helpful (e.g. reduced spatial sense, forgetfulness, low resilience, learning experiences fixed to specific learning situations etc). The use of psychological tests which take into account the neuropsychological specifics of patients with addictions and which determine the client's/patient's deficits and resources are often helpful.

The absence of ego resources often leads to housing difficulties. A standard finding in the care of the homeless is that certain clients in assisted living facilities prove themselves over months and years to be capable of living independently but, following relocation to an independent flat, suffer an acute crisis, often related to alcohol relapse. As a consequence, some patients often lose their flats. These crises can be explained by the client's sudden loss of compensatory measures, such as the loss of stable social networks and regular contacts to important attachment figures, and sudden changes in daily structure, namely the collapse of a supportive environment.

Example:
After three months of withdrawal therapy, Mr W. has moved to a residential facility of the Caritas. A couple of months afterwards, he finds work at a construction site. He finds it very easy to stay abstinent. Daily alcohol tests show that his alcohol level is at 0.0‰. Within the housing community, Mr W. seems very balanced and calm and his housemates value him for his "calm nature". Indeed Mr W. is very quiet. Every night he spends time in the television room. Occasionally, he takes part in group activities. After one and a half years, the team of carers decides that Mr W., who seems to be stabilised, can move to a supported accommodation flat. Half a year later, the time has come. Shortly before relocating, Mr W. starts to feel nervous. On the first night in his new flat, Mr W. suffers from a severe relapse which lasts several days. Epileptic

seizures set in and he needs to go to hospital. Therapeutic support only brings short-term relief. Mr W. continues to drink, loses his job and stops paying rent. Half a year later, he needs to move back to the home. Here Mr W. continues with the daily rhythm that he had before. He finds it easy to stay abstinent, is content and quickly finds work again.

After a year of abstinence, and in the hope that the continuation of psychotherapy will have a stabilising effect, a second attempt to relocate Mr W. to a local residential community flat is planned.

On the first day, Mr W. relapses again and the drama of two years ago recurs. Mr W. moves back to the home where he calms down and becomes abstinent again. However, in the meantime, Mr W. suffers a heart attack. The heart attack is compensated with high dosages of different medication but Mr W. won't be able to work again. Nevertheless a further attempt to move him to a flat is undertaken which ends in the same was as previous attempts and Mr W.'s condition worsens.

After further heart problems and epileptic seizures, Mr W. undergoes rehabilitation, and decides to relocate to a senior residence.

Mr W.'s case is thought-provoking. If care and psychotherapy had realistically judged the case, much distress could have been prevented.

Generally, in the case of type IV patients with reduced performance ability, questions always need to be raised about the real feasibility of supportive therapy and its limitations. Additionally, personal resources need to be assessed (see salutogenic diagnosis) as they provide information about the potential for development. In most cases, therapy can't replace the creation of structure but only serves to support the client in terms of helping to maintain his level of motivation.

Which "compensations" are really effective, depends on the ego deficits and ego strengths ("resistance resources") which are present on psychological, physical and social levels. Experience has shown that the securing of positive social conditions is crucial, so that we can speak of "stabilisation through social stimulation" (SSS). An improvement of relationships has stabilising effects on the alcohol dependent as rewarding relationships at the same time act as an impetus for motivation:

- stable relationship to carers
- new (non-alcohol-related) friendships
- receiving visitors to the flat
- living as part of a community e.g. flat-sharing community
- residential homes
- home help services
- custodianship (in particular to ensure the security of the flat – e.g. paying rent and bills)
- regular outpatient appointments
- motivational groups (AA, International Blue Cross …)
- recreational activities (e.g. pets, "garden therapy")
- occupational therapy projects
- projects for the long-term unemployed

- Disulfiram adjustment (with existing motivation)
- daily structure
- efficient (that is quick and empathic) crisis intervention in case of relapses
- life skills training etc.

Helmut Hesse, an experienced pedagogical co-worker in the sociotherapeutic residential home for CMA[29] in Remscheid, Germany, has summarized five central points in his article "Effective factors in sociotherapy" (Hesse 2004):

- rigid daily structures
- a decent living environment worthy of human beings
- community life
- a climate of alcohol abstinence
- identification, and support, of individual skills and abilities

These factors, which were defined in regard to the CMA, also apply for type IV groups:

10.9.5.6 Stabilisation through social stimulation (SSS)

It is known that dependence, apart from physiological and psychological factors, is mainly influenced by social factors (Feuerlein 1998).

Type IV dependents often live within a social "drinking and smoking milieu", in which the mutual consumption of alcohol and nicotine has a stabilising effect on the group. Drinking and smoking are linked to group status and this has a direct effect on brain functions[30]. Group membership and thus the security of the individual within his social group is strongly associated with collective drinking and smoking. Despite the presence of high levels of motivation for therapy, these mechanisms can cause relapses, especially when the individual returns to his familiar environment. Without the establishment of resources, the individual will always be at risk of relapse and will be lonely as he is unable to form alternative relationships. This "atrophy of the social atom" destabilises an individual's identity, which has far-reaching consequences. On the other hand, some type IV dependents manage to become abstinent for rest of their lives due to their successful integration into dry and stable social environments and sometimes don't even need withdrawal treatment.

Example:
Mr B. has spent the last 20 years living in unstable conditions most of which he has spent "under the bridge", that is as a homeless person. During the day, the 60-year old visits various soup kitchens and watering holes with his companions in misfortune. At one point, as he was feeling unwell, he is taken to the emergency shelter of a Caritas home where he decides to stay permanently. Although his performance is clearly reduced, he takes over diverse jobs in the residential community. Yet, every afternoon he disappears for

29 Chronisch mehrfach beeinträchtigte Abhängigkeitskranke (CMA): ‚chronically multiply impaired alcohol dependents'

30 Experiments with primates have shown that social dominance stops the development of an addiciton. "This suggests that environmental conditions, like social isolation or living in a community, modify the cerebral metabolism and consequently the behaviour." (Schmidt 2005; Bauer 2006, 2007).

Fig. 120 Stabilising measures in type IV alcohol dependents

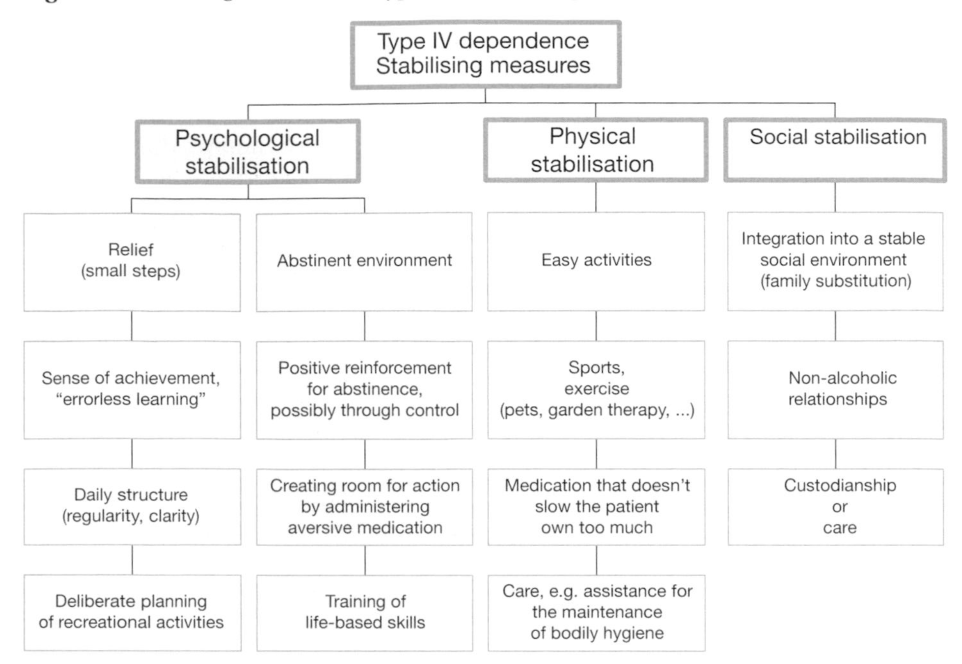

one or two hours and drinks "his two beers" or his "spritzer" in the beer garden close by.
Although he has reduced his drinking since moving to the Caritas home, he still continues to drink a reduced amount every day. Several sanctions, such as being banned from entering the residential home, have not changed his behaviour at all. For two years, he continues with this behaviour. One day, however, Mr. B. decides "out of the blue" to drink a soft drink instead of the "spritzer". Suddenly, without any withdrawal therapy, Mr B. stops drinking and continues to live without alcohol until his death. This shows that the integration into the house's social network and the resulting creation of structure have lead to as "miracle healing".

The relationship between social integration and emotional stability has also been described by Maslow's theory of the hierarchy of needs, although the hierarchy needs to be modified for alcohol dependent patients and especially for type IV patients. It tends to be the case that physiological needs e.g. food intake and personal hygiene become secondary to the point of negligence at a certain stage in the progression of dependence.

On the other hand, many type IV patients re-establish their self-regulatory skills (their needs assuming thereby their natural priority) when social integration takes place, enabling the dependent to go without alcohol.

The link between social impairment and limited individual self-regulation can be explained by deficits in the frontal cortex. Strategy development and modification, problem solving, application of know-how, and especially the implementation of social norms (social self-monitoring), are located in the frontal lobes (see section on ECF-executive cognitive functioning). From an evolutionary perspective, the frontal lobe started to develop when individuals started to live in social groups. Life in "social" organisations is mentally represented by the frontal lobe (Kolb and Whishaw 1996). This enables the compensation of performance deficits by an integration into intact and helpful social structures. Further, this changes the value of social integration for the overall situation of the individual. The stronger the actual disintegration, the more social integration is needed to active and integrate other areas of personality.

In his hypothesis, Maslow (1954) suggests that human needs are organised within a hierarchy and that those needs can be satisfied independently from each other ("dilatory satisfaction"). After the individual's physiological and safety needs are relatively satisfied, social and value-related needs can develop. The higher needs in this hierarchy only come into focus once the lower needs in the pyramid have been met. Therefore the aim of personality development is to make room for self-actualization and to guide the shaping of a person's life. These motives might vary in regard to dependence-related disintegration:

10.9.5.7 Compliance

The term "compliance" (cooperation in social work or therapeutic settings) presupposes verbal understanding and the ability to translate what has been discussed in therapy into behaviour or behavioural concepts which can be integrated into real life. Within this context, the following questions need to be considered:

- To what extent can I (as a social worker) rely on "conversations", do I need other mediums of communication?
- How valid are "therapies" which use conversation as their prime medium?
- To what extent can I rely on verbal agreements and trust them as the basis of therapy?
- To what extent can I rely on the client's verbal self-portrayal? (Confabulations?)
- To what extent do I know how I/ my environment define(s) motivation?

After successful withdrawal, type I patients show high levels of "compliance" which, however, quickly decrease after acute symptoms disappear (Burger and Marx 2001). Compliance in type II patients tends to fluctuate with psychosocial crises and increases when crises are handled.

Compliance in type III dependents depends on the psychological state of the alcohol dependent and therefore fluctuates severely. Compliance is weaker in depressive or (hypo)manic phases. Furthermore, the alcohol dependent may show signs of a "pseudo motivation" which is either rooted in emotion-

Fig. 121 A triangle model illustrating dependence conditions

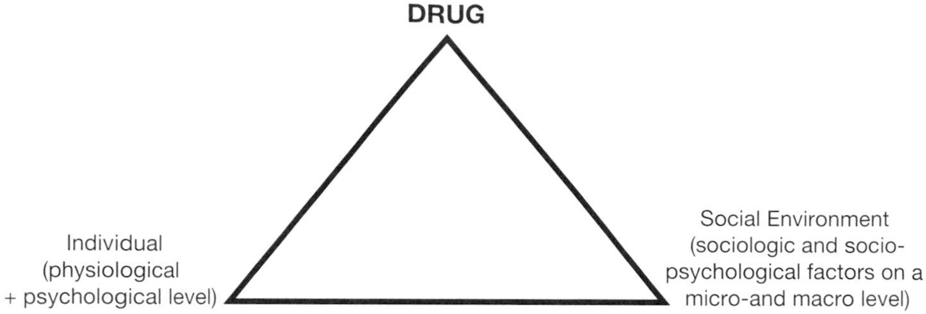

DRUG

Individual (physiological + psychological level)

Social Environment (sociologic and socio-psychological factors on a micro-and macro level)

al stress or in the super ego. If suffering is reduced (e.g. disappearance of withdrawal symptoms or stabilisation of basic dysfunctions), compliance may also decrease. Only those aims that have been rationalised by the super ego remain unaffected by biorhythmic changes which severely impact body-soul dynamics. Usually sociotherapeutic stabilisation (via the creation of structures) and/or crisis interventions will be needed to manage crises until basic dysfunctions can be treated again.

Example:
Mr F. episodically suffers from depression during which he drinks bottles of Vodka. As he doesn't eat, he loses lots of weight. After 20 years of homelessness, he is very deprived of social contacts. He has been living in a council flat for a year and receives help from an alcohol outpatient clinic and sociotherapeutic care centre. As soon as he starts feeling better, he develops hypomanic behaviour and starts to do adult education courses which quickly overwhelm him. This is usually quickly followed by a depressive episode and an alcohol relapse. During these periods of heavy drinking and depression, Mr F. shows signs of personal neglect and he stops taking care of his flat. He is not able to keep in touch with his contact person. The contact person tries to maintain or even increase communication (visits, phone calls) until such time as it is possible to admit Mr F. into outpatient care again. After physiological withdrawal, the setting is expanded again (contact group, regular support meetings and visits to the outpatient clinic and the creation of activities that provide a daily structure etc.). The aim of therapy is to extend Mr F.'s periods of abstinence and to ensure adequate adjustment to mood stabilising medication (e.g. carbamazepine), which has not been possible so far due to his relapses. A long-term goal for these clients could be concomitant psychotherapy.

Verbal accessibility
The limited understanding of verbal information due to cognitive deficits may be more pronounced than usual in type IV dependents, especially in the first

Fig. 122 Social structure of motivation

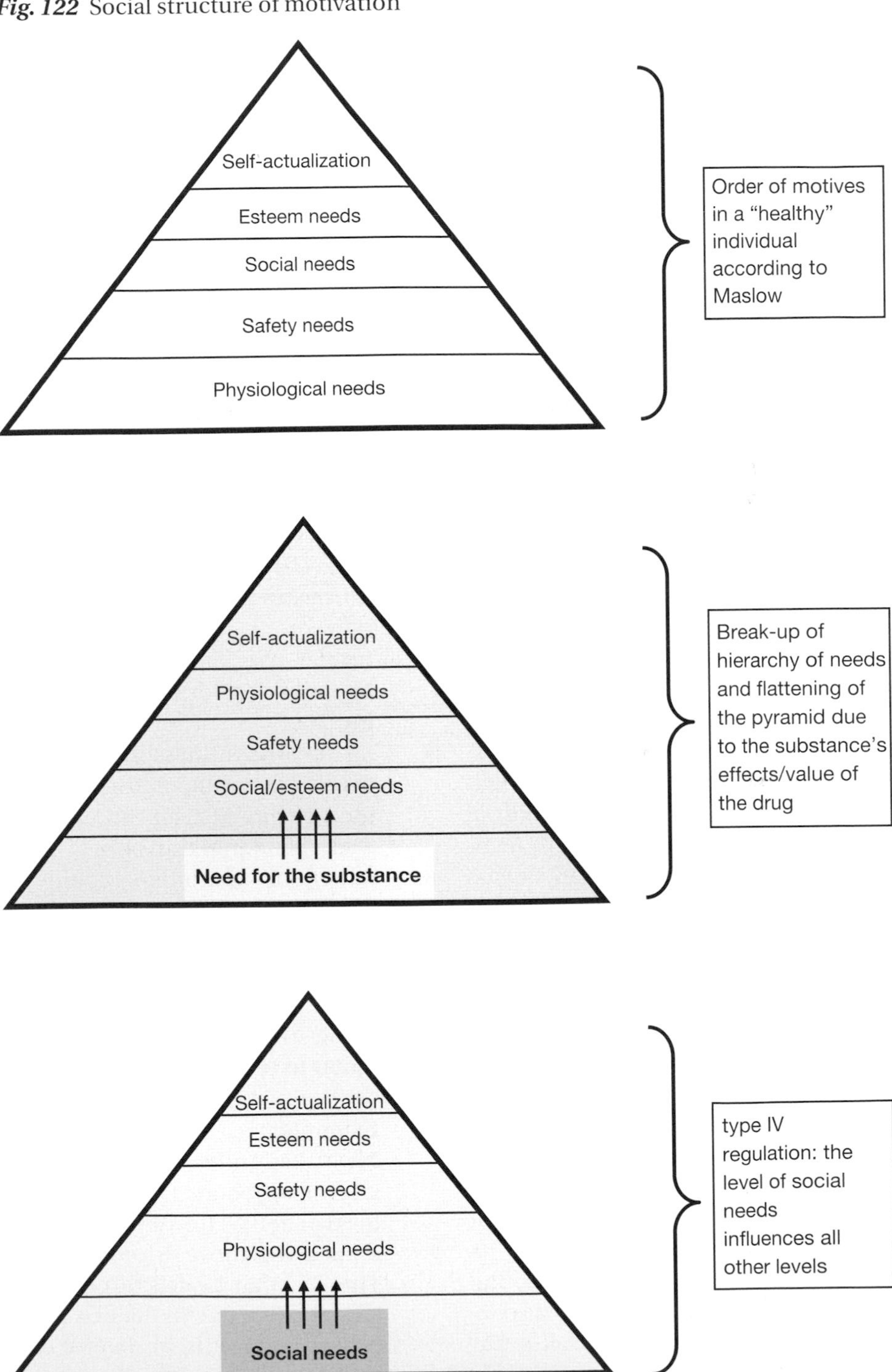

weeks and months of abstinence. The status of mental capacities such as understanding, concentration and memory need to be checked. Besides existing deficits, chronic alcohol dependents also show damage to many other complex cerebral functions (both reversible and irreversible). Only few persons form this group have normal patterns in computer tomography (16%). Atrophic changes were detected in the frontal and parietal brain as well as enlargements of the ventricles. 50% of all alcohol dependents show deviations from the norm. Alcohol dependents who are older than 50, show reduced brain circulation.

14% to 20% show signs of the Korsakow syndrome which includes impairments in memory spontaneity, concentration and intelligence (caused by lesions in the thalamus). The speech faculty is still intact despite deficits in other performance areas e.g. spatial orientation which leads to serious misjudgements. Furthermore, the right hemisphere of the cortex (location of spatial orientation) is more severly damaged in alcohol dependents (Steingass 1998).

Example:
Mr K. regularly meets with his counsellor. He is usually on time and waits in the waiting room before an appointment. Yet he is often irritated if other clients speak to him whilst he is waiting. He is especially annoyed when phone calls or other matters interrupt the therapy session. Although he tries to hide his annoyance, the counsellor notices it and discovers that its cause is Mr K.'s impaired ability to concentrate. Mr K. tries hard to follow his counsellor and not to lose track of his thoughts. When he is distracted, he falls into a mental "hole" and finds it difficult to pick up the thread again. Now the counsellor also understands why Mr K. always uses a notebook in which he records all appointments and agreements.

It is important to optimize one's speech when talking to type IV patients with cognitive impairments (which can be permanent). This means the following:

- short, lucid sentences, which are suggestively repeated
- no overly complicated information
- regular checking of understanding (allowing for misunderstandings)
- taking forgetfulness into account (writing down appointments, written agreements, repeating…) => wall calendar in the room
- telephone reminders could be used
- compensatory methods (memos at the pin board, calendar, mobile phone time-manager, accompanying to the local ministry, flatmates to remind him etc)

Example:
Mr N. has suffered from epilepsy since childhood. Despite having lived in homes for 10 years, he has managed to move to a council flat. The fact that he fell through the 'social safety net' in the first place is due not least to his fear of officialdom.

Whenever something had to be done via official channels, Mr N. reacted by withdrawing. An analysis of his behaviour showed that he felt intellectually and linguistically inept in such situations. As a former pupil of a special school, he was afraid to admit his reading, writing and comprehension difficulties. Now, whenever he has to attend a meeting with officialdom, Mr N. asks a carer to come with him.

With regards to type IV patients who have recently been through withdrawal, it is often difficult to determine whether deficits in concentration, memory (forgetfulness) or incomprehension of verbal information existed before the development of the dependence (thus making them irreversible), or whether they have been caused by alcohol abuse (possibly reversible). It has been shown that adequate support can improve existing deficits (memory training, responsibility for small tasks, sense of achievement …). For example the method **"errorless learning"** (in contrast to "trial and error") has been shown to be beneficial for this subgroup of alcohol dependents (information is repeated more frequently and presented in such ways that positive reinforcement can set in directly) (Streubel 1998).

Nootropics can help to compensate reversible performance deficits. On the other hand, there is always a risk of highly dosed psychotropic drugs slowing down the compensatory processes of the brain and the organism generally. This is why motivating these patients to become active should be regarded as an important matter (see next chapter).

Example:
Mr Z. lives in a home for formerly homeless people. There are few opportunities for therapy in this home. Residents of this institution often go to a pub together. On occasions when Mr Z. tries to refrain from drinking, he finds it very difficult to find alternative activities. Although his television is constantly switched on, he is not able to concentrate on the programmes. He can only read the newspaper for a short time and he can't set any goals for himself, nor can he organise daily activities. Sooner or later, he joins the others in drinking again. Previously, Mr Z. used to live in a home where alcohol was prohibited. There he took part in biking tours, was involved in projects and was employed as a handy man in the home. He misses this kind of daily structure in his new home. His health has deteriorated since moving to the new place and he has lost touch with his friends from his "old" home.
He gets along well with the home manager and together they are considering which changes to his lifestyle can be made and whether he should relocate to another home.

When individuals who are reduced in performance abilities, start to become active again, their "compliance" level changes because cognitive performance usually improves with increased well-being and the absence of damaging substances. The constitutive deficit in self-regulation (e. g. separation from an alcohol-permissive environment) will continue to exist and needs to be institutionally bridged through the support of a helping ego. If this solution is possible, "compliance" is likely to improve as well.

Example:
Mr H. lives in an assisted housing project. Before moving here, he lived in a home for alcohol dependents for a few years. Mr H. drinks regularly but not as much as he used to. He used to work on a voluntary basis as a porter in his old home three times a week, meant that he had to control his alcohol consumption. In view of the fact that he has not worked for ten years and feeling the duties of a porter are too much for him, it is unlikely that he will find employment through the normal job market. The daily and weekly structure provides him with so much security that he is virtually able to drink controllably. He himself states that he needs those responsibilities and that without these structures he would relapse. The home has learned to cope with him being episodically overchallenged in complex situations.

10.9.5.8 Overview of pedagogical context variables

As verbal and intellectual capacities in alcohol dependents are temporarily or permanently impaired, it makes sense that non-verbal intervention strategies are more important for the therapy of chronically affected dependents than verbal interventions. Suggestions, influenced by Gestalt therapy/Gestalt pedagogical theory (Petzold 1985), are:

- **A stimulating, communication-enhancing environment.**
  "Life is arousal ... stimulation promotes social contact, arousal, energy and life." (Perls)

Examples:
- bright rooms
- common rooms (e.g. shared instead of private kitchens)
- group activities
- group exercises or games
- possibility to receive visitors
- possibility to retreat
- pets
- plants
- contact to nature etc.

- **Promotion of "awareness", disclosure of different means of perception.**
  Making the individual aware of his environment e.g. "Have you noticed that the lilacs in the garden have started to blossom?" "Have you read in the newspaper, that today ...", directing attention towards the individual's inner life: e.g. "What did you dream about last night?"

- **Promotion of self-regulation and personal responsibility.**
  Many of the affected individuals are convinced about their own helplessness (often as a result of their hospitalisation) and therefore reject co-determination. Hospitalisation leads to **passivity** and **resignation**.
  Activating clients' inner resources towards greater self-regulation

and towards taking an active part in co-determining their own lives is usually a long and arduous process and requires **repeated efforts** and, above all, creativity on the part of the people in the client's social environment who will need to find out what the client is capable of doing, and what he would like to do. (e.g. by initiating special projects: games evening, helping in organising an event, decoration of the common room, responsibility for certain tasks such as watering the plants, setting the table, taking care of a pet etc.).

- **Increasing solidarity and cooperation.**
  In a social environment, cooperation is an important key to activating resources in socially deprived individuals. There is an art to knowing how to gradually "entice out " hospitalised individuals who are used to isolation, so that they have a chance to adopt a different role i.e. **active role** within contexts which are more or less familiar to them. Taking part in "excursions" is often too challenging at the beginning but eating ice cream together might be a possibility, as it is a relatively short, time-limited activity. Cooperating on certain **"projects"** (e.g. arranging a room, organising a party, cooking together etc.) is only gradually realisable. The feeling of **solidarity** experienced through helping out a **weaker group member** is very beneficial (e.g. showing a flat-mate how to cook or accompanying someone who is frightened of going to the dentist).

10.9.5.9 Over-challenge, "motivation"

Due to their appearance/biography, type IV patients are said to have no motivation to become abstinent. In the regards to this group's ego deficits, the question needs to be asked whether the common concept of motivation (provided that such a concept actually exists) can and should be applied to these individuals. Reduced motivation, an impaired ability to identify, and implement, appropriate behaviour are all consequences of the underlying performance impairment. Some everyday situations are very stressful for type IV patients, a fact that is often ignored. For example going to the doctor's, or a local authority office, or seeking out a counselling centre: tasks that are thought to be very easy to handle. This feeling of being over-challenged is both due to negative learning experiences and cognitive deficits (e.g. not being able to quickly or sufficiently understand forms or complicated information, and embarrassment due to dyslexia etc.). Often severe social anxiety, which individuals previously suppressed with alcohol, and which still manifest in times of abstinence, plays a role as well.

> **Example:**
> Mr B. lives in a housing community for alcohol dependents. Shortly after moving in, he decorated his room in a homely way. This is where he spends most of his time. He only appears in the common room, where he usually watches television, for short periods. He rarely leaves the flat. Only after his first alcohol relapse does he start talking about his social anxiety. Up to then, nobody knew that he

had to take a cab in order to go to the doctor's because he was afraid of the people on the street insulting him about his appearance. Most social interactions make Mr B. anxious. For many decades he has "treated" his anxiety with alcohol (sedation).

"Motivation" (if this term actually exists in a neutral sense) in this patient group should only be assessed after deficits have disappeared. Furthermore, type IV patients are often motivated by stable relationships which compensate their ego-weakness. In this context, the concept of motivation is an **interactive phenomenon** between counsellor/supporter/doctor on the one side, and the client on the other side. Furthermore, whether the client is exclusively responsible for his own "motivation", and whether determining external factors have been sufficiently taken into consideration, are questions that need to be critically assessed, especially in relation to patients with a severe reduction in performance and self-regulation (ego strength).

In regard to patients who have been admitted to sociotherapeutic care facilities, Steingass (2001), an expert practitioner, sums up as follows:

> **Due to organic changes in the brain, many residents are no longer able to critically evaluate themselves, their condition or their situation and are no longer able to make far-reaching decisions or long-term plans. Due to this fact, it is of little help to demand detailed explanations or commitments concerning an "acceptance of the disease", "readiness to stay abstinent", "motivation for treatment" or voluntary participation from alcohol dependents, or to base treatment upon these.**

10.9.5.10 Case studies of long-term abstinent type IV patients

The following section will introduce three examples of type IV alcohol dependents who received treatment in a sociotherapeutic care facility or addiction therapy centre on one or more occasions in their lives, and who have managed to stay abstinent (stabilisation) in the long term. These are individuals whose social and psychological conditions and later biographies have been so dramatic that they have led to definite social exclusion (prison, homelessness, long-term unemployment). For a long time, all three cases matched the cliché of homeless alcoholics who no one believes are capable of living abstinently. Yet, we are convinced that these examples are *no exceptions*, but represent individuals who were helped to escape their dependence through adequate support/therapy. In regard to the first case, the aversive medication disulfiram (Disulfiram) was successfully been administered, which was facilitated by the care setting.

In all cases, social disintegration was replaced by new social networks (Caritas community, theatre group, new partner...), which in a certain sense help to create structure and to develop social competence.

10.9.5.10.1 Norbert T., Type IV

N.T. was born in 1962 in Vienna as the third of four children. At birth, an undersupply of oxygen was diagnosed as a result of which he is classified as belonging to the type IV subgroup. Like his brother, Mr T. was underweight at birth and spent some time in an incubator. His underdevelopment was probably alcohol-related (only the youngest brother, who doesn't show any signs of underdevelopment, has no alcohol problem). Mr T. has two half-sisters who also live with the family. His father and mother were both severely alcohol-dependent. He had a good relationship with his grandmother who he visited every day after school. His brother, J., lived at the grandmother's and was therefore never directly confronted with the alcoholism of his parents. When the children came home from school, their mother was usually severely intoxicated ("five out of seven days a week"). His father worked as a labourer in the metal industry. When Mr T. was twelve years old, his father lost his job due to alcohol-related problems and was only employed subsequently by temporary employment agencies.

Due to his brother, A., displaying behavioural problems (aggression towards his classmates), the social services department intervened. When Mr T. was eleven years old, social services decided that all the children should be admitted to residential care. At the same time, his mother was diagnosed with liver cirrhosis which necessitated hospitalisation. Mr T. and his sister, G., moved to a Caritas children's home and his brother, A., moved to a home for difficult children. His parents lost their flat and became homeless. During this time, only his older brother, stayed in touch with Mr T. and his sister. A bit later, his grandmother died and Mr J. had to move to a home as well.

At the age of twelve, Mr T. experienced his first alcohol intoxication as a result of a drinking contest with his siblings and had to be admitted to a children's hospital for detoxification. Like his brother A., Mr T. had to go to special school where he displayed similar aggressive behavioural patterns. "I threw a table at my teacher and a compass at my brother…" However, his teachers were eventually able to curb his aggressive outbursts by means of positive reinforcement.

At the age of 15, Mr T. and his sister relocated to different hostels for apprentices where it was common for residents to drink a considerable amount of alcohol. Mr T. quit his apprenticeship as a chimney sweeper after two months ("It wasn't any fun anymore"). He subsequently finds and completes an apprenticeship as a tyre vulcanizer. Due to bureaucratic problems, Mr T. does not receive his certificate of apprenticeship. After finishing the apprenticeship he wanted to transfer to a craftsmen's hostel but he got into trouble for contravening the house rules. Spontaneously, "without thinking much about it", he decided to leave. At that time, at the age of 18, he was already drinking five bottles of beer per day. Mr T. subsequently found his homeless parents who at that time were living in derelict houses. From age 18 to 21 years, he lived with his parents as a homeless person. Short imprisonments followed. Mr T.'s mother died of an embolism (sequelae of liver cirrhosis) in 1983 and the same week his father fell down the staircase of a dilapidated house. As the result of a blood clot with months of subsequent hospitalisation, his father is left disabled and needs constant care. He has suffered a severe loss of memory and is no longer able to remember his own children.

At this time, brother A. gave up his flat and moved in with his girlfriend. Mr

T. and his father moved in together after the latter was discharged from hospital. Mr T. took care of his father until his death in 1987. Mr T. was able to keep the flat until 1990. Other residents started complaining about Mr T.'s alcohol excesses, upon which he moved out and, after a short stay in a home in Meldemannstrasse, ended up in a newly opened community hostel for men in Vienna. Here he stayed for one and a half years and then had the opportunity of moving to an independent, "start-up" flat. Mr T. had to subsequently leave this flat due to continued excessive alcohol consumption. He received his first course of therapy at Baumgartner Hoehe Psychiatric Hospital. In 1993, he moved to the sociotherapeutic home, "Vinzenzhaus", where he lived relapse-free (three "slips") for two years and worked for one year as a seasonal worker for the refuse collection services. In 1994, he moved into a Caritas "start-up" flat. Here he relapsed more often as he was not subject to any tests or check-ups but the relapses are nowhere near as bad as previously.

In 1996, Mr T. joined the Caritas community, started serving at the altar and became a volunteer sacristan, something that he has continued to do to this day. Mr T. received the sacrament of confirmation in 1997. In 1998, he joined a theatre group where he worked as a lighting technician. The same year he received a council flat and took over the cat of the previous tenant.

Mr T. tried to repeatedly to find a job but all attempts failed due to his persistent excessive alcohol consumption. Although Mr T. has reduced his drinking, any attempts to completely control it regularly fail. In 2001, Caritas suggests he undergo further long-term therapy, which he completed at Ybbs Therapy Centre.

In 2002, Mr T. almost lost his council flat due to the fact that he had failed to pay the rent. Social-work based interventions prevented an eviction. In 2003, he found himself in another housing crisis. For months, Mr T had been voluntarily going without unemployment benefit because he couldn't face going to the employment centre. Further interventions were needed and implemented which resulted in Mr T. managing to keep his flat.

On the advice of his carer, Mr T. contacted the outpatient department for alcohol dependents in Vienna General Hospital in November 2003. An inpatient therapy is decided against due to the problematic anamnesis. Mr T. finds marginal employment which is stopped after four months. In his anger about this, Mr T. starts to drink again despite taking Disulfiram which results in a serious vegetative collapse. Mr T. voluntarily goes to hospital for one night for observation. After this, he starts drinking again for a few weeks and then contacts the outpatient department again where he his put back on Disulfiram, at his own request.

As a result of preceding events, the therapy setting is changed. In addition to his appointments at the outpatient department, Mr T. meets his therapist fortnightly where his alcohol problem is continually addressed. Behavioural therapeutic reinforcements are used to enhance therapy. In the first year, he receives a reward for every check up appointment he keeps and for long phases of abstinence. Furthermore, tangible therapy goals are formulated. The combination of motivation-enhancing strategies and Disulfiram was very effective.

During this time, Mr T. was socially more active and contact with his sister and her parents-in-law improved.

In 2004, Mr T. started working at a project, which was extended in 2005. In February 2006, he started driving lessons. After having finished the project in May 2006, he found work with a construction company. At the same time, he terminated his intake of Disulfiram without which he has managed to stay abstinent up until now (2010). In April 2010, Mr T. celebrated six years of abstinence.

10.9.5.10.2 Peter N., Type IV

Mr N. was born in Vienna in 1949. Due to epilepsy, he is classified as a type IV alcohol dependent. Despite antiepileptic medication and regular check-ups he suffers from grand mal seizures every few weeks.

Mr N. grew up in an extremely uncommunicative family. Nobody ever talked about emotions and in later life Mr N. also rather "quiet" and prefers to stay in the background. He completed an apprenticeship as a house painter and decorator. He was once married and has three children. When intoxicated, Mr N.'s personality seems to change, which explains his previous criminal convictions. This could be the reason why his wife left him. His three children consequently live with their mother.

Mr N. describes himself as a "loner". So is his brother, who is five years older and socially marginalised due to his excessive alcohol consumption. His brother lost his job and was imprisoned for committing grievous bodily harm. Yet, Mr N. sees his brother as a role model. At the age of 30, a family tragedy occurred. Severely intoxicated, Mr N.'s brother threatens his mother, Mr N. intervened with a knife whereupon his brother fell onto the knife and died. Mr N. was imprisoned for six years and was torn between feelings of guilt and anger during this period of time.

Following his release from prison, Mr N. lived on the street for ten years, slept on park benches and drank two litres of wine a day, which increased the frequency of his epileptic seizures. A fractured leg led to hospital admission, where he was advised to undergo alcohol detoxification and rehabilitation which he started in 1995 (the first and only course of detoxification and rehabilitation in his life). In April 1996, he transferred to a Caritas care home. Although Mr N. is very shy, he was well integrated in the housing community, taking on responsibility for caring for the plants and cleaning the house. After a few months of doing the cleaning, he finds a permanent niche in the housing community as a cook, a job which he has continued to do without interruption until today (2007). During this time, he has never relapsed. An especially moving event was the reunion of Mr N. with his son when the latter was admitted to the organisation's emergency shelter for the homeless and father and son – both homeless – met again after not seeing each other for decades.

It is interesting that, even during the first three years, Mr N. was really determined to permanently stay in the home and neither wanted to move to a transitional nor a permanent flat. His argument was that he thought he would relapse if he moved out of the safe environment of the home. After a struggle, Mr N. was finally granted, as an exception, the right to stay in the transitional home forever. He moved to a single room on the top floor and decorated his room in a homely fashion. His self-sufficiency was a mystery to the carers. He rarely went out and he saved all his money. Conflicts only arose when he was being stressed by his colleagues in the kitchen.

After three years, a "miracle" happened. Mr. N told his carer that he was now ready to move to an independent flat, which was consequently arranged. After four years in the home, he was able to live in his own flat, but still cooked for the home three times a week. Mr N. managed to stay abstinent during this phase and, all in all, he has managed to stay abstinent for thirteen years to this date.

10.9.5.10.3 Karl H., Type IV

Mr H. was born in Vienna in 1952 as the oldest of three children. His grandfather (presumably) and father were alcohol-dependent. His father was disabled after World War II and his mother was an epileptic. Mr H. himself also suffers from epilepsy and is thus classified as a type IV patient. He didn't realise he had epilepsy until adulthood, as his parents never talked about it. He grew up in cramped and socially restricted conditions. His brother killed himself in the 1980s and his sister works as a civil servant and is divorced.

His performance in elementary school dropped in the third grade, and as a result of being caught stealing, he subsequently spent two years in a children's home. At the age of twelve he moved back to Vienna. At this time he started to read many books which offered him an alternative world into which he could escape. At the age of 14, he ran away from his parent's home and lived with various men until he was picked up by the police, and sent to a juvenile detention centre, where he was sexually and violently assaulted. Mr H. describes himself at this time as very fearful and as having a victim personality. Nevertheless, Mr H. managed to complete his apprenticeship as a printer and bookbinder.

After having undergone traumatic experiences in several homes, especially in the juvenile detention centre, Mr H. tried to avoid the imminent draft to military service. He pretty much lived "on the street" and at different friends' and acquaintances' places between the ages of 18 to 30.

After he left the juvenile detention centre at the age of 18, Mr H. became drunk for the first time at a friends' party – "I just couldn't get enough". He lived off occasional jobs and became part of the artist scene, which made it easier for him to get alcohol. During the following years, he got used to drinking alone, especially as a means of forgeting his troublesome situation. He drank up to four litres of beer or two litres of wine per day, usually at pubs and train stations. As a result, he suffered from grand mal seizures which lead to several hospital admissions.

At the age of 30, experiencing a physical and psychological decline, he decided to join Alcoholics Anonymous and managed to quit drinking. Only after three years did he suffer his first relapse, which lasted one month and he also had small relapses, lasting up to two days, in the years to come. He stayed with the Alcoholics Anonymous for 17 years. He never considered undergoing in-patient therapy and, in retrospect, he still doesn't think it was necessary.

Through the support of the AA, Mr H. found the strength to confront the military service commission only to find out that he didn't qualify anyway because of his medical history. During his periods of abstinence, Mr H. had developed personality traits which up to now had (apparently) not been effective. "Not running away, but standing your ground". He discovered his talent for "discipline" and "conscientiousness". He started to work as a printer and bookbinder and worked his way up to the head of the department.

At the age of 35, he got married and two years later his son was born. Five years later, the couple divorced. His wife's health problems during pregnancy and after the child's birth caused severe anxiety in Mr H., which he tried to handle by withdrawing from the relationship. He suffered from several small relapses, which led to the break-up of the marriage. After a while he lost his job as well.

In this time of crisis, Mr H. made contact with the church again. Since the age of six, he had been active in the church, serving at the altar and a sacristan, which he finds very supportive. In a charismatic Franciscan project ("House of Peace"), he is able to connect with a larger community and manages to stay abstinent again with the help of their support. Since then (1996), Mr H. has not suffered a single relapse. Since 1998 he has been in a serious relationship, got married in 2001 and became a father again. He works as a gardener in a small town in Lower Austria and is relapse-free to this day (2010).

Appendix 1

Appendix 1
Lesch Alcoholism Typology – Questionnaire

Lesch Alcoholism Typology – Questionnaire

Lesch Alcoholism Typology 3.0.22

Personal Data

Patient's number: ____________________

Patient ID: ____________________

Surname: ____________________

First Name: ____________________

Date of examination: ____________________

Sex:
- O Male
- O Female

Date of birth: ____________________

Age (in years): ____________________

Maiden name: ____________________

Street: ____________________

ZIP-code: ____________________

City: ____________________

Phone nr. (patient): ____________________

E-mail: ____________________

Phone nr. (relatives) ____________________

Outpatient:
- O No
- O Yes

Place of admission: ____________________

Height (cm): ____________________

Weight (kg): ____________________

Time of observation (how many months is the patient known to the examiner): ____________________

Diagnosis ICD 10:
- ☐ A strong desire or sense of compulsion to take the substance
- ☐ Difficulties in controlling substance-taking behaviour in terms of its onset, termination, or levels of use
- ☐ A physiological withdrawal state when substance use has ceased or been reduced.
- ☐ Evidence of tolerance
- ☐ progressive neglect of alternative pleasures or interests
- ☐ Persisting with substance use despite clear evidence of overtly harmful consequences

Diagnosis ICD 10:
- O No
- O Yes

Lesch Alcoholism Typology 3.0.22

Social and family history

Patient's data up to the age of 14:

Date of examination:	______________________
Mother's age at patient's birth:	______________________
Alcohol addictions among 1st degree relatives?	O No O Yes
Nicotine addictions among 1st degree relatives?	O No O Yes
Severe chronic diseases in the family (or household):	O No O Yes
Parent's attitude towards the patient when s/he was a child (patient's view):	O Loved O Not loved O Judgement not possible
Who raised the patient:	O Parents O Grandparents O Other family members O Frequently changing people
Psychiatric diseases in the patient's family (other than alcohol):	O No O Yes
If applicable, which:	______________________
Did the patient suffer from severe physical disabilities:	O No O Yes
Did the patient suffer from other severe diseases:	O No O Yes

Patient's data after the age of 14:

Marital status:	O Single O Living with a partner O Divorced O Widowed
Partner's attitude towards the patient:	O Inconspicuous O Dominant O Insecure / Resigning O Dismissive

Lesch Alcoholism Typology – Questionnaire

Lesch Alcoholism Typology 3.0.22

Examination's report

Date of examination: ______________________

Admission/Examination:
- O Voluntary
- O Involuntary

Pretreatment:
- O None
- O Outpatient
- O Once inpatient
- O Repeatedly inpatient

Inpatient treatment, how often? ______________________

Onset of alcohol dependence (age): ______________________

Onset of alcohol abuse (age): ______________________

Onset of somatic withdrawal symptoms (age): ______________________

Onset of tolerance decrease (age): ______________________

Drinking pattern:
- O Constant
- O Periodically changing
- O Changing in irregular intervals

Criminal acts before admission:
- O None
- O Alcohol related crime
- O Other crimes

Type of crime (1):
- O Disturbance of the peace
- O Bodily harm
- O Damage of property
- O Sex offence
- O Traffic offences
- O Others

If applicable, which (1): ______________________

Type of crime (2):
- O Disturbance of the peace
- O Bodily harm
- O Damage of property
- O Sex offence
- O Traffic offences
- O Others

If applicable, which (2): ______________________

Type of crime (3):
- O Disturbance of the peace
- O Bodily harm
- O Damage of property
- O Sex offence
- O Traffic offences
- O Others

If applicable, which (3): ______________________

Injuries under the influence of alcohol:
- O None
- O Once
- O Repeated

Lesch Alcoholism Typology 3.0.22

Examination's report (Fortsetzung)

Self assessment (last 3 months):
- O Abstinent
- O Moderate drinking
- O Heavy drinking
- O Judgement not possible

Loss of control (last 3 months):
- O Never
- O Ocassionally
- O Frequently
- O Permanently
- O Judgement not possible

Periods of abstinence:
- O Less than 1 month
- O 1 month to 6 months
- O 6 months to 1 year
- O More than 1 year
- O Judgement not possible

Assessment of patient's drinking behavior by others (relatives, doctor):
- O Abstinent
- O Adapted drinking
- O Not tolerated drinking
- O Judgement not possible

Self-treatment with hypnotics and benzodiacepines:
- O None
- O Regular
- O Irregular

Alcohol is currently used against (multiple answers possible):
- ☐ Anxiety
- ☐ Depressed mood
- ☐ Agitation
- ☐ Withdrawal symptoms (tremor, sweats, anxious and depressed states)
- ☐ Sleep disturbance
- ☐ To approve well-being
- ☐ Other

Relationship between drinking and smoking:
- O No
- O Yes

If applicable, which: ______________________

Relationship between drinking and drug abuse:
- O No
- O Yes

If applicable, which: ______________________

Drug abuse during last 3 months:
- O No
- O Yes

If applicable, which: ______________________

Lesch Alcoholism Typology – Questionnaire

Lesch Alcoholism Typology 3.0.22

Typology

This page defines the Lesch Typology.

Date of examination: ______________________

Symptoms before the age of 14 having a severe negative impact on childhood development:

Perinatal traumata:
- O No
- O Yes

Cerebral traumata:
- O No cerebral trauma
- O Contusio (unconscious for longer than 6 hours and/or neurological focal signs)

Other cerebral diseases:
- O No
- O Yes

Bedwetting after the age of 3:
- O No
- O Yes

Nail biting (>6 months):
- O No
- O Yes

Stuttering (>6 months):
- O No
- O Yes

Symptoms before and after the age of 14:

Seizures (grand mal):
- O None
- O Only during withdrawal
- O Also outside withdrawal

Symptoms after the age of 14:

Polyneuropathy:
- O None
- O Mild (pain and disturbed sensitivity)
- O Severe (missing Achilles reflex, calf-muscle atrophy, stocking-like numbness)

Somatic withdrawal syndrome:
- O Not existing
- O Mild withdrawal syndrome
- O Severe withdrawal syndrome and/or up to delirium tremens

Assessment of comorbidity:

Periodicity of drinking behavior:
- O No periodicity detectable
- O Periodicity detectable

Depressed mood:
- O None
- O Reactive depression
- O Affective mood disorders (ICD 10 - F3, DSM IV - 296.xx)

Sleep disturbances without alcohol intake:
- O No sleep disturbance
- O Interrupted sleep and/or very early awakening >4 weeks (independent of alcohol or withdrawal)
- O Major difficulties to fall asleep

Suicidal or parasuicidal tendencies:
- O Never
- O Only under influence of alcohol or during withdrawal
- O Independent of alcohol and withdrawal

Lesch Alcoholism Typology 3.0.22

Laboratory

Under the influence of alcohol at the time of examination: O No O Yes

If applicable, breathalyzer test: ____________________

Average daily alcohol intake of the last week in units (1 unit = 0.3 l beer, 1/8 l wine, 20 cl spirit)) ____________________

% CDT (cutoff <= 2.5%) ____________________

Laboratory:

	Current status:		**After 3 months sobriety:**		**Change:**
(*) ASAT (GOT):		U/l		U/l	
(*) ALAT (GPT):		U/l		U/l	
(*) gamma-GT:		U/l		U/l	
(*) Bilirubine:		mg/dl		mg/dl	
(*) Platelets:		G/l		G/l	
(*) MCV:		fl		fl	
Glucose:		mg/dl		mg/dl	
Cholesterol:		mg/dl		mg/dl	
Triglycerides:		mg/dl		mg/dl	
Red Blood Cells:		T/l		T/l	
Creatinine:		mg/dl		mg/dl	
Uric Acid:		mg/dl		mg/dl	

For scientific purpose:

Homocysteine:		µmol/l		µmol/l	
Leptine:		µmol/l		µmol/l	
Ghreline:		µmol/l		µmol/l	
proBNP:		pg/ml		pg/ml	

Lesch Alcoholism Typology 3.0.22

Liver

Symptoms:

Jaundice:
- O No
- O Yes

Ascites:
- O No
- O Yes

Spider hemangiomata:
- O No
- O Yes

Sonography:

Steatosis:
- O No
- O Yes

Hepatomegaly:
- O No
- O Yes

Splenomegaly:
- O No
- O Yes

Hepatitis B Serology (HbS-Ag):
- O Negative
- O Positive

HCV Antibody:
- O Negative
- O Positive

Additional information: ______________________

Lesch Alcoholism Typology 3.0.22

Additional Information

Date of examination: ______________________

Gastrointestinal or pancreatic diseases:
- O None
- O Mild
- O Severe

Other somatic diseases:
- O None
- O Functional
- O Severe

Which: ______________________

Cognitive impairment:
- O None
- O Slight
- O Severe
- O Judgement not possible

Additional important information:

Appendix 2

Appendix 2
Lesch European Smoker Classification

EUROPEAN SMOKER CLASSIFICATION

Patient- Initials ☐☐

Gender m ☐ f ☐

Age ☐

Name of questioner

Date of examination

☐.☐.☐

Please document

the personel data of your patient on the enclosed paper,

which, on reasons of data protection, should remain to you.

Authors:
M.Kunze
O.M.Lesch
R.Schoberberger
Dr.H.Walter

Biometry und Statistics:
A.Klingler

Treating physician:

Patient: ☐ outpatient ☐ inpatient

☐ Psychiatry

☐ special addicition center

☐ Pneumology

☐ Surgery

☐ Oncology

☐ Cardiology/ Angiology

☐ General practitioner

☐ Rehabilitation centre

☐ other:

which:

First contact ☐

The patient is known since:

☐ weeks

☐ months

☐ years

History of smoking

Onset of regular smoking:	☐ <10years ☐ 11-14years ☐ >15years

Patients self assessment:

Symptoms of dependence according ICD10:

A strong desire or sense of complusion to smoke a cigarette ☐	Evidence of tolerance, such that increased doses are required in order to achieve effects originally produced by lower doses ☐
Difficulties in controlling substance use in terms of onset, termination, or levels of use ☐	Progressive neglect of alternative pleasures or interests in favor of substances use ☐
Physical withdrawal ☐ (Mood disturbances, autonomous nervous system or strong desire, aggression and use of tobacco with the aim to soft these symptoms).	Continued substance use despite clear evidence of overtly harmful physical or psychological consequences ☐

Strong nicotine withdrawal syndrome	☐ yes ☐ no

Withdrawal syndrome is characterized by: (multiple answers possible)	
	☐ Mood disturbances, e.g. depression
	☐ vegetarian syndrom, e.g. sweeting
	☐ strong desire
	☐ aggressiv behaviour
	☐ others

Kind of pretreatment for nicotine withdrawal		
	☐ none	☐ out-patient
	☐ in-patient	☐ frequently in-patient

Since when did/do you want to stop smoking or to reduce the number of cigarettes?	☐ there is no intention ☐ during the last year ☐ 1 year or longer
Motivation for examination	☐ self-motivation ☐ disease ☐ others
Longest non-smoking period	☐ more than 1year ☐ 6 month - 1 year ☐ 1-6 months ☐ less than 1 month ☐ no episode without smoking
Do you smoke regularly (e.g. a cigarette every 30 minutes) if it is possible?	☐ yes ☐ no
Are there periods where you have no craving for nicotine, and are there situations when you even smoke more than usual?	☐ yes ☐ no

Smoking is used mainly in case of: (multiple answers possible)	☐ anxiety	☐ depression
	☐ agitation	☐ Sleep-disturbances
	☐ interrupted sleep	☐ stress
	☐ boredom	☐ Digestions-problems
	☐ increase of weight	☐ other
	☐ social reasons	
	☐ habit	which:

For females only: **Did you stop smoking during pregnancy?**	☐ yes	☐ no
	☐ never pregnant	

None prescribed sleeping pills or sedatives	☐ yes
	☐ no

Packyears:
average Quantity of the packs
per day x quantity of smoking years
(e.g. 30 Cig. since 40 years:
1,5 Pack./d x 40a = 60 pack-years) ☐

Familyhistory

Dependents in 1st degree relatives (parents, children, brothers)	☐ yes ☐ no	**If yes, addicted to which substance?** (multiple answers possible) ☐ alcohol ☐ tobacco ☐ others
Marital status of patient	☐ Single ☐ divorced	☐ living with a partner ☐ widowed
Parent´s attitude towards the patient as a child (patient´s view)	☐ positive	☐ not positive ☐ no judgment possible
Who brought up the patient?	☐ mainly father ☐ grandparents ☐ out of family	☐ mainly mother ☐ other family members ☐ changing persons
Psychiatric diseases in 1st degree relatives? (parents, children, brother)	☐ yes ☐ no	

Subgroups

Perinatal damage, which lead to developmental disturbances	☐ yes	☐ non
Cerebral traumata **Concussion: < 6 h unconscious** **Contusion: > 6 h unconscious or neurological focus**	☐ concussion ☐ no cerebral traumata	☐ contusion
other cerebral diseases, which had lead to developmental disturbances	☐ yes	☐ no
Epilepsy	☐ yes	☐ no
Enuresis nocturna after the age of 3 years	☐ yes (longer than 6 months)	☐ no ☐ occasionally
Nail biting strongly disturbing	☐ yes (longer than 6 months)	☐ no ☐ occasionally
Stuttering strongly disturbing	☐ yes (longer than 6 months)	☐ no ☐ occasionally
Periodicity of smoking behavior	☐ no periodicity detectable	☐ periodicity detectable

Lesch European Smoker Classification

How soon do you smoke your first cigarette after you wake up in the morning?	☐ within 5 minutes ☐ 6-30 minutes ☐ 31-60 minutes ☐ after 60 minutes
Do you find it difficult not to smoke in places where it is forbidden - for example, in church, library, etc.?	☐ yes ☐ no
Which cigarette would be hardest to refrain from?	☐ the first one in the morning ☐ any other
How many cigarettes do you smoke per day?	☐ 10 or less ☐ 11-20 ☐ 21-30 ☐ 31 or more
Do you smoke more frequently in the morning than during the rest of the day?	☐ yes ☐ no
Do you smoke when you have to stay bed for some days because you are ill?	☐ yes ☐ no
Sleep disorders	☐ yes ☐ no
Major depression in history	☐ yes ☐ no
Suicidal tendencies and attempts	☐ yes ☐ no

Other diseases:

Alcohol dependence	☐ yes	☐ no		
If yes: Lesch´s typology	☐ Type I	☐ II	☐ III	☐ IV
Liver diseases		☐ no	☐ light	☐ strong
Gastrointestinal diseases, (pancreatitis)		☐ no	☐ light	☐ strong
Bronchical/Pulmonary diseases		☐ no	☐ light	☐ strong
Cancer		☐ no	☐ light	☐ strong
Cardiovasculare diseases		☐ no	☐ light	☐ strong
Skin diseases		☐ no	☐ light	☐ strong
Metabolisation disturbances		☐ no	☐ light	☐ strong
Osteoporose		☐ no	☐ light	☐ strong
If one of the above mentioned diseases is declared with light or strong, please enter here the kind of the disease:				

If any other somatic diseases, which:

	☐ no	☐ light	☐ strong
	☐ no	☐ light	☐ strong

How strong was the desire for smoking in the last 30 days before your present examination

I had a great aversion against smoking

Please mark the degree of the desire intensity of craving.
(It is possible to mark intervalues, e.g. 29).

I don't care about smoking

I had great desire to smoke

Have there ever been moods/situations or periods within the last 12 months before the present examination, in which you never had a desire for nicotine?

no ☐

yes ☐

please declare which situations or moods:

In which situations and moods did you feel a desire for smoking (in the smoking periods) within the last 12 months before the present examination?

Please declare how strong (severe) the **desire** for smoking was. Then mark with a cross, if you have **usually smoked in this mood/situation** or not.

	desire for cigarettes				followed by smoking	
moods and situations	no	low	strong	very strong	yes	no
when I felt lonley	☐	☐	☐	☐	☐	☐
when I felt low-spirited	☐	☐	☐	☐	☐	☐
when I was in a depressed mood	☐	☐	☐	☐	☐	☐
when I wanted to get closer to someone I like	☐	☐	☐	☐	☐	☐
when I wanted to increase my sexual feelings	☐	☐	☐	☐	☐	☐
when I thought it does not matter to smoke a few cigaretts	☐	☐	☐	☐	☐	☐
when I was in good mood	☐	☐	☐	☐	☐	☐
when I was content and relaxed	☐	☐	☐	☐	☐	☐
when I wanted myself to comfortable	☐	☐	☐	☐	☐	☐

Continuation

Please declare how strong (severe) the **desire** for smoking was. Then mark with a cross, if you have usually smoked in this **mood/situation** or not.

	desire for cigarettes				followed by smoking	
mood situation	no	low	strong	very strong	yes	no
when I had troubles at work, e.g. with collegues	☐	☐	☐	☐	☐	☐
when I was at a party where people smoked	☐	☐	☐	☐	☐	☐

Do you wake up at night and have to smoke, to continue sleep?	☐ never ☐ rarely ☐ frequently per week
Are there any situations or **periods with strong desire for food, especially for sweets?**	☐ never ☐ rarely ☐ frequently per week
To which stress or load are you exposed?	☐ Physical hard work ☐ time-pressure ☐ conflicts ☐ multiple stress ☐ other which:

Comments:

This questionnaire was created with the scientific support of:

K. Aigner, Krankenhaus d. Elisabethinen, Linz
H. Brath, Krankenhaus Lainz, Wien
E. Groman, Nikotininstitut Wien
E. Hammer, Betriebsärztin Firma Swarovski, Wattens
R. Hainz, praktischer Arzt, Wien
R. Heschl, Rehabilitationszentrum Bad Ischl, Bad Ischl
I. Homeier, Pulmologisches Zentrum, Wien
A. Lichtenschopf, Rehabilitationszentrum Weyer
H. Lindner, Universitätsklinik f. Psychiatrie, Wien
M. Lobendanz, Landeskrankenhaus Salzburg
R. Matys, Kaiserin Elisabeth Spital, Wien
W. Reinisch, Betriebsarzt, Wien
A. Riegler, Universitätsklinik f. Psychiatrie, Wien
K. Ramskogler, Universitätsklinik f. Psychiatrie, Wien
F. Wimberger, Krankenhaus der Elisabethinen, Linz

Many thanks!

Literature

AAP Position paper (2005) J Periodontol 76:1601–1622.

Adams DR. (1990) An early counseling intervention program for problem drinkers contrasting group and individual delivery formats (group treatment). Unpublished doctoral dissertation, the University of British Columbia, Canada.

Adams JW. (1978) Psychoanalysis of drug dependence. In Feuerlein W. (Hrsg.) (1981) Sozialisationsstörungen und Sucht, Entstehungsbedingungen, Folgen, therapeutische Konsequenzen. Wiesbaden: Akademische Verlagsgesellschaft.

Addolorato G, Capristo E, Leggio L, Ferrulli A, Abenavoli L, Malandrino N, Farnetti S, Domenicali M, D'Angelo C, Vonghia L, Mirijello A, Cardone S, Gasbarrini G. (2006) Relationship between ghrelin levels, alcohol craving and nutritional status in current alcoholics. Alcohol Clin Exp Res 30:1933–7.

Aharan CH, Ogilvie RD, Partington JT. (1967) Clinical indications of motivation in alcoholic patients. Quaterly Journal of Studies on Alcohol 28:486–492.

Ait-Daoud N, Lynch WJ, Penberthy JK, Breland AB, Marzani-Nissen GR, Johnson BA. (2006) Treating smoking dependence in depressed alcoholics. Alcohol Res Health 29/3:213–20.

Ait-Daoud N, Wiesbeck GA, Bienkowski P, Li MD, Pfützer RH, Singer MV, Lesch OM, Johnson BA. (2005) Comorbid Alcohol and Nicotine Dependece: From the Biomolecular Basis to Clinical Consequences. Alcohol Clin Exp Res 29/8:1541–9.

Alden L. (1980) Preventive strategies in the treatment of alcohol abuse: A review and a proposal. In Davidson P and Davidson S. Behavioral medicine: Changing health lifestyles. New York: Brunner/Mazel:256–278.

Alden LE. (1988) Behavioral self-management controlled-drinking strategies in a context of secondary prevention. Journal of Consulting and Clinical Psychology 56:280–286.

Aliyev NN. (1993) Trail of interferon in chronic alcoholism. Psychiatry Research 54:307–308.

American Psychiatric Association. (1994) DSM IV. Diagnostic and statistical manual of mental disorders. Fourth Edition.

Angst J, Gamma A, Endrass J, Rössler W, Ajdacic-Gross V, Eich D, Herrell R, Merikangas KR. (2006) Ist the association of alcohol use disorders with major depressive disorder a consequence of undiagnosed bipolar-II disorder? Eur Arch Psychiatry Clin Neurosci 256:452–457.

Angst J. (1973) The course of monopolar depression and bipolar psychosis. Psychiatria, Neurologia, Neurochirurgica 76/6:489.

Anke M, Bojack B, Krämer G, Seißelberg K. (2003) Deeskalationsstrategien in der psychiatrischen Arbeit. Psychosoziale Arbeitshilfen 23, Bonn: Psychiatrieverlag.

Annis HM and Liban CB. (1979) A follow-up study of male halfway-house residents and matched non-resident controls. Journal of Studies on Alcohol 40:63–69.

Anthenelli R. (2004) Smoking cessation in smokers motivated to quit. Presented at: American College of Cardiology Scientific Sessions: March 7–10, 2004; New Orleans, LA.

Anthenelli RM, Smith TL, Craig CE, Tabakoff B, Schuckit MA. (1995) Platelet monoamine oxidase activity levels in subgroups of alcoholics: diagnostic, temporal, and clinical correlates. Biological Psychiatry 38:361–368.

Anton RF, Moak DH, Latham P. (1995) The Obsessive Compulsive Drinking Scale: a self-rated instrument for the quantification of thoughts about alcohol and drinking behaviour. Alcohol Clin Exp Res 19:92–99.

Anton RF, O'Malley SS, Ciraulo DA, Cisler RA, Couper D, Donovan DM, Gastfriend DR, Hosking JD, Johnson BA, LoCastro JS, Longabaugh R, Mason BJ, Mattson ME, Miller WR, Pettinati HM, Randall CL, Swift R, Weiss RD, Williams LD, Zweben A, COMBINE Study Research Group. (2006) Combined pharmacotherapies and behavioral interventions for alcohol dependence: the COMBINE study: a randomized controlled trial. JAMA 295/17:2003–17.

Antonovsky A. (1997) Salutogenese. Zur Entmystifizierung der Gesundheit. (A. Franke & N. Schulte, Übers.) Tübingen: Dgvt-Verlag (Original 1987).

Aramakis VB, Hsieh CY, Leslie FM, Metherate R. (2000) A critical period for nicotine-induced disruption of synaptic development in rat auditory cortex. The Journal of Neuroscience 20/16:6106–6116.

Arend H. (1999) Alkoholismus – Ambulante Therapie und Rückfallprophylaxe. Weinheim/Basel: Beltz.

Arendt F. (1994) Impairment in memory function and neurodegenerative changes in the cholinergic forebrain system induced by chronic intake of ethanol. J Neural Transm 44:173–187.

Arenz-Greiving I. (2001) Traditionelle Selbsthilfe – ein Auslaufmodell? In: Wienberg/Driessen (Hrsg.): Auf dem Weg zur vergessenen Mehrheit. Innovative Konzepte für die Versorgung von Menschen mit Alkoholproblemen. Bonn: Psychiatrieverlag.

Arkwright PD, Beilin LJ, Rouse I, Armstrong BK, Vandongen R. (1982) Effect of alcohol use and other aspects of lifestyle on blood pressure levels and prevalence of hypertension in a working population. Circulation 66:60–66.

Aveyard P and West R. (2007) Managing smoking cessation. BMJ 335:37–41.

Azrin NH, Sisson RW, Meyers R, Godley M. (1982) Alcoholism treatment by disulfiram and community reinforcement therapy. Journal of Behavior Therapy and Experimental Psychiatry 13:105–112.

Baan R, Straif K, Grosse Y, Secretan B, El Ghissassi F, Bouvard V, Altieri A, Cogliano V; WHO International Agency for Research on Cancer Monograph Working Group. (2007) Carcinogenicity of alcoholic beverages. Lancet Oncol 8:292–293.

Babor T, De Hoffman MI, Boca F, Hesselbrock V, Meyer R, Dolinsky Z, Rounsaville B. (1992) Types of alcoholics. I. Evidence for an empirically derived typology based on indicators of vulnerability and severity. Arch Gen Psychiatry 49:599–608.

Babor TF and Del Boca FK. (2003) Treatment Matching in Alcoholism. Cambridge: University Press.

Babor TF and Meyer RE. (1986) Typologies of Alcoholics: Overview. In M. Galanter (ed.), Recent Developments in Alcoholism. New York, NY: Plenum Publishing Corp 5:105–111.

Babor TF. (1996) The classification of alcoholics: typology theories from the 19th century to the present. Alcohol Health & Research World 20:6–14.

Baer U. (1991/2005) Sozialtherapie. Versuch einer Begriffsbestimmung. In Baer & Frick-Baer (Hrsg.): Bausteine einer kreativen Sozio- und Psychotherapie. Ausgewählte Beiträge 1991 bis 2005. Neunkirchen-Vluyn: Affenkönig.
Baer U. (2004/2005) Zur inhaltlichen Unterscheidung zwischen Soziotherapie und Psychotherapie. In Baer & Frick-Baer (Hrsg.): Bausteine einer kreativen Sozio- und Psychotherapie. Ausgewählte Beiträge 1991 bis 2005. Neunkirchen-Vluyn: Affenkönig.
Baer U. (2005) Die fünf Ebenen des Sozialen und die Landschaft der Soziotherapie. In Baer & Frick-Baer (Hrsg.): Bausteine einer kreativen Sozio- und Psychotherapie. Ausgewählte Beiträge 1991 bis 2005. Neunkirchen-Vluyn: Affenkönig.
Bailer UF, Frank GK, Henry SE, Price JC, Meltzer CC, Becker C, Ziolko SK, Mathis CA, Wagner A, Barbaric-Marsteller NC, Putnam K, Kaye WH. (2007) Serotonin transporter binding after recovery from eating disorders. Psychopharmacology 195/3:315–324.
Bailer UF, Frank GK, Henry SE, Price JC, Meltzer CC, Mathis CA, Wagner A, Thornton L, Hoge J, Ziolko SK, Becker CR, McConaha CW, Kaye WH. (2007) Exaggerated 5-HT 1A but normal 5-HT 2A receptor activity in individuals III with anorexia nervosa. Biol Psychiatry 61:1090–1099.
Bailer UF, Frank GK, Henry SE, Price JC, Meltzer CC, Weissfeld L, Mathis CA, Drevets WC, Wagner A, Hoge J, Ziolko SK, McConaha CW, Kaye WH. (2005) Altered brain serotonin 5-HT 1A receptor binding after recovery from anoresia nervosa measured by positron emission tomography and [Carbonyl11C]way-100635. Arch Gen Psychiatry 62:1032–1041.
Bailer UF, Price JC, Meltzer CC, Mathis CA, Frank GK, Weissfeld L, McConaha CW, Henry SE, Brooks-Achenbach S, Barbaric N, Kaye WH. (2004) Altered 5-HT 2A Receptor Binding after Recovery from bulimia-type anorexia nervosa: relationship to harm avoidance and drive for thinness. Neuropsychopharmacology 29:1143–1155.
Baischer W, Brichta A, Pfeffel F, Hajji M, Leitner H, Lesch OM, Müller Ch. (1995) Infection with hepatitis B or C virus of peripheral blood mononuclear cells in serologically negative chronic alcoholic patients. Journal of Hepatology 23/4:181.
Baker TB, Udin H, Vogler RE. (1975) The effects of videotaped modelling and confrontation on the drinking behaviour of alcoholics. International Journal of the Addictions 10:779–793.
Baldwin S, Heather N, Lawson A, Robertson I, Mooney J, Graggins F. (1991) Comparison of effectiveness: Behavioral and talk-based alcohol education courses for court-referred young offenders. Behavioural Psychotherapy 19:157–172.
Bales RF. (1991/1946) Cultural differences in rates of alcoholism. Quarterly Journal of Studies on Alcohol 6:480–499.
Balfour DJ and Ridley DL. (2000) The effects of nicotine on neural pathways implicated in depression: a factor in nicotine addiction? Pharmacol Biochem Behav 66/1:79–85.
Balint M. (1970) Therapeutische Aspekte der Regression. Stuttgart: Klett.
Barz J, Sprung R, Freudenstein P, Bonte W, Nimmerrichter A, Lesch OM, Jacob B. (1988) Investigations on methanol kinetics in alcoholics. Blutalkohol 25/3:163–71.
Basu D, Ball Sa, Feinn R, Gelernter J, Kranzler HR. (2004) Typologies of drug dependence: comparative validity of a multivariat and four univariat models. Drug Alcohol Depend 73:289–300.

Batra A. (2005) Tabakabhängigkeit. Wissenschaftliche Grundlagen und Behandlung. Stuttgart: Kohlhammer Verlag.

Bauer J. (2006) Prinzip Menschlichkeit. Warum wir von Natur aus kooperieren. Hamburg: Hofmann und Campe.

Bauer J. (2006) Warum ich fühle, was du fühlst. Intuitive Kommunikation und das Geheimnis der Spiegelneurone. München: Heyne.

Bauer J. (2007) Das Gedächtnis des Körpers. Wie Beziehungen und Lebensstile unsere Gene steuern. München: Piper.

Baumgartner Ch, Zeiler K, Auff E, Dal Bianco P, Holzner F, Lesch OM, Deecke L. (1988) Begünstigt Alkoholismus die Manifestation von Schlaganfällen? Wiener klinische Wochenschrift 100/4:99–107.

Baumgartner I. (2003) Pastoralpsychologie. Düsseldorf: Patmos.

Beck U. (2003) Risikogesellschaft. Auf dem Weg in eine andere Moderne. Frankfurt am Main: SuhrkampVerlag.

Beelmann A. (2006) Wirksamkeit von Präventionsmaßnahmen bei Kindern und Jugendlichen. Zeitschrift für Klinische Psychologie und Psychotherapie 35/2:151–162.

Beiglböck W, Feselmayer S, Honemann E. (2006) Handbuch der klinisch-psychologischen Behandlung. 2. erweiterte und überarbeitete Auflage. Wien New York: Springer.

Beiglböck W, Feselmayer S, Marx R. (1999) Nikotinentwöhnung bei Alkoholkranken – Eine Einführung ins Thema. Wiener Zeitschrift für Suchtforschung 22/2:3–7.

Benkelfat C, Murphy D, Hill J, George DT, Nutt D, Linnoila M. (1991) Ethanol like properties of the serotonergic partial agonist m-chlorophenylpiperazine in chronic alcoholic patients. Archives of General Psychiatry 48:383.

Benowitz NL, Porchet H, Sheiner L, Jacob III P. (1988) Nicotine absorption and cardiovascular effects with smokeless tobacco use: comparison with cigarettes and nicotine gum. Clin Pharmacol Ther 44:23–28.

Benyamina A et al. (2009) Association between MTHFR 677C-T polymorphism and alcohol dependence according to Lesch and Babor typology. Addict Biol. Sep; 14(4): 503–5

Beresford TP, Arciniegas DB, Alfers J, Clapp L, Martin B, Beresford HF, Du Y, Liu D, Shen D, Davatzikos C, Laudenslager ML. (2006a) Hypercortisolism in alcohol dependence and its relation to hippocampal volume loss. J Stud Alcohol 67/6:861–7.

Beresford TP, Arciniegas DB, Alfers J, Clapp L, Martin B, Du Y, Liu D, Shen D, Davatzikos C. (2006) Hippocampus volume loss due to chronic heavy drinking. Alcohol Clin Exp Res 30/11:1866–70.

Berlakovich GA, Windhager T, Freundorfer E, Lesch OM, Steininger R, Mühlbacher F. (1999) Carbohydrate Deficient Transferrin for Detection of Alcohol Relapse after Orthotopic Liver Transplantation for Alcoholic Cirrhosis. Transplantation 67/9:1231–1235.

Berner P, Lesch OM, Walter H. (1986) Alcohol and depression. Psychopahtology 19/2:177–183.

Berner P. (1986) Psychiatrische Systematik. Bern Stuttgart Wien: Huber.

Besson J, Aeby F, Kasas A, Lehert P, Potgieter A. (1998) Combined efficacy of acamprosate and disulfiram in the treatment of alcoholism: a controlled study. Alcohol Clin Exp Res 22/3:573–9.

Best JA, Thomson SJ, Santi SM. (1988) Preventing cigarette smoking among school children. Annual Review of Public health 9:161–201.

Bien TH and Burge R. (1990) Smoking and drinking: A review of the literature. International Journal of Addiction 25:1429–1454.

Blanc M and Daeppen JB. (2005) Does disulfiram still have a role in alcoholism treatment? Rev Med Suisse 1/26:1728–1733.

Bleich S, Bayerlein K, Reulbach U, Hillemacher T, Bonsch D, Mugele B, Kornhuber J, Sperling W. (2004) Homocysteine levels in patients classified according to Lesch's typology. Alcohol &Alcoholism 39/6:493–8.

Bleich S, Bleich K, Kropp S, Bittermann HJ, Degner D, Sperling W, Rüther E, Kornhuber J. (2001) Moderate alcohol consumption in social drinkers raises plasma, homocystein levels: a contradiction to the ‚french paradox'. Alcohol and Alcoholism 36:189–192.

Bleuler M. (1972) Die schizophrenen Geistesstörungen im Lichte langjähriger Kranken- und Familiengeschichten. Stuttgart: Thieme.

Bleuler M. (1983) Lehrbuch der Psychiatrie. 15. Auflage, Berlin Heidelberg New York: Springer.

Boening J, Lesch OM, Spanagel R, Wolffgramm J, Narita M, Sinclair D, Mason B, Wiesbeck G. (2001) Pharmacological Relapse Prevention in Alcohol Dependence: From Animal Models To Clinical Trials. Alcohol Clin Exp Res 25/5:127–131.

Boffetta P and Hashibe M. (2006a) Alcohol and Cancer. Lancet Oncol 7:149–156.

Boffetta P, Hashibe M, La Vecchia C, Zatonski W, Rehm J. (2006b) The burden of cancer attributable to alcohol drinking. Int J Cancer 119:884–887.

Bohman MS, Sigvardsson S, Cloninger CR. (1981) Maternal inheritance of alcohol abuse. Cross-fostering analysis of adopted women. Arch Gen Psychiatr 38:965.

Bolego C, Poli A, Paoletti R. (2002) Smoking and gender. Cardiovasc Res 53:568–576.

Bonneux L. (2007) Cardiovascular risk models. BMJ 335:107–108.

Bönsch D, Bayerlein K, Reulbach U, Fiszer R, Hillemacher T, Sperling W, Kornhuber J, Bleich S. (2006) Different allele-distribution of MTHFR 677 C -> T and MTHFR -393 C -> A in patients classified according to subtypes of Lesch's typology. Alcohol and Alcoholism 41/4:364–367.

Bonte W. (1987) Begleitstoffe alkoholischer Getränke. Lübeck: Verlag Max Schmidt-Römhild.

Boruin CM, Mann BJ, Cone LT, Henggeler SW, Fucci BR, Blaske DM, Williams RA. (1995) Multisystemic Treatment of Serious Juvenile Offenders: Long-term Prevention of Criminality and Violence. Journal of Consulting and Clinical Psychology 63:569–578.

Bowers TG und Al-Redha MR. (1990) A comparison of outcome with group/marital and standard/individual therapies with alcoholics. Journal of Studies on Alcohol 51:301–309.

Bradley KA, Kivlahan DR, Bush KR, McDonell And MB, Fihn SD; Ambulatory Care Quality Improvement Project Investigators (2001) Variations on the CAGE alcohol screening questionnaire: strengths and limitations in VA general medical patients. Alcohol Clin Exp Res 25:1472–1478.

Brady KT, Myrick H, Henderson S, Coffey SF. (2002) The use of divalproex in alcohol relapse prevention: a pilot study. Drug Alcohol Depend 67/3:323–30.

Brandsma JM, Maultsby MC, Welsh RJ. (1980) The outpatient treatment of alcoholism: A review and comparative study. Baltimore MD: University Park Press.

Brenner MH. (1975) Trends in alcohol consumption and associated illness. Some effects of economic changes. American Journal of Public Health 65/12):1279–1292.

Brody AL, Mandelkern MA, London ED, Olmstead RE, Farahi J, Scheibal D, Jou J, Allen V, Tiongson E, Chefer SI, Koren AO, Mukhin AG. (2006) Cigarette smoking saturates brain alpha 4 beta 2 nicotinic acetylcholine receptors. Arch Gen Psychiatry 63/8:907–15.

Brown GL and Linnoila MI. (1990) CSF serotonin metabolite (5-HIAA) studies in depression, impulsivity and violence. The Journal of Clinical Psychiatry 51:31–41.

Brown J, Babor TF, Litt M, Kranzler H. (1994) The Type A/Type B distinction. Subtyping alcoholics according to indicators of vulnerability and severity. Babor T, Hesselbrock V, Meyer R, Shoemaker W. Types of Alcoholics. Ann NY Acad Sci 708:23–33.

Brown RA. (1980) Conventional education and controlled drinking education courses with convicted drunken drivers. Behavior Therapy 11:632–642.

Bruun K. (1963) Outcome of different types of treatment of alcoholics. Quarterly Journal of Studies on Alcohol 24:280–288.

Burger Ch, Marx R. (2001) Psychotherapiemotivation, generalisierte Kompetenzerwartung und Kontrollüberzeugungen zu Krankheit und Gesundheit von männlichen Alkoholikern klassifiziert nach der Typologie von Lesch. Wiener Zeitschrift für Suchtforschung 24/2:23–40.

Butler R and Goldstein H. (1973) Smoking in Pregnancy and Subsequent Child Development. British Medical Journal 4:573–575.

Buydens-Branchey L, Branchey MH, Noumair D, Lieber CS. (1989) Age of alcolism onset. II: Relationship to susceptibility to serotonin precursor availibility. Archives of General Psychiatry 46:231–236.

Caddy GR and Lovibond SH. (1976) Self-regulation and discriminated aversive conditioning in the modification of alcoholics' drinking behavior. Behavior Therapy 7:223–230.

Cahalan D. (1970) Problem Drinkers. San Francisco, Calif: Jossey-Bass.

Cahill K, Stead LF, Lancaster T. (2007) Nicotine receptor partial agonists for smoking cessation (Review). The Cochrane Library 1:1–25.

Cahill K, Ussher M. (2007) Cannabinoid type 1 receptor antagonists (rimonabant) for smoking cessation. Cochrane Database Syst Rev. 2007 Jul 18;(3):CD005353.

Cardoso Neves JM, Barbarosa A, Ismail F, Pombo S. (2006) NETER Alcoholic Typology (NAT). Alcohol and Alcoholism 41/2:133–139.

Cardoso RA, Brozowski SJ, Chavez-Noriega LE, Harpold M, Valenzuela CF, Harris RA. (1999) Effects of ethanol on recombinant human neuronal nicotinic acetylcholine receptors expressed in Xenopus oocytes. J Pharmacol Exp Ther 289/2:774–80.

Carpenter RA, Lyons CA, Miller WR. (1985) Peer-managed self-control program for prevention of alcohol abuse in American Indian high school students: A pilot evaluation study. International Journal of the Addictions 20:299–310.

Carr A. (1992) Endlich Nichtraucher! Der einfachste Weg mit dem Rauchen Schluss zu machen. Wilhelm Goldmann.

Carroll KM, Nich C, Ball SA, McCance E, Frankforter TL, Rousanaville BJ. (2000) One-Year follow-up of disulfiram and psychotherapy for cocain-alcohol users: Sustained effects of treatment. Addiction 95/9:1335–1349.
Caspi A and Moffitt TE. (2006) Gene-environment interactions in psychiatry: joining forces with neuroscience. Nat Rev Neurosci 7/7:583–90.
Caspi A, Sugden K, Moffitt TE, Taylor A, Craig IW, Harrington H, McClay J, Mill J, Martin J, Braithwaite A, Poulton R. (2003) Influence of life stress on depression: moderation by a polymorphism in the 5-HTT gene. Science 301/5631:386–9.
Chan AW, Pristach EA and Welte JW. (1994) Detection by the CAGE of alcoholism or heavy drinking in primary care outpatients and the general population. Journal of Substance Abuse 6:123–135.
Chaney ER, O'Leary MR, Marlatt GA. (1978) Skill training with alcoholics. Journal of Consulting and Clinical Psychology 46:1092–1104.
Chantenoud L, Parazzini F, Di Cintio E, Zanconato G, Benzi G, Bortolus R, La Vecchia C. (1998) Paternal and maternal smoking habitus before conception and during the first trimester: relation to spontaneous abortion. Annals of Epidemiology 8/8:520–6.
Chapman PLH and Huygens I. (1988) An evaluation of three treatment programmes for alcoholism: An experimental study with 6- and 18-month follows-ups. British Journal of addiction 83:67–81.
Cheer JF, Wassum KM, Sombers LA, Heien ML, Ariansen JL, Aragona BJ, Phillips PE, Wightman RM. (2007) Phasic dopamine release evoked by abused substances requires cannabinoid receptor activation. J Neurosci 27/4:791–5.
Chick J, Anton R, Checinski K, Croop R, Drummond DC, Farmer R, Labriola D, Marshall J, Moncrieff J, Morgan MY, Peters T, Ritson B. (2000) A multicentre, randomized, double-blind, placebo-controlled trial of naltrexone in the treatment of alcohol dependence or abuse. Alcohol Alcohol 35/6:587–93.
Chick J, Gough K, Wojeciech F, Kershaw P, Hore B, Mehta B, Ritson B, Ropner R, Torley D. (1992) Disulfiram treatment of alcoholism. British Journal of Psychiatry 161:84–89.
Chick J. (1995) Acamprosate as an aid in the treatment of alcoholism. Alcohol Alcohol 30/6:785–7.
Chick J. (2004) Disulfiram: cautions on liver function; how to supervise. Addiction 99/1:25.
Chudley AE, et al. (2005) Fetal alcohol spectrum disorder: Canadian guidelines for diagnosis. CMAJ, Mar. 1, 172(5 suppl).
Cloninger CR, Bohman M, Sigvardsson S. (1981) Inheritance of alcohol abuse: cross-fostering analyses of adopted men. Arch Gen Psychiatry 38:861–8.
Cloninger CR, Sigvardsson S, Gilligan SB, von Knorring AL, Reich T, Bohman M. (1988) Genetic heterogeneity and the classification of alcoholism. Adv Alcohol Subst Abuse 7/3-4:3–16.
Cloninger CR. (1987) Neurogenetic adaptive mechanisms in alcoholism. Science 236:410–416.
Coe JW, Brooks PR, Vetelino MG, Wirtz MC, Arnold EP, Huang J, Sands SB, Davis TI, Lebel LA, Fox CB, Shrikhande A, Heym JH, Schaeffer E, Rollema H, Lu Y, Mansbach RS, Chambers LK, Rovetti CC, Schulz DW, Tingley FD 3rd, O'Neill BT. (2005) Varenicline: an alpha4beta2 nicotinic receptor partial agonist for smoking cessation. J Med Chem 48/10:3474–7.

Coghlan GR. (1979) The investigation of behavioural self-control theory and techniques in a short-term treatment of male alcohol abusers. Unpublished doctoral dissertation, State University of New York at Albany.

Cohen C, Kodas E, Griebel G. (2005) CB1 receptor antagonists for the treatment of nicotine addiction. Pharmacol Biochem Behav 81/2:387–95.

Cohen C, Perrault G, Voltz C, Steinberg R, Soubrie P. (2002) SR141716, a central cannabinoid (CB(1)) receptor antagonist, blocks the motivational and dopamine-releasing effects of nicotine in rats. Behav Pharmacol 13:451–463.

Cole A and Kmietowicz Z. (2007) BMA calls for action on "epidemic" of alcohol related problems. BMJ 334:1343.

Coleman D. (2006) Soziale Intelligenz. München: Droemer.

Collins AC. (1990) Interactions of ethanol and nicotine at the receptor level. Recent Developments in Alcoholism 8:221–231.

Colombo G, Agabio R, Fa M, Guano L, Lobina C, Loche A, Reali R, Gessa GL. (1998) Reduction of voluntary ethanol intake in ethanol-preferring sP rats by the cannabinoid antagonist SR-141716. Alcohol Alcohol 33/2:126–30.

Colombo G, Serra S, Vacca G, Carai MA, Gessa GL. (2005) Endocannabinoid system and alcohol addiction: pharmacological studies. Pharmacol Biochem Behav 81/2:369–80.

Connors GJ, Tarbox AR, Faillace LA. (1992) Achieving and maintaining gains among problem drinkers: Process and outcome results. Behavior Therapy 23:449–474.

Conrad KJ, Hultman CI, Pope AR, Lyons JS, Baxter WC, Daghestani AN, Lisiecki JP, Elbaum PL, McCarthy M, Manheim LM. (1998) Case managed residential care for homeless addicted veterans: Results of a true experiment. Medical Care 1:40–53.

Cooney NL, Kadden RM, Litt MD, Gerter H. (1991) Matching alcoholics to coping skills or interactional therapies: Two-year follow-up results. Journal of Consulting and Clinical Psychology 59:598–601.

Cooper ML, Frone M, Russell M, Mudar P. (1995) Drinking to regulate positive and negative emotions: a motivational model of alcohol use. Journal of Personality and Social Psychology 69:990–1005.

Cornelius JR, Salloum IM, Mezzich J, Cornelius MD, Fabrega H, Ehler JG, Ulrich RF, Thase ME, Mann JJ. (1995) Disproportionate suicidality in patients with comorbid major depression and alcoholism. American Journal of Psychiatry 152:358–364.

Covey LS, Glassman AH, Jiang H, Fried J, Masmela J, Loduca C, Petkova E, Rodriguez K. (2007) A randomized trial of bupropion and/or nicotine gum as maintenance treatment for preventing smoking relapse. Addiction 102/8:1292–302.

Coyle JT. (2006) Substance use disorders and Schizophrenia: a question of shared glutamatergic mechanisms. Neurotox Res 10/3–4:221–33.

Cramon DY. (1988) Planen und Handeln. In: Cramon/Zihl (Hrsg.): Neuropsychologische Rehabilitation, Berlin: Springer.

Cravo ML, Gloria LM, Selhub J, Nadeau MR, Camilo ME, Resende MP, Cardoso JN, Leitao CN, Mira FC. (1996) Hyperhomocysteinemia in chronic alcoholism: correlation with folate, vitamin B-12, and vitamin B-6 status. The American Journal of Clinical Nutrition 63:220–224.

Cravo, ML and Camilo, ME. (2000) Hyperhomocysteinemia in chronic alcoholism: relations to folic acid and vitamins B6 and B12 status. Nutrition 16: 296–302.

Crews FT and Braun CJ. (2003) Binge ethanol treatment causes greater brain damage in alcohol-preferring P rats than in alcohol-non-preferring NP rats. Alcoholism: Clinical and Experimental Research 27/7:1075–82.

Crews FT, Braun CJ, Hoplight B, Switzer RC, Knapp DJ. (2000) Binge ethanol consumption causes differential brain damage in young adolescent rats compared with adult rats. Alcoholism: Clinical and Experimental Research 24/11:1712–23.

Crews FT, Collins MA, Dlugos C, Littleton J, Wilkins L, Neafsey EJ, Pentney R, Snell LD, Tabakoff B, Zou J, Noronha A. (2004) Alcohol-induced neurodegeneration: when, where and why? Alcohol Clin Exp Res 28/2:350–64.

Cuculi F, Kobza R, Ehmann T, Erne P. (2006) ECG changes amongst patients with alcohol withdrawal seizures and delirium tremens. Swiss Med Wkly 136:223–227.

Dahlgren L and Willander A. (1989) Are special treatment facilities for female alcoholics needed? A controlled 2-year follow-up study from a specialized female unit (EWA) versus a mixed male/female facility. Alcoholism: Clinical and Experimental Research 13/4:499–504.

Damasio AR. (2003) Der Spinoza Effekt. Wie Gefühle unser Leben bestimmen. List Verlag.

Danysz W, Parsons CG, Jirgensons A, Kauss V, Tillner J. (2002) Amino-alkyl-cyclohexanes as a novel class of uncompetitive NMDA receptor antagonists. Curr Pharm Des 8/10:835–43.

Dauer S. (1999) Zu Wechselwirkungen von Gesundheit und Arbeitslosigkeit. In: Dauer S, Henning H. (Hrsg): Arbeitslosigkeit und Gesundheit. Halle: Mitteldeutscher Verlag:12–23.

Davidson DM. (1989) Cardiovascular effects of alcohol. West J Med 151:430–439.

De Bree A, Verschuren WMM, Kromhout D, Kluitmans LAJ, Blom HJ. (2002) Homocysteine determinants and to what extent homocysteine determines the risk of coronary heart disease. Pharmacological Reviews 54:599–618.

De Sousa A and De Sousa A. (2004) A one-year pragmatic trial of naltrexone vs disulfiram in the treatment of alcohol dependence. Alcohol Alcohol 39/6:528–31.

De Vito RA. (1970) Toward a Psychodynamic Theory of Alcoholism. In Wetzer E. (1995) Determinanten des Suchtverhaltens und der Rückfallsituation bei Alkoholkranken typologiesiert nach Lesch. Diplomarbeit aus dem Hauptfach Psychologie. Wien.

De Witte P, Littleton J, Parot P, Koob G. (2005) Neuroprotective and abstinence-promoting effects of acamprosate: elucidating the mechanism of action. CNS Drugs 19/6:517–37.

Deev A, Shestov D, Abernathy J, Kapustina A, Muhin N, Irving S. (1998) Association of alcohol consumption to mortality in middle-ages U.S. and Russian men and women. Annals of Epidemiology 8:147–153.

Del Boca FK and Hesselbrock MN. (1996) Gender and alcoholic subtypes. Alcohol Health Res World 20:56–66.

Del Boca FK. (1994) Sex, gender and alcoholic typologies. Babor T, Hesselbrock V, Meyer R, Shoemaker W. Types of Alcoholics. Ann NY Acad Sci 708:34–48.

Demir B, Ucar G, Ulug B, Ulusoy S, Sevinc I, Batur S. (2002) Platelet monoamine oxidase acitivity in alcoholism subtypes: relationships to personality and executive functions. Alcohol Alcohol 37:597–602.

Denson R, Nanson JL, McWatters MA. (1975) Smoking mothers more likely to have hyperactive (ADHD) children. Canadian Psychiatric Asociation Journal 20:183–187.

Després JP, Golay A, Sjöström L. (2005) Effects of Rimonabant on Metabolic Risk Factors in Overweight Patients with Dyslipidemia. The new England Journal of Medicine 353:2121–2134.

Devlin AM, Clarke R, Birks J, Grimley Evans J, Halsted CH. (2006) Interactions among polymorphisms in folate-metabolizing genes and serum total homocysteine concentrations in a healthy elderly population. American Journal of Clinical Nutrition 83:708–713.

Diaz FJ, Jane M, Salto E, Pardell H, Salleras L, Pinet C, De Leon J. (2005) A brief measure of high nicotine dependance for busy clinicians and large epidemiological surveys. Australian and New Zealand Journal of Psychiatry 39:161–168.

Dilling H, Mombour W, Schmidt MH. (1991) Internationale Klassifikation psychischer Störungen. Verlag Hans Huber Bern Göttingen Toronto (WHO).

Ditman KS, Crawford GG, Forgy EW, Moskowitz H, Mac Andrew C. (1967) A controlled experiment on the use of court probation for drunk arrests. American Journal of Psychatry 124:160–163.

Dörner K, Plog U, Teller C, Wendt F. (2002) Irren ist menschlich. Lehrbuch der Psychiatrie und Psychotherapie. Bonn: Psychiatrie-Verlag.

Dostojewskij FM. (2001) Der Spieler. Patmos Verlag.

Driessen M, Meier S, Hill A, Wetterling T, Lange W, Junghanns K. (2001) The course of anxiety, depression and drinking behaviours after completed detoxification in alcoholics with and without comorbid anxiety and depressive disorders. Alcohol and Alcoholism 36/3:249–255.

Driessen M, Schulte S, Luedecke C, Schaefer I, Sutmann F, Ohlmeier M, Kemper U, Koesters G, Chodzinski C, Schneider U, Broese T, Dette C, Havemann-Reinicke U, and the TRAUMAB-Study group. (2008)Trauma and PTSD in patients with alcohol, drug or dual dependence: a multi-center study. Alcohol Clin Exp Res.;32(3):481–8.

Dubois B, Slachevsky A, Litvan I,Pillon B. (2000) The FAB: A frontal assessment battery at bedside. Neurology; 55: 1621–1626

Dvorak A, Pombo S, Ismail F, Barbosa A, Cardoso JM, Figueira ML, Walter H, Lesch OM (2006) Tipologias da dependência do álcool e o seu significado para a terapêutica médica. Acta Psiquiátrica Portuguesa 52/2:1693–1705.

Dvorak A, Ramskogler K, Hertling I, Walter H, Lesch OM (2003) Alcohol dependence and depressive Syndromes. International Clinical Psychopharmacology 18/1:47–53.

Dyer AR, Stamler J, Berkson DM, Lepper MH, McKean H, Shekelle RB, Lindberg HA, Garside D. (1977) Alcohol consumption, cardiovascular risk factors, and mortality in two Chicago epidemiologic studies. Circulation 56:1067–1074.

Edwards G und Guthrie S. (1967) A controlled trial of inpatient and outpatient treatment of alcohol dependency. Lancet 1:555–559.

Edwards NB, Simmons RC, Rosenthal TL, Hoon PW, Downs JM. (1988) Doxepin in the treatment of nicotine withdrawal. Psychomatics 29:203–206.

Eisenbach-Stangl I. (1991) Eine Gesellschaftsgeschichte des Alkohols. Produktion, Konsum und soziale Kontrolle alkoholischer Rausch- und Genußmittel in Österreich 1918–1984. Frankfurt: Campus Verlag.

Eisenbach-Stangl I. (1994) Die neue Nüchternheit. Epidemiologie legalen und illegalen Drogengebrauchs von Kindern, Jugendlichen und jungen Erwachsenen in Österreich. In: Janig H./Rathmayr B. (Hg.): Wartezeit. Studien zu den Lebensverhältnissen Jugendlicher in Österreich. Wien: Österreichischer Studienverlag:189–216.

Eisermann G. (1973) Die Lehre von der Gesellschaft Ein Lehrbuch der Soziologie. 2. Auflage, Enke Ferdinand Verlag.

Ends EJ and Page CW. (1957) A study of three types of group psychotherapy with hospitalized inebriates. Quarterly Journal of Studies on Alcohol 18:263–277.

Engel U and Hurrelmann K. (1993) Was Jugendliche wagen. Juventa.

Engel U and Hurrelmann K. (1998) Was Jugendliche wagen. Eine Längsschnittstudie über Drogenkonsum, Stressreaktionen und Delinquenz im Jugendalter. Weinheim: Juventa.

Erfurth A, Gerlach A L, Michael N, Boenigk I, Hellweg I, Signoretta S, Akiskal K, Akiskal H S (2005) Distribution and gender effects of the subscales of a German version of the temperament autoquestionaire briefTEMPS-M in a university student population. Journal of Affective Disorders 85, 71–76

Eriksen L, Björnstad S, Götestam KG. (1986b) Social skills training in groups for alcoholics: One-year treatment outcome for groups and individuals. Addictive Behaviors 11:309–330.

Eriksen L. (1986a) The effect of waiting for inpatient treatment after detoxification: An experimental comparison between inpatient treatment and advice only. Addictive Behaviors 11:389–398.

Evans SM, Levin FR, Brooks DJ, Garawi F. (2007) A pilot double-blind treatment trial of memantine for alcohol dependence. Alcohol Clin Exp Res 31/5:775–82.

Ewing JA. (1984) Detecting alcoholism. The CAGE questionnaire. Journal of American Medical Association 252:1905–1907.

Eysenck HJ. (1973) Personaltiy and the maintenance of the smoking habit. Dunn WL. Smoking Behavior: Motives and Incentives. Toronto Wiley:113–136.

Fabian-Fine R, Skehel P, Errington ML, Davies HA, Sher E, Stewart MG, Fine A. (2001) Ultrastructural distribution of the alpha7 nicotinic acetylcholine receptor subunit in rat hippocampus. The Journal of Neuroscience 21/20:7993–8003.

Fachausschuss Soziotherapie des AHG Wissenschaftsrates (Hrsg.) (2000): Soziotherapie chronisch Abhängiger – ein Gesamtkonzep.t Verhaltensmedizin heute. Geesthacht: Neuland.

Fagerström KO and Schneider NG. (1989) Measuring nicotine dependence: a review of the Fagerström Tolerance Questionnaire. J Behav Med 12/2:159–182.

Fengler J. (2004) Süchtige und Tüchtige – Erkennen und Bewältigen von Burn-out in der Arbeit mit Abhängigen. In: Steingass (Hrsg): Geht doch. Soziotherapie chronisch mehrfach beeinträchtiger Abhängiger. Geesthacht: Neuland.

Fenichel O. (2005) Psychoanalytische Neurosenlehre. Band I, II und III. Psychosozial-Verlag.

Ferrell WL and Galassi JP. (1981) Assertion training and human relations training in the treatment of chronic alcoholics. International Journal of the Addictions 16:959–968.

Ferry LH. (1999) Non-nicotine pharmacotherapy for smoking cessation. Prim Care 26:653–669.

Feuerlein W, Küfner H, Soyka M. (1998) Alkoholismus – Missbrauch und Abhängigkeit. 5. Aufl. Stuttgart/New York: Thieme.
Feuerlein W. (1975) Alkoholismus – Missbrauch und Abhängigkeit, Entstehung – Folgen – Therapie. 1. Auflage. Thieme.
Feuerlein W. (1981) Sozialisationsstörungen und Sucht, Entstehungsbedingungen, Folgen, therapeutische Konsequenzen. Wiesbaden: Akademische Verlagsgesellschaft.
Feuerlein W. (1989) Wenn Alkohol zum Problem wird. TRIAS, Thieme Hippokrates Enke.
Fichter MM and Quadflieg N. (2001) Prevalence of mental illness in homeless men in Munich, Germany: results from a representative sample. Acta Psychiatrica Scandinavica 103:94–104.
Fichter MM, Quadflieg N, Greifenhagen A, Koniarczyk M, Wölz J. (1997) Alcoholism among homeless men in Munich, Germany. Eur Psychiatry 12:64–74.
Fiedler P. (1998) Persönlichkeitsstörungen. Weinheim: Beltz Psychologie Verlags-Union.
Fiore MC, Bailey WC, Cohen SJ, Dorfman SF, Goldstein MG, Gritz ER, Heyman RB, Jaen CR, Kottke TE, Lando HA, Mecklenberg RE, Mullen PD, Nett LM, Robinson L, Stizer ML, Tommasello AC, Villejo L, Wewers ME. (2000) Treating Tobacco Use and Dependence. Clinical Practice Guideline. Rockville, MD: US Department of Health and Human Services, Public Health Service.
Fiore MC, Jaén CR, Baker TB, et al. (2008) Treating Tobacco Use and Dependence: 2008 Update. Clinical Practice Guideline. Rockville, MD: US Department of Health and Human Services, Public Health Service.
Fischer G. (2002) Therapie mit Opioiden. Facultas Verlag.
Forel A. (1930) Die Trinksitten, ihre hygienische und soziale Bedeutung. Sozialst. Abstinentenbund d. Schweiz.
Forel A. (1935) Rückblick auf mein Leben. Zürich; Mémoires. Neuchâtel 1941; Out of my life and work. New York.
Formigoni MLOS und Neumann BRG. (1995) Treatment of drug and alcohol dependents through brief intervention: The first Brazilian experience. In Monteiro MG und Inciardi JA. Brasil-United States binational research. Sao Paulo, Brasil: CEBRID.
Foroud T, Bucholz KK, Edenberg HJ, Goate A, Neuman RJ, Porjesz B, Koller DL, Rice J, Reich T, Bierut LJ, Cloninger CR, Nurnberger JI, Li TK Jr., Conneally PM, Tischfield JA, Crowe R, Hesselbrock V, Schuckit M, Begleiter H. (1998) Evidence for linkage of an alcohol-related phenotype to chromosome 16. Alcohol ClinExp Res 22:2035–42.
Foucault M. (1980) Power/Knowledge: Selected Interviews and Other Writings 1972–77. New York: Pantheon.
Foy DW, Nunn Bl, Rychtarik RG. (1984) Broad-spectrum behavioural treatment for chronic alcoholics: Effects of training controlled drinking skills. Journal of Consulting and Clinical Psychology 52:213–230.
Frank GK, BailerUF, Henry SE, Drevets W, Meltzer CC, Price JC, Mathis CA, Wagner A, Hoge J, Ziolko S, Barbaric-Marsteller N, Weissfeld L, Kaye WH. (2005) Increased dopamine D2/D3 receptor binding after recovery from anorexia nervosa measured by positron emission tomography and [11C] raclopride. Biol Psychiatry 58:908–912.
Frank H. (2002) Risikokinder. Wiener Zeitschrift für Suchtforschung 25/1–2:83–92.

Franke A, Elsesser K, Sitzler F, Algermissen G, Kötter S. (1998) Gesundheit und Abhängigkeit bei Frauen: eine salutogenetische Verlaufsstudie. Cloppenburg: Runge.

Freedberg EJ and Johnston WE. (1978) The effects of assertion training within the context of a multi-modal alcoholism treatment program for employed alcoholics. Substudy No. 796. Toronto, Ontario: Addiction Research Foundation.

Freud S. (1905) 3 Abhandlungen zur Sexualtheorie. Fischer Verlag.

Freud S. (1952–1968) Gesammelte Werke in 18 Bänden, London Frankfurt: Fischer Verlag.

Frieboes RM. (2005) Grundlagen und Praxis der Soziotherapie. Richtlinien, Begutachtung, Behandlungskonzepte, Fallbeispiele, Antragsformulare. Stuttgart: Kohlhammer.

Friedrich F, Grünberger J, Blüml V, Kogoj D, Vissoky B, Walter H, Lesch O (2010) Vigilanzprüfung bei Alkoholabhängigkeit mittels Pupillometrie. Publication in preparation

Fromme K and Kruse MI. (2003) Socio-cultural and individual influences on alcohol use and abuse by adolescents and young adults. In Johnson BA, Ruiz P, Galanter M (Eds.) Handbook of Clinical Alcoholism Treatment:26–36, Lippincott Williams & Wilkins: Baltimore, MD.

Frost L and Vestergaard P. (2004) Alcohol and risk of atrial fibrillation or flutter: a cohort study. Arch Intern Med 164:1993–1998.

Fuller RK and Roth HP. (1979) Disulfiram for the treatment of alcoholism: An evaluation in 128 men. Annals of Internal Medicine 90:901–904.

Fuller RK, Branchey L, Brightwell Dr, Derman RM, Emrick CD, Iber FL, James KE, Lacoursiere RB, Lee KK, Lowenstam I, Maany I, Neiderheiser D, Nocks JJ, Shaw S. (1986) Disulfiram treatment of alcoholism: A Veterans Administration cooperative study. Journal of the American Medical Association 256:1449–1455.

Gallant DM, Bishop MP, Faulkner MA, Simpson L, Cooper A, Lathrop D, Brisolara AM, Bossetta JR. (1968) A comparative evaluation of compulsory (group therapy and/or Disulfiram) and voluntary treatment of the chronic alcoholic municipal court offender. Psychosomatics 9:306–310.

Garbutt JC, Kranzler HR, O'Malley SS, Gastfriend DR, Pettinati HM, Silverman BL, Loewy JW, Ehrich EW; Vivitrex Study Group. (2005) Efficacy and tolerability of long-acting injectable naltrexone for alcohol dependence: a randomized controlled trial. JAMA 293/13:1617–25.

Garbutt JC, West SL, Carey TS, Lohr KN, Crews FT. (1999) Pharmacological treatment of alcohol dependence: A review of the evidence. Journal of the American Medical Association 281:1318–1325.

Gastpar M, Bonnet U, Böning J, Mann K, Schmidt LG, Soyka M, Wetterling T, Kielstein V, Labriola D, Croop R. (2002) Lack of efficacy of naltrexone in the prevention of alcohol relapse: results from a German multicenter study. J Clin Psychopharmacol 22:592–598.

Gdovinová Z. (2006) Cerebral blood flow velocity and erythrocyte deformability in heavy alcohol drinkers at the acute stage and two weeks after withdrawal. Drug and Alcohol Dependence 81/3:207–213.

Geerlings P and Lesch OM. (1999) Introduction: craving and relapse in alcoholism: neurobio-psychosocial understanding. Alcohol Alcohol 34/2:195–6.

Gerrein JR, Rosenberg CM, Manohar V. (1973) Disulfiram maintenance in outpatient treatment of alcoholism. Archives of General Psychiatry 28:798–802.

Giancola PR and Moss HB. (1998) Executive functioning in alcohol use disorders. Recent development in alcoholism:14227–14251.

Gilligan SB, Reich T, Cloninger CR. (1987) Etiologic heterogeneity in alcoholism. Gen Epidemiol 4:395–414.

Ginner J. (2006) Stellenwert der Sozialarbeit in der Alkoholikerinnen-Therapie nach Otto Lesch. Entwicklung von Erfolgskriterien für einen transdisziplinären Therapieansatz aus der Sicht der im Wohnheim Winden/Melk betreuten Menschen. Fachhochschule für Sozialarbeit St. Pölten.

Glassman AH, Stetner F, Walsh BT, Raizman PS, Fleiss JL, Cooper TB, Covey LS. (1988) Heavy smokers, smoking cessation, and clonidine: results of a double-blind, randomized trial. JAMA 259:2863–2866.

Glotzbach LD. (1984) Effects of outpatient treatment upon alcoholism severity in male alcoholics. Unpublished doctoral dissertation, University of Missouri.

Goldstein LB, Adams R, Alberts MJ, Appel LJ, Brass LM, Bushnell CD, Culebras A, Degraba TJ, Gorelick PB, Guyton JR, Hart RG, Howard G, Kelly-Hayes M, Nixon JV, Sacco RL. (2006) Primary prevention of ischemic stroke. Stroke 37:1583–1633.

Gonzales DH, Rennard SI, Billing CB, Reeves KR. (2006) A pooled analysis of varenicline, an alpha4beta2 nicotinic receptor partial agonist versus bupropion for smoking cessation. Presented at Society for Research on Nicotine and Toobacco, February 2006.

Gregor K, Zvolensky M, McLeish A, Bernstein A, Morissette SB. (2008) Anxiety Sensitivity and Perceived Control over Anxiety-related Events: Associations with Smoking Outcome Expectancies and Perceived Cessation Barriers among Daily Smokers. Nicotine & Tobacco Research 10/4:627–635.

Greving JP et al. (2007) Alcohol beverages and risk of renal cell cancer. British Journal of Cancer, 97 (3): 429–433

Grünberger J, Lesch OM, Linzmayer L. (1988) Bestimmung von vier Alkoholikertypen mit Hilfe der statischen und licht-evozierten dynamischen Pupillometrie. Wiener Zeitschrift für Suchtforschung 11/4:29–34.

Grünberger J, Linzmayer L, Saletu B, Lesch OM. (1989) Klinische psychophysiologische Diagnostik bei ambulanten Alkoholikern: Statische und lichtevozierte dynamische Pupillometrie. Wiener Zeitschrift für Suchtforschung 12/1–2:53–62.

Grünberger J, Linzmayer L, Walter H, Stöhr H, Saletu-Zyhlarz G, Grünberger J, Lesch OM. (1998) Psychophysiological Diagnostics in Alcohol Dependency: Fourier Analysis of Pupillary Oscillations and the Receptor Test for Determination of Cholinergic Deficiency. Alcohol Alcohol 33/5:341–348.

Grünberger J. (2007) Humaner Strafvollzug. Am Beispiel Sonderanstalt Mittersteig. Wien New York: Springer.

Gsellhofer B, Fahrner EM, Weiler D, Vogt M, Hron U. (1993) Deutsche Version: IFT (Institut für Therapieforschung) und J. Platt (Hahnemann University); nach dem amerikanischen Original von T. McLellan, 5. Ed., 1992, und der europäischen Version EuropASI von A. Kokkevi, Ch. Hartgers, P. Blanken, E.-M. Fahrner, G. Pozzi, E. Tempesta & A. Uchtenhagen, 1993.

Guydish JR. (1987) Self control bibliotherapy as a secondary prevention strategy with heavy-drinking college students. Unpublished doctoral dissertation, Washington State University.

Haag F. (1976) Sozialtherapie. In: Hahn P. (Hrsg) Die Psychologie des 20. Jahrhunderts, Bd. 9. München.

Haaga JG and FaithM. (1997) Consumption of alcohol and mortality in Russia. The Lancet 350/9082:956.

Hall SM, Reus VI, Munoz RF, Sees KL, Humfleet G, Hartz DT, Frederick S, Triffleman E. (1998) Nortriptyline and cognitive-behavioral therapy in the treatment of cigarette smoking. Arch Gen Psychiatry 55:683–689.

Haller R. (2007) (Un) Glück der Sucht. Wie Sie Ihre Abhängigkeiten besiegen. Ecowin Verlag GmbH.

Hanewinkel R, Burow F, Ferstl R. (1996) Verhaltenstherapeutische Primär- und Sekundärprävention des Rauchens am Beispiel einer Interventionsstudie an Schulen. In: Reinecker S, Schmelzer D. (Hrsg.) Verhaltenstherapie, Selbstregulation, Selbstmanagement, Göttingen: Hogrefe:417–433.

Harris KB and Miller WR. (1990) Behavioral self-control training for problem drinkers: Components of efficacy. Psychology of Addictive Behaviors 4:82–90.

Hart CL, Smith GD, Hole DJ, Hawthorne VM. (1999) Scottish men with 21 years of follow up results from a prospective cohort study of causes, coronary heart disease, and stroke: Alcohol consumption and mortality from all. BMJ 318:1725–1729.

Hartmann S, Aradottir S, Graf M, Wiesbeck G, Lesch OM, Ramskogler K, Wolfersdorf, Alling C, Wurst FM. (2007) Phosphatidylethanol as a sensitive and specific biomarker – comparison with gamma-glutamyl transpeptidase, mean corpuscular volume and carbohydrate-deficient transferrin. Addiction Biology 121:81–84.

Hasdai D, Garratt KN, Grill DE, Lerman A, Holmes DR Jr. (1997) Effect of smoking status on the long-term outcome after successful percutaneous coronary revascularization. N Engl J Med 336:755–761.

Hashimoto JG and Wiren KM. (2008) Neurotoxic consequences of chronic alcohol withdrawal: expression profiling reveals importance of gender over withdrawal severity. Neuropsychopharmacology 33/5:1084–96.

Hasin D. et al., 1997 D. Hasin, B.F. Grant, L. Cottler, J. Blain, L. Towlw, B. Ustun and N. Sartorius, Nosological comparisons of alcohol and drug diagnoses: a multisite, multi-instrument international study, *Drug and Alcohol Dependence* **47** (1997), pp. 217–226

Hass W and Petzold HG. (1999) Die Bedeutung der Forschung über soziale Netzwerke, Netzwerktherapie und soziale Unterstützung für die Psychotherapie – diagnostische und therapeutische Perspektiven. In: Petzold, Märtens: Wege zu effektiven Psychotherapien. Psychotherapieforschung und Praxis. Band 1. Opladen: Leske u. Budrich:193–272.

Haustein KO. (2000) Rauchen, Nikotin und Schwangerschaft. Geburtshilfe und Frauenheilkunde 60/1:11–19.

Havassy BE, Hall SM, Wasermann DA. (1991) Social support and relapse: Commonalities among alcoholics, opiate users and cigarette smokers. Addictive Behaviors 16:235–245.

Heath AC, Bucholz KK, Madden PAF, Dinwiddie SH, Slutske WS, Statham DJ, Dunne MP, Whitfield J, Martin N. (1997) Genetic and environmental contributions to alcohol dependence risk in a national twin sample consistency of findings in men and women. Psychological Medicine 27:1381–1396.

Heatherton TF, Kozlowski LT, Frecker RC, Fagerström KO. (1991) The Fagerström Test for Nicotine Dependence: a revision of the Fagerström Tolerance Questionnaire. Br J Addict 86:1119–27.

Heatherton TF, Kozlowski LT, Frecker RC, Rickert W, Robinson J. (1989) Measuring the heaviness of smoking: using self-reported time to the first cigarette of the day and number of cigarettes smoked per day. Br J Addict 84:791–9.

Heigl FS and Heigl-Evers A. (1991) Basale Störungen bei Abhängigkeit und Sucht und ihre Therapie. In Heigl-Evers A, Helas I, Vollmer HC. Suchttherapie, psychoanalytisch, verhaltenstherapeutisch. Göttingen: Vandenhoeck & Ruprecht:128–139.

Heigl-Evers A und Standke G. (1991) Die Beziehungsdynamik Patient-Therapeut in der psychoanalytisch-orientierten Diagnostik. In Heigl-Evers A, Helas I, Vollmer HC. Suchttherapie, psychoanalytisch, verhaltenstherapeutisch. Göttingen: Vandenhoeck & Ruprecht:43–56.

Heigl-Evers A, Standke G, Wienen G. (1981) Sozialisation und Sucht – psychoanalytische Aspekte. In Feuerlein W. Sozialisationsstörungen und Sucht, Entstehungsbedingungen, Folgen, therapeutische Konsequenzen. Wiesbaden: Akademische Verlagsgesellschaft:51–61.

Heilig M and Koob GF. (2007) A key role for corticotropin-releasing factor in alcohol dependence. Trends Neurosci 30(8):399–406.

Heinz A, Mann K, Weinberger DR, Goldman D. (2001) Serotonergic dysfunction, negative mood states, and response to alcohol. Alcohol Clin Exp Res 25:487–495.

Heltzel R. (2000) Teamsupervision in der Psychiatrie. In: Pühl (Hrsg.): Handbuch der Supervision 2.2. Aufl. Berlin: Edition Marhold.

Henkel D. (1998) „Die Trunksucht ist die Mutter der Armut" – zum immer wieder fehlgedeuteten Zusammenhang von Alkohol und Armut in Deutschland vom Beginn des 19. Jahrhunderts bis zur Gegenwart. In D. Henkel (Hrsg) Sucht und Armut. Alkohol, Tabak, illegale Drogen. Opladen: Westdeutscher Verlag:13–79.

Henningfield JE, Fant RV, Buchhalter AR, Stitzer ML. (2005) Pharmacotherapy for Nicotine Dependence. CA Cancer J Clin 55:281–299.

Henningfield JE, Fant RV, Gopalan L. (1998) Non-nicotine medications for smoking cessation. J Respir Dis 19:33–42.

Hermann M, Kindermann I, Müller S, Georg T, Kindermann M, Böhm M, Herrmann W. (2005) Relationship of plasma homocysteine with the severity of chronic heart failure. Clinical Chemistry 51:1512–1515.

Hernandez-Avila CA, Song C, Kuo L, Tennen H, Armeli S, Kranzler HR. (2006) Targeted versus daily naltrexone: secondary analysis of effects on average daily drinking. Alcohol Clin Exp Res 30/5:860–5.

Hertling I, Ramskogler K, Dvorak A, Klingler A, Saletu-Zyhlarz G, Schoberberger R, Walter H, Kunze M, Lesch OM. (2005) Craving and other characteristics of the comorbidity of alcohol and nicotine dependence. European Psychiatry 20:442–450.

Hertling I, Ramskogler K, Riegler A, Walter H, Mader R, Lesch OM. (2001) Alkoholverlangen und Rückfallprophylaxe. Wiener klinische Wochenschrift 113/19:717–726.

Hertling I, Ramskogler K, Riegler A, Walter H, Mader R, Lesch OM. (2001) Craving for alcohol and prevention of relapse. Wien Klin Wochenschr 113/19:717–26.

Hertling I, Ramskogler K, Riegler A, Zoghlami A, Walter H, Lesch OM. (2001) Enzugsbehandlung von alkoholabhängigen Patienten, Wiener Zeitschrift für Suchtforschung 24/1:41–46.

Hertling I, Walter H, Fischer DE, Lindner H, Ramskogler K, Lesch OM. (2002) Behandlung der chronischen Alkoholabhängigkeit. Gibt es Untergruppen für Psychotherapie mit Hypnose. In: Burkhard P, Kraiker C. (Hrsg.) Hypnose in Medizin und Zahnmedizin. Hypnose und Kognition, Band 19:107–116.

Hesse H. (2004) Wirkfaktoren der Soziotherapie. In: Steingass (Hrsg.) Geht doch! Soziotherapie chronisch mehrfach beeinträchtigter Abhängiger. Neuland: Geeshacht.

Hesselbrock MN, Hesselbrock VM, Del Boca F. (2001) Typology of alcoholism, gender and 20-year mortality. Alcohol Clin Exp Res 25:151A.

Hesselbrock VM and Hesselbrock MN. (2006) Are there empirically supported and clinically useful subtypes of alcohol dependence? Addiction 101/1:97–103.

Hester RK and Delaney HD. (1997) Behavioral self-control program for windows: Results of a controlled clinical trial. Journal of Consulting and Clinical Psychology 65:686–693.

Hester RK and Miller WR. (2003) Handbook of Alcoholism and Treatment Approaches. Effective Alternatives – Third Edition, Allyn & Bacon.

Hickson M, D'Souza AL, Muthu N, Rogers TR, Want S, Rajkumar C, Bulpitt CJ. (2007) Use of probiotic Lactobacillus preparation to prevent diarrhoea associated with antibiotics: randomised double blind placebo controlled trial. BMJ 335:80.

Hill EM, Stoltenberg SF, Bullard KH, Li S, Zucker RA, Burmeister M. (2002) Antisocial alcoholism and serotonin-related polymorphisms: association tests. Psychiatr Genet 12/3:143–53.

Hillemacher T and Bleich S. (2008) Neurobiology and treatment in alcoholism – recent findings regarding Lesch's typology of alcohol dependence. Alcohol Alcohol. 2008 May-Jun;43(3):341–6. Epub 2008 Mar 13. Review.

Hillemacher T, Bayerlein K, Wilhelm J, Frieling H, SperlingW, Kornhuber J, Bleich S. (2006) Prolactin Serum Levels and Alcohol Craving – An Analysis Using Lesch's Typology Neuropsychobiology 53:133–136.

Hillemacher T, Bleich S, Frieling H, Schanze A, Wilhelm J, Sperling W, Kornhuber J, Kraus T. (2007) Evidence of an association of leptin serum levels and craving in alcohol dependence. Psychoneuroendocrinology 32/1:87–90.

Hillemacher T, Kraus T, Rauh J, Wei J, Schanze A, Frieling H, Wilhelm J, Heberlein A, Gröschl M, Sperling W, Kornhuber J, Bleich S. (2007) Role of Appetite-Regulating Peptides in Alcohol Craving: An Analysis in Respect to Subtypes and Different Consumption Patterns in Alcoholism. Alcohol Clin Exp Res 31/6:950–954.

Hoff EC and McKeown CE. (1953) An evaluation of the use of tetraethylthiuram disulfide in the treatment of 560 cases of alcohol addiction. American Journal of Psychiatry 109:670–673.

Hölter SM, Danysz W, Spanagel R. (1996) Evidence for alcohol anti-craving properties of memantine. Eur J Pharmacol 314/3:R1–2.
Hörmann K and Riedel F. (2005) Alkohol und Mundhöhle/Pharynx einschließlich schlafbezogener Atmungsstörungen. In: Singer M und Teyssen S. Alkohol und Alkoholfolgekrankheiten, Grundlagen-Diagnostik-Therapie. Berlin: Springer.
Hughes J, Stead L, Lancaster T. (2004) Antidepressants for smoking cessation. Cochrane Database Syst Rev 4:CD000031.
Hughes JR. (2000) New treatments for smoking cessation. CA Cancer J Clin 50:143–151.
Hull CL. (1943) Principles of behaviour. New York: Appleton-Century-Crafts.
Hultberg B, Berglund M, Andersson A, Fran K. (1993) Elevated plasma homocysteine in alcoholics. Alcohol Clin Exp Res 17:687–689.
Hurrelmann K. (2006) Gesundheitssoziologie. Eine Einführung in sozialwissenschaftliche Theorien von Krankheitsprävention und Gesundheitsförderung. 6. Aufl. Weinheim/München: Juventa Verlag.
Hurst W, Gregory E, Gussman T. (1997) Alcoholic Beverage Taxation and Control Policies. International Survey, Brewers Association of Canada, Ontario.
Hüseyin U, Çagdas Ö, Ahmet K, Ertan Ö, Nese Ç. (2005) Acute alcohol intake and wave dispersion in healthy men – Original Investigation. The Anatolian Journal of Cardiology 5:289–293.
Huss M. (1852) Chronische Alkoholkrankheit. Stockholm.
Hussain MZ and Harinath M. (1972) Helping alcoholics abstain: An implantable substance. American Journal of Psychiatry 129:363.
Hwang BH, Wang GM, Wong DT, Lumeng L, Li TK. (2000) Norepinephrine uptake sites in the locus coeruleus of rat lines selectively bred for high and low alcohol preference: a quantitative autoradiographic binding study using [3H]-tomoxetine. Alcohol Clin Exp Res 24/5:588–94.
Hwang BH, Wang GM, Wong DT, Lumeng L, Li TK. (2000) Norepinephrine Uptake Sites in the Locus Coeruleus of Rat Lines Selectively Bred for High and Low Alcohol Preference: A Quantitative Autoradiographic Binding Study Using [3H]-Tomoxetine. Alcohol Clin Exp Res 24/5:588–594.
Innerhofer P, Schuster B, Klicpera Ch, Lobnig H, Weber G. (1993) Psychosoziale Probleme im Erwachsenenalter. Wien: WUV-Universitätsverlag.
J Clin Psychiatry Monograph 2003; 18/1 „Treatment of Tobacco Dependence".
Jackson P and Oei TPS. (1978) Social skills training and cognitive restructuring with alcoholic. Drug and Alcohol Dependence 3:369–374.
Jacobson NO and Silfverskiold NP. (1973) A controlled study of a hypnotic method in the treatment of alcoholism with evaluation by objective criteria. British Journal of Addiction 68:25–31.
Javors M, Tiouririne M, Prihoda T. (2000) Platelet serotonin uptake is higher in early onset than in late-onset alcoholics. Alcohol Alcohol 35:390–393.
Jellinek EM. (1960) The disease concept of alcoholism. Hillhouse. New Brunswick RI.
Jessor SL and Jessor R. (1978) Die Entwicklung Jugendlicher und der Beginn des Alkoholkonsums. In Vogler E, Revenstorf D. Alkoholmissbrauch, sozialpsychologische und lerntheoretische Ansätze. Fortschritte der Klinischen Psychologie 13. München-Wien-Baltimor: Urban & Schwarzenberg:19–43.

Joca SR, Ferreira FR, Guimaraes FS. (2007) Modulation of stress consequences by hippocampal monoaminergic, glutamatergic and nitrergic neurotransmitter systems. Stress 10/3:227–49.
John U, Veltrup C, Driessen M, Wetterling T, Dilling H. (2000) Motivationsarbeit mit Alkoholabhängigen. Lambertus Verlag.
Johnsen J and Morland J. (1991) Disulfiram implant: A double-blind placebo controlled follow-up on treatment outcome. Alcohol Clin Exp Res 15:532–536.
Johnsen J, Stowell A, Bache-Wig JE, Stenstrud T, Ripel A, Morland J. (1987) A double-blind placebo controlled study of male alcoholics given a subcutaneous disulfiram implantation. British Journal of Addiction 82:607–613.
Johnson BA (2004) Role of the serotonergic system in the neurobiology of alcoholism: implications for treatment. CNS Drugs 18/15:1105–18.
Johnson BA and Ait-Daoud N. (2000) Neuropharmacological treatments for alcoholism: scientific basis and clinical findings. Psychopharmacology 149:327–344.
Johnson BA, Ait-Daoud N, Akhtar FZ, Javors MA. (2005) Use of oral topiramate to promote smoking abstinence among alcohol-dependent smokers: a randomized controlled trial. Arch Intern Med 165/14:1600–5.
Johnson BA, Ait-Daoud N, Akhtar FZ, Ma JZ. (2004) Oral topiramate reduces the consequences of drinking and improves the quality of life of alcohol-dependent individuals: a randomized controlled trial. Arch Gen Psychiatry 61/9:905–12.
Johnson BA, Ait-Daoud N, Bowden CL, DiClemente CC, Roache JD, Lawson K, Javors MA, Ma JZ. (2003) Oral topiramate for treatment of alcohol dependence: a randomised controlled trial. Lancet 361/9370:1677–85.
Johnson BA, Mann K, Willenbring ML, Litten RZ, Swift RM, Lesch OM, Berglund M. (2005) Challenges and opportunities for medications development in alcoholism: an international perspective on collaborations between academia and industry. Alcohol Clin Exp Res 29/8:1528–1540.
Johnson BA, Roache JD, Javors MA, DiClemente CC, Cloninger CR, Prihoda TJ, Bordnick PS, Ait-Daoud N, Hensler J. (2000) Ondansetron for reduction of drinking among biologically predisposed alcoholic patients: a randomized controlled trial. Journal of the American Medical Association 284:963–971.
Johnson BA, Ruiz P, Galanter M. (2003) Handbook of Clinical Alcoholism Treatment. Lippincott Williams & Wilkins.
Johnson BA. (2000) Serotonergic agents and alcoholism treatment: Rebirth of the subtype concept – a hypothesis. Alcohol Clin Exp Res 24:1597–1601.
Johnson BA. (2004) Progress in the development of topiramate for treating alcohol dependence: from a hypothesis to a proof-of-concept study.Alcohol Clin Exp Res 28/8:1137–44.
Johnson BA. (2008) Update on neuropharmacological treatments for alcoholism: Scientific basis and clinical findings. Biochemical Pharmacology 75(1):34–56.
Johnson FG. (1970) A comparison of short-term treatment effects of intravenous sodium amytal-methedrine and LSD in the alcoholic. Canadian Psychiatric Association Journal 15:493–497.
Jones Sl, Kanfer R, Lanyon Ri. (1982) Skill training with alcoholics: A clinical extension. Addictive Behaviors 7:285–290.

Jorch G. (2001) Privates Symposium der Stiftung Kindergesundheit im Dr. v. Haunerschen Kinderspital der Universität München.

Jorenby DE, Leischow SJ, Nides MA, Rennard SI, Johnston JA, Hughes AR, Smith SS, Muramoto ML, Daughton DM, Doan K, Fiore MC, Baker TB. (1999) A controlled trial of sustained-release bupropion, a nicotine patch, or both for smoking cessation. N Engl J Med 340:685–691.

Kadden RM, Litt MD, Cooney NL, Kabela E, Getter H. (2001) Prospective matching of alcoholic clients to cognitive-behavioral or interactional group therapy. J Stud Alcohol 62:359–64.

Kadden RM. (1996) Project MATCH: Treatment Main Effects and Matching results. Alcoholism: Clinical and Experimental Research 20/8:196a–197a.

Kampman KM, Pettinati HM, Lynch KG, Whittingham T, Macfadden W, Dackis C, Tirado C, Oslin DW, Sparkman T, O'Brien CP. (2007) A double blind, placebo controlled pilot trial of Quetiapine fort he treatment of Type A and Type B alcoholism. J Clin Psychopharmacol 27/4:344–351.

Kapusta ND, Plener PL, Schmid R, Thau K, Walter H, Lesch OM. (2007) Multiple substance use among young males. Pharmacol Biochem Behav 86:306–311.

Kapusta ND, Ramskogler K, Hertling I, Schmid R, Dvorak A, Walter H, Lesch OM. (2006) Epidemiology of substance use in a representative sample of 18-year-old males. Alcohol Alcohol 41:188–192.

Katschnig H. (1977) Epidemiologie und primäre Soziogenese psychischer Erkrankungen. In Alois Becker und Ludwig Reiter (Hrsg) Psychotherapie als Denken und Handeln. München: Kindler.

Kauhanen J, Kaplan GA, Goldberg DE, Salonen JT. (1997) Beer binging and mortality: results from the kuopio ischaemic heart disease risk factor study, a prospective population based study. BMJ 315:846–851.

Kelly AB, Halford WK, Young RM. (2000) Maritally distressed women with alcohol problems: The impact of a short-term alcohol focused intervention on drinking behaviour and marital satisfaction. Addiction 95/10:1537–1549.

Kennedy PJ. (1989) The effect of moderate drinking skill training on alcohol-related knowledge, attitude and behaviour. Unpublished doctoral dissertation, University of Minnesota.

Kenyon SH, Nicolaou A, Gibbons WA. (1998) The effect of ethanol and its metabolites upon methionine synthase activity in vitro. Alcohol 15:305–309.

Kernberg OF, Dulz B, Sachsse U. (2000) Handbuch der Borderline-Störungen. Stuttgart New York: Schattauer.

Kernberg OF. (1979) Borderline-Störungen und pathologischer Narzissmus. 3. Auflage Frankfurt/Main: Suhrkamp.

Kersting-Dürrwächter G and Mielck A. (2001) Unfälle von Vorschulkindern im Landkreis Böblingen – Unfallursachen und Risikogruppen. Gesundheitswesen 63:335–342.

Kessler RC, Crum RM, Warner LA, Nelson CB, Schulenberg J, Anthony JC. (1997) Lifetime co-occurrence of DSM-III-R alcohol abuse and dependence with other psychiatric disorders in the National Comorbidity Survey. Arch Gen Psychiatry 54:313–321.

Ketelsen R und Pieters V. (2004) Prävention durch Nachbereitung – Maßnahmen der tertiären Prävention. In: Ketelsen et al. (Hrsg.) Seelische Krise und Aggressivität. Bonn: Psychiatrieverlag.

Ketelsen R, Schulz M, Zechert C. (2004) Seelische Krise und Aggressivität. Der Umgang mit Deeskalation und Zwang. Bonn: Psychiatrieverlag.

Keupp H and Rerrich D. (1982) Psychosoziale Praxis. Wien München Baltimore.

Kiefer F, Helwig H, Tarnaske T, Otte C, Jahn H, Wiedemann K. (2005) Pharmacological relapse prevention of alcoholism: clinical predictors of outcome. Eur Addict Res 11:83–91.

Kiefer F, Jahn H, Jaschinski M, Holzbach R, Wolf K, Naber D, Wiedemann K. (2001a) Leptin: a modulator of alcohol craving? Biol Psychiatry 49:782–787.

Kiefer F, Jahn H, Wiedemann K. (2005) A neuroendocrinological hypothesis on gender effects of naltrexone in relapse prevention treatment. Pharmacopsychiatry 38/4:184–6.

Kiefer F, Jahn H, Wolf K, Kampf P, Knaudt K, Wiedemann K. (2001b) Free-choice alcohol consumption in mice after application of the appetite regulating peptide leptin. Alcohol Clin Exp Res 25:787–789.

Kiefer F, Jiménez-Arriero MA, Klein O, Diehl A, Rubio G. (2007) Cloninger's typology and treatment outcome in alcohol-dependent subjects during pharmacotherapy with naltrexone. Addiction Biology 13:124–129.

Kienast T, Lindenmeyer J, Löb M, Löber S, Heinz A. (2007) Alkoholabhängigkeit. Ein Leitfaden zur Gruppentherapie. In der Serie Batra A und Buchkremer G. Störungs-spezifische Psychotherapie. Kohlhammer Verlag.

Kim DJ, Yoon SJ, Choi B, Kim TS, Woo YS, Kim W, Myrick H, Peterson BS, Choi YB, Kim YK, Jeong J. (2005) Increased fasting plasma ghrelin levels during alcohol abstinence. Alcohol Alcohol 40/1:76–9.

Kish GB, Ellsworth RB, Woody MM. (1980) Effectiveness of an 84-day and a 60-day alcoholism treatment program. Journal of Studies on Alcohol 41:81–85.

Kivlahan DR, Marlatt GA, Fromme K, Coppel DB, Williams E. (1990) Secondary prevention with college drinkers: Evaluation of an alcohol skills training program. Journal of Consulting and Clinical Psychology 58:805–810.

Klein M. (1972) Das Seelenleben des Kleinkindes und andere Beiträge zur Psychoanalyse. Reinbeck bei Hamburg: Rowohlt.

Klesges RC, Meyers AW, Klesges LM, La Vasque ME. (1989) Smoking, body weight, and their effects on smoking behaviour: a comprehensive review of the literature. Psychol Bull 106:204–230.

Klesges RC, Winders SE, Meyers AW, Eck LH, Ward KD, Hultquist CM, Ray JW, Shadish WR. (1997) How much weight gain occurs following smoking cessation? A comparison of weight gain using both continuous and point prevalence abstinence. J Consult Clin Psychol 65:286–291.

Knight RP. (1937) Zur Dynamik und Therapie des chronischen Alkoholismus. Internationale Zeitschrift für Psychoanalyse 23:429–442.

Knorring AL, Bohman Mv, Knorring Lv, Oreland L. (1985) Platelet MAO activity as biological marker in subgroups of alcoholism. Acta psychiat scand 72:511–558.

Kolb B and Whishaw IQ. (1996) Neuropsychologie. 2. Aufl. Heidelberg Berlin Oxford: Spektrum Akademischer Verlag.

Koller G and Soyka M. (2001) Biological and genetic markers of alcoholism – a psychiatric perspective In: Wurst FW. (Hrsg.) New and Upcoming Markers of Alcohol Consumption, Springer, Darmstadt:3–16.

König B. (1998) Alkoholabhängigkeit – Selektiert nach Rechtsbrechern, eingewiesen nach §21 Abs.2 StGB und freiwillig stationär aufgenommenen Patienten. Diplomarbeit aus dem Hauptfach Psychologie.

Koob GF and Le Moal M. (2006) Neurobiology of Addiction. 1. Auflage, Academic Press – Elsevier.

Koob GF, Roberts AJ, Schulteis G, Parsons LH, Heyser CJ, Hyytiä P, Merlo-Pich E, Weiss F. (1998) Neurocircuitry targets in ethanol reward and dependence. Alcohol Clin Exp Res 22:3–9.

Koppi S, Eberhardt G, Haller R, König P. (1987) Calcium-channel-blocking agent in the treatment of acute alcohol withdrawal--caroverine versus meprobamate in a randomized double-blind study. Neuropsychobiology 17/1–2:49–52.

Körkel J und Kruse G. (1997) Mit dem Rückfall leben. Bonn: Psychiatrie-Verlag.

Körkel J, Langguth W, Schellberg B. (2001) Jenseits des Abstinenzfundamentalismus – das „Ambulante Gruppenprogramm zum kontrollierten Trinken“ (AkT). In: Wienberg/Driessen (Hrsg.): Auf dem Weg zur vergessenen Mehrheit. Innovative Konzepte für die Versorgung von Menschen mit Alkoholproblemen. Bonn: Psychiatrieverlag.

Körkel J. (1992) Der Rückfall des Suchtkranken. Berlin: Springer.

Korninger C, Roller RE, Lesch OM. (2003) Gamma-Hydroxybutyric Acid in the Treatment of Alcohol Withdrawal Syndrome in Patients Admitted to Hospital. Acta Medica Austriaca 3:83–86.

Kranzler H, Lappalainen J, Nellissery M, Gelernter J. (2002) Association study of alcoholism subtypes with a functional promoter polymorphism in the serotonin transporter protein gene. Alcohol Clin Exp Res 26/9:1330–5.

Kranzler HR, Burleson JA, Brown J, Babor TF. (1996) Fluoxetine treatment seems to reduce the beneficial effects of cognitive behavioral therapy in type B alcoholics. Alcohol Clin Exp Res 20:1534–1541.

Kranzler HR, Burleson JA, Del Boca FK, Babor TF, Korner P, Brown J, Bohn MJ. (1994) Buspirone treatment of anxious alcoholics. A placebo-controlled trial. Archives of General Psychiatry 51:720–731.

Kraus T, Schanze A, Groschl M, Bayerlein K, Hillemacher T, Reulbach U, Kornhuber J, Bleich S. (2005) Ghrelin levels are increased in alcoholism. Alcohol Clin Exp Res 29/12:2154–7.

Kries RV. (2001) Langzeitwirkungen des Rauchens in der Schwangerschaft auf die spätere Gesundheit. Privates Symposium der Stiftung Kindergesundheit im Dr. v. Haunerschen Kinderspital der Universität München.

Kruesi MJ, Fine S, Valladares L, Phillips RA Jr, Rapoport JL. (1992) Paraphilias: a double-blind crossover comparison of clomipramine versus desipramine. Arch Sex Behav 21/6:587–93.

Kruesi MJP, Hibbs ED, Zahn TP, Keysor CS, Hamburger SD, Bartko JJ, Rapoport JL. (1992) A 2-year prospective followup study of children and adolescents with disruptive behaviour disorders. Archives of General Psychiatry 49:429–435.

Krupitsky EM, Rudenko AA, Burakov AM, Slavina TY, Grinenko AA, Pittman B, Gueorguieva R, Petrakis IL, Zvartau EE, Krystal JH. (2007) Antiglutamatergic strategies for ethanol detoxification: comparison with placebo and diazepam. Alcohol Clin Exp Res 31/4:604–611.

Krystal JH, Webb E, Cooney NL, Kranzler HR, Charney DS. (1994) Specifity of ethanollike effects elicited by serotonergic and noradrenergic mechanisms. Archives of General Psychiatry 51:898–911.

Krystal JH, Cramer JA, Krol WF, Kirk GF, Rosenheck RA; Veterans Affairs Naltrexone Cooperative Study 425 Group. (2001) Naltrexone in the treatment of alcohol dependence. N Engl J Med 345/24:1734–1739.

Kuntz H. (2000) Der rote Faden in der Sucht. Neue Ansätze in Theorie und Praxis. Weinheim Basel: Beltz.

Lal S. (1969) Metronidazole in the treatment of alcoholism: A clinical trial and review of the literature. Quarterly Journal of Studies on Alcohol 30:140–151.

Lallemand F, Ward RJ, De Witte P. (2007) Nicotine increases ethanol preference but decreases locomotor activity during the initial stages of chronic ethanol withdrawal. Alcohol Alcohol 42/3:207–218.

Lallemand F, Ward RJ, Dravolina O, De Witte P. (2006) Nicotine-induced changes of glutamate and arginine in naive and chronically alcoholised rats: an in vivo microdialysis study. Brain Res 1111/1:48–60.

Lampert T und Burger M. (2004) Rauchgewohnheiten in Deutschland – Ergebnisse des telefonischen Gesundheitssurveys. Das Gesundheitswesen 66:511–517.

Lazarus RS and Launier R. (1978) Stress–related transactions between person and environment. In Pervin LA, Lewis M. Perspectives in International Psychology. New York: Plenum:287–327.

Le Foll B, Melihan-Cheinin P, Rostoker G, Lagrue G; Working Group of AFSSAPS. (2005) Smoking cessation guidelines: evidence-based recommendations of the French Health Products Safety Agency. Eur Psychiatry 20/5–6:431–41.

Leggio L, Kenna GA, Fenton M, Bonenfant E, Swift RM, (2009) Typologies of Alcohol Dependence. From Jellinek to Genetics and Beyond. Neuropsychology Review, Volume 19, Number 1/März 2009: 115–129

Ledermair O. (1988) Rauchen und Schwangerschaft. Wiener Medizinische Wochenschrift 138/6–7:138–139.

Lee HY, Li SP, Park MS, Bahk YH, Chung BC, Kim MO. (2007) Ethanol's effect on intracellular signal pathways in prenatal rat cortical neurons is GABAB1 dependent. Synapse 61/8:622–8.

Lee JE et al.(2007) Alcohol intake and renal cell cancer in a pooled analysis of 12 prospective studies. Journal of the National Cancer Institute, 99 (10): 801–810

Leitner A, Gierth L, Lentner S, Platz WE, Rommelspacher H, Schmidt L, Lesch OM. (1994) Untergruppen Alkoholkranker. Gibt es biologische Marker? Harmann- und Norharman-Befunde. In: P. Baumann (Hrsg.): Biologische Psychiatrie der Gegenwart:636–640.

LeMarquand D, Pihl RO, Benkelfat C. (1994) Serotonin and alcohol intake, abuse, and dependence: Clinical evidence. Biological Psychiatry 36/5:326–337.
Lempp R (1978) Frühkindliche Hirnschädigung und Neurose: Die Bedeutung eines frühkindlichen exogenen Psychosyndroms für die Entstehung kindlicher Neurosen und milieureaktiver Verhaltensstörungen. 3. überarb. u. erw. Auflage. Bern Stuttgart Wien: Verlag Hans Huber
Lenz B, Hillemacher T, Kornhuber J, Bleich S. (2007) Alkohol aus der Sicht der Hirnforschung. Ärztekrone 20:20–21.
Lenz G and Küfferle B. (2002) Klinische Psychiatrie. Grundlagen, Krankheitslehre und spezifische Therapiestrategien. 2. Auflage, Facultas Verlag.
Lerman C, Niaura R, Collins BN, Wileyto P, Audrain-McGovern J, Pinto A, Hawk L, Epstein LH. (2004) Effect of bupropion on depression symptoms in a smoking cessation clinical trial. Psychol Addict Behav 18:362–366.
Lesch OM and Walter H. (1996) New 'State' Markers for the Detection of Alcoholism. Alcohol Alcohol 31/1:59–62.
Lesch OM and Walter H. (1996) Subtypes of alcoholism and their role in therapy. Alcohol Alcohol Suppl 1:63–7.
Lesch OM and Walter H. (2004) Milnacipran in relapse prevention of alcohol dependent patients – an open trial. The International Journal of Neuropsychopharmacology 7/1:308–309.
Lesch OM and Nimmerrichter A. (1993) Pharmakotherapie des chronischen Alkoholismus. In: Möller HJ. (Hrsg.) Therapie psychiatrischer Erkrankungen, Ferdinand Enke Verlag:634–645.
Lesch OM and Soyka M. (2005) Typologien der Alkoholabhängigkeit und ihre Bedeutung für die medikamentöse Therapie. In: Riederer P, Laux G, Pöldinger W (eds.) Neuro-Psychopharmaka, Bd. 6, 2. Aufl. Wien New York: Springer:332–348.
Lesch OM and Walter H. (1984) Chronischer Alkoholismus und Mortalität. Gemeindenahe Psychiatrie, Heft 1 und 2, Nr. 17/18:46–54.
Lesch OM and Walter H. (1984) Neuere Wege der Diagnostik und Therapie des chronischen Alkoholismus. Gemeindenahe Psychiatrie, Heft 1 und Heft 2, Nr. 17/18:19–39.
Lesch OM and Walter H. (1994) Neue Ansätze in der Therapie Alkoholabhängiger, New Approaches in Therapy of Alcohol Addicts. Psychiatria Danubina 6/1–2:63–81.
Lesch OM and Walter H. (2004) Theorien zur Entstehung süchtigen Verhaltens: Alkoholismus. Springer-Kremser M, Löffler-Stastka H, Kopeinig-Kreissl M (Hrsg.) Psychische Funktionen in Gesundheit und Krankheit – MCW Block 20.
Lesch OM, Ades J, Badawy A, Pelc I, Sasz H. (1993) Alcohol Dependence – Classificatory Considerations, Alcohol Alcohol 2:127–131.
Lesch OM, Benda N, Gutierrez K, König B, Ramskogler K, Riegler A, Semler B, Zyhlarz G, Walter H, Mader R. (1997) Addictive Behaviors on Bipolar Patients, Classificatory Issues. Psiquiatria Na Prática Médica 10/6:14–21.
Lesch OM, Benda N, Gutierrez K, Walter H. (1997) Craving in Alcohol Dependence-Pharmaceutical Interventions. In: Judd LL, Saletu B, Filip V. (Eds.) Basic and Clinical Science of Mental and Addictive Disorders. Bibliotheca Psychiatrica 167/12:136–147.

Lesch OM, Bonte W, Grünberger J. (1988) Eine Typologie des chronischen Alkoholismus – Neue Basisdaten für Forschung und Therapie. In: Ladewig D (Hrsg.) Drogen und Alkohol, ISPA Press Lausanne:119–134.

Lesch OM, Bonte W, Walter H, Musalek M, Sprung R. (1990) Verlaufsorientierte Alkoholismusdiagnostik. In: Schwoon DR, Krausz M. (Hrsg.) Suchtkranke – Die ungeliebten Kinder der Psychiatrie. Ferdinand Enke Verlag:81–91.

Lesch OM, Dietzel M, Musalek M, Walter H, Zeiler K. (1988) The course of alcoholism. Long – Term prognosis in different types. Forensic Sci Int 36/1–2:121–38.

Lesch OM, Dietzel M, Musalek M, Walter H, Zeiler K. (1989) Therapiekonzepte und Therapieziele im Lichte langfristiger Katamnesen (therapierelevante Untergruppen Alkoholkranker). In: Heimann H, Mayer K, Schied HW. (Hrsg.) Psychiatrische und neurologische Aspekte des Alkoholismus heute, Gustav Fischer Verlag:267–284.

Lesch OM, Dietzel M, Musalek M, Walter H, Zeiler K. (1990) Therapiekonzepte und Therapieziele im Lichte langfristiger Katamnesen. In: Kunze M, Schoberberger R. (Hrsg.) Psychosomatik 2000. Neue Aspekte, Dr. Peter Müller Verlag, Wien:161–178.

Lesch OM, Dietzel-Rogan M, Musalek M, Rajna P, Rustem-Begovich A, Schjerve M, Walter H. (1985) Soziale Integration paraphrener Langzeitpatienten bei niedrigdosierter Depotneuroleptikamedikation. Psychiatrische Praxis 12:63–68.

Lesch OM, Dvorak A, Hertling I, Klingler A, Kunze M, Ramskogler K, Saletu-Zylharz G, Schoberberger R, Walter H. (2004) The Austrian Multicentre Study on Smoking: Subgroups of Nicotine Dependence and their Craving. Neuropsychobiology 50:78–88.

Lesch OM, Grünberger J, Rajna P. (1983) Das Model „Burgenland". In: Mader R. (Hrsg.) Alkohol- und Drogenabhängigkeit, Neue Ergebnisse aus Theorie und Praxis:155–189.

Lesch OM, Grünberger J, Rajna P. (1985) Outpatient Treatment of Alcohol Addicts – the Burgenland Model. Medicine and Law, Springer Verlag 4:71–76.

Lesch OM, Hertling I, Ramskogler K, Riegler A, Dvorak A, Walter H. (2006) Gender differences in smoking. Women's Mental Health – A central European Collaborative Research Discourse, Halbreich U, Gaszner P, Saletu B (Eds.):32–37.

Lesch OM, Kefer J, Lentner S, Mader R, Marx B, Musalek M, Nimmerrichter A, Preinsberger H, Puchinger H, Rustembegovic A, Walter H, Zach E. (1990) Diagnosis of Chronic Alcoholism – Classificatory Problems. Psychopathology 23/2:88–96.

Lesch OM, Lang A, Rajna R. (1980) Bericht über den Einfluss eine Behandlungsstruktur auf das Suchtverhalten der burgenländischen Patienten, die in der Zeit zwischen dem 1. Jänner 1973 und dem 31. Dezember 1975 im Anton-Proksch-Institut aufgenommen waren. Wiener Zeitschrift für Suchtforschung, Jahrgang 3:7–14.

Lesch OM, Lentner S, Mader R, Musalek M, Nimmerrichter A, Walter H. (1989) Medication and Drug Abuse in Relation to Road Traffic Savety (A Study, representative for the Country of Austria). Pharmatherapeutica 5:338–354.

Lesch OM, Lentner-Jedlicka S, Walter H. (1984) Umgang mit Alkoholkranken und anderen Süchtigen. Wiener klinische Wochenschrift 96/21:790–796.

Lesch OM, Lesch E, Dietzel M, Musalek M, Walter H, Zeiler K. (1986) Chronischer Alkoholismus – Alkoholfolgekrankheiten – Faktoren, die die Lebenserwartung beeinflussen. In: Sammelband der Van Swieten Tagung, Verlag der österreichischen Ärztekammer:92–98.

Lesch OM, Musalek M, Walter H, Dietzel M. (1992) Le Pronostic de l'Alcoolisme Chronique, alcoologie. Revue de la société francaise d'alcoologie, tome 14/1–92:5–13.

Lesch OM, Musalek M, Wessely P, Zeiler K. (1986) Neurologische und psychiatrische Akutmaßnahmen, Abschnitt Psychiatrie. Wien: Facultas Universitätsverlag:160–163.

Lesch OM, Passweg V, Saletu M, Marx B, Rommelspacher H, Walter H. (1995) Alcoholics Type II – Is there a biological marker for the efficiency of psychotherapy for anxiety. In: Bölcs E, Guttmann G, Martin M, Mende M, Kanitschar H, Walter H. (Eds.) Hypnosis Connecting Disciplines. Proceedings of the 6th European Congress of Hypnosis in Psychotherapy and Psychosomatic Medicine,Vienna, August 14–20, 1993:18–20.

Lesch OM, Riegler A, Gutierrez K, Hertling I, Ramskogler K, Semler B, Zoghlami A, Benda N, Walter H. (2001) The European Acamprosate trials: conclusions for research and therapy. J of Biomedical Science 8/1:89–95.

Lesch OM, Platz W, Soyka M, Walter H. (2010) Die medikamentöse Therapie von Missbrauch und Abhängigkeiten (Tabak, Alkohol und illegale Drogen). In: Riederer P and Laux G (eds.) Grundlagen der Neuro-Psychopharmakologie. Ein Therapiehandbuch. Wien New York: Springer:537–555

Lesch OM, Walter H, Antal J, Heggli DE, Kovacz A, Leitner A, Neumeister A, Stumpf I, Sundrehagen E, Kasper S. (1996) Carbohydrate Deficient Transferrin As a Marker for Alcohol Intake: A Study with Healthy Subjects. Alcohol Alcohol 31/3:265–271.

Lesch OM, Walter H, Antal J, Kanitz RD, Kovacs A, Leitner A, Marx B, Neumeister A, Saletu M, Semler B, Stumpf I, Mader R. (1996) Alcohol Dependence. Is Carbohydrate Deficient Transferrin a Marker for Alcohol Intake? Alcohol Alcohol 31/3:257–264.

Lesch OM, Walter H, Bonte W, Grünberger J, Musalek M, Sprung R. (1991) Etiology of Subgroups in Chronic Alcoholism and different Mechanisms in Transmitter Systems. In: Norman Palmer T. (Ed.) Alcoholism:A Molecular Perspective. Nato Asi Series A: Life Sciences. Plenum Press New York 206:145–160.

Lesch OM, Walter H, Freitag H, Heggli DE, Leitner A, Mader R, Neumeister A, Passeg V, Pusch H, Semler B, Sundrehagen E, Kasper S. (1996) Carbohydrate Deficient Transferrin as a Screening Marker for Drinking in a General Hospital Population. Alcohol Alcohol 31/3:249–256.

Lesch OM, Walter H, Mader R, Musalek M, Zeiler K. (1988) Chronic Alcoholism in Relation to attempted or Effected Suicide – A Long-Term-Study. Psychiatr & Psychobiol 3:181–188.

Lesch OM, Walter H, Rommelspacher H. (1996) Alcohol abuse and alcohol dependence. In: Weller MPI, van Kammen DP. (Eds.), Rommelspacher H, Schuckit M. (Guest Eds.) "Drugs of Abuse" Baillière's Clinical Psychiatry 2/3, Baillière's Clinical Psychiatry, Baillière Tindall, LondonPhiladelphia Sydney Tokio Toronto:421–444.

Lesch OM. (1985) Chronischer Alkoholismus – Typen und ihr Verlauf – eine Langzeitstudie. Thieme Copythek, Georg Thieme Verlag Stuttgart New York, 235 Seiten, 116 Tabellen.

Lesch OM. (1991) Chronic Alcoholism: Subtypes useful for Therapy and Research. In: T. Norman Palmer (Ed.) Alcoholism: A Molecular Perspective. Nato Asi Series A: Life Sciences, Plenum Press, New York, Vol 206:353–356.

Lesch OM. (1992) Towards a Standardisation for the Methodology in Treatment Research of Alcohol Abuse and Alcoholism. Clinical Neuropharmacology 15/1A:307–308.

Lesch OM. (1997) La disintossicazione nei pazienti alcol-dipendenti. Il trattamento della dipendenza e della crisi d'astinenza. Intensità dei sintomi e terapia. I quattri tipidi alcolismo. Medicina delle Tossicodipendenze. Italian Journal of the Addictions V/1–2:34–39.

Lesch OM. (2007) Raucherentwöhnung – Tipps zur Prävention und Therapie in der Praxis. Uni-Med Verlag.

Lesch OM. (2009) Die Diagnose Abhängigkeit im DSM V und ICD-11 zum jetzigen Stand der Forschung. Addiction in DSM V and ICD-11 State of the Art. Fortschr Neurol Psychiat; 77: 507–512

Levy MS, Livingstone BL, Collins DM. (1967) A clinical comparison of disulfiram and calcium carbimide. American Journal of Psychiatry 123:1018–1022.

Ling W, Weiss DG, Charuvastra VC, O'Brien CP, Blakis M, Wang R, Savage C, Roszell D, Way EL, McIntyre J. (1983) Use of disulfiram for alcoholics in methadone maintenance programs: A Veterans Administration cooperative study. Archives of General Psychiatry 40:851–861.

Linnoila M, Virkkunen M, Scheinin M, Nuutila A, Rimon R, Goodwin FK. (1983) Low cerebrospinal fluid 5-hydroxyindolacetic concentration differentiates impulsive from nonimpulsive violent behavoir. Life Science 33:2609–2614.

Liskow B, Campbell J, Nickel EJ, Powell BJ. (1995) Validity of the CAGE questionnaire in screening for alcohol dependence in a walk-in (triage) clinic. Jounral of Studies on Alcohol 56:277–281.

Litten R and Allen J. (1992) Measuring Alcohol Consumption. New Jersey: The Humana Press Inc Totowa.

Litten RZ and Allen JP. (1998) Advances in the development of medications for alcoholism treatment. Psychopharmacology 139:20–33.

Longabaugh R, McCrady B, Fink E, Stout R, McAuley T, Doyle C, McNeill D. (1983) Cost-effectiveness of alcoholism treatment in partial vs. inpatient settings: Six-month outcomes. Journal of Studies on Alcohol 44:1049–1071.

Longabaugh R. (1996) Matching Relational vs. individual treatment focus to patients. Alcohol Clin Exp Res 20/8:248a–249a.

Longo LP, Campbell T, Hubatch S.(2002) Divalproex sodium (Depakote) for alcohol withdrawal and relapse prevention. J Addict Dis 21/2:55–64.

Lopez-Moreno JA, Gonzalez-Cuevas G, Navarro M. (2007) The CB1 cannabinoid receptor antagonist rimonabant chronically prevents the nicotine-induced relapse to alcohol. Neurobiol Dis 25/2:274–83.

Löser H. (1995) Alkoholembryopathie und Alkoholeffekte. Stuttgart.

Lovibond SH. (1975) Use of behaviour modification in the reduction of alcohol-related road accidents. In: Götestam KG, Melin GL, Dockens WS. Applications of behaviour modification. New York: Academic Press:399–406.

Lovinger DM. (1997) Serotonin's role in alcohol's effect on the brain. Alcohol Health and Research World 21/2:114–120.

Ludwig A, Levine J, Stark L, Lazar R. (1969) A clinical study of LSD treatment in alcoholism. American Journal of Psychiatry 126:59–69.

Ma JZ, Ait-Daoud N, Johnson BA. (2006) Topiramate reduces the harm of excessive drinking: implications for public health and primary care. Addiction 101/11:1561–8.

Maher JJ. (2007) Alcoholic steatohepatitis: management and prognosis. Curr Gastroenterol Rep 9/1:39–46.
Majewski F. (1987) Die Alkohol Embryopathie. Frankfurt/Main: Umwelt & Medizin Verlagsgenossenschaft mbH.
Majewski F. (1987) Die Alkoholembryopathie – eine häufige und vermeidbare Schädigung. In: Majewski F. (Hrsg.). Die Alkoholembryopathie – Ein Leitfaden der Stiftung für das behinderte Kind zur Förderung von Vorsorge und Früherkennung. Frankfurt:109–123.
Makin J und Fried PA. (1991) A comparison of active and passive smoking during pregnancy: long term effects. Neurotoxicology and Teratology 13/1:5–12.
Malcolm R, Anton RF, Randall CL, Johnston A, Brady K, Thevos A. (1992) A placebo-controlled trial of buspirone in anxious inpatient alcoholics. Alcohol Clin Exp Res 16:1007–1013.
Malec E, Malec T, Gagne MA, Dongier M. (1996a) Buspirone in the treatment of alcohol dependence: a placebo.controlled trial. Alcohol Clin Exp Res 20:307–312.
Malec TS, Malec EA, Dongier M. (1996b) Efficacy of buspirone in alcohol dependence: a review. Alcohol Clin Exp Res 20:853–858.
Malka R, Fouquet P, Vachorfrance G. (1983) Alcoologie. Masson, Paris.
Malla A. (1988) An outcome study comparing refusers and acceptors of treatment for alcoholism. Canadian Journal of Psychiatry 33:183–187.
Malyutina S, Bobak M, Kurilovitch S, Gafarov V, Simonova G, Nikitin Y, Marmot M. (2002) Relation between heavy and binge drinking and all-cause and cardiovascular mortality in Novosibirsk, Russia: a prospective cohort study. The Lancet 360:1448–1454.
Mandl M. (2002) Kognitive Defizite und Beharrungstendenzen bei chronischem Alkoholismus. Diss. Universität Wien.
Mann K, Lehert P, Morgan MY. (2004) The efficacy of acamprosate in the maintenance of abstinence in alcohol-dependent individuals: results of a meta-analysis. Alcohol Clin Exp Res 28/1:51–63.
Mann K, Stetter F, Batra A, Mundle G, Opitz H, Petersen D, Schroth G. (1988) Hirnorganische Veränderungen bei Alkoholabhängigen. Ergebnisse der Tübinger CT- und NMR-Studie. Wiener Zeitschrift für Suchtforschung Jg. 11/4:35–40.
Mann K. (2004) Pharmacotherapy of alcohol dependence: a review of the clinical data. CNS Drugs 18/8:485–504.
Mannelli P and Pae CU. (2007) Medical comorbidity and alcohol dependence. Current Psychiatry reports 9/3:217–224.
Manzanares J, Ortiz S, Oliva JM, Pérez-Rial S, Palomo T. (2005) Interactions between cannabinoid and opioid receptor systems in the mediation of ethanol effects. Alcohol Alcohol 40/1 :25–34.
Maremmani I, Pacini M, Popovic D, Romano A, Maremmani AG, Perugu G, Deltoto J, Akiskal K, Akiskal H. (2009) Affective temperaments in heroin addiction. J Affect Disord. 117 (3): 186–92
Markou A, Kosten TR, Koob GF. (1998) Neurobiological similarities in depression and drug dependence: a self-medication hypothesis. Neuropsychopharmacology 18:135–174.

Marmot MG, Elliott P, Shipley MJ, Dyer AR, Ueshima HU, Beevers DG, Stamler R, Kesteloot H, Rose G, Stamler J. (1994) Alcohol and blood pressure: the INTERSALT study. BMJ 308:1263–1267.

Maslow AA. (1954) Motivation and Personality. Harper.

Mason BJ, Kocsis JH, Ritvo EC, Cutler RB. (1996) A double-blind, placebo-controlled trial of desipramine for primary alcohol dependence stratified on the presence or absence of major depression. JAMA 13/275/10:761–7.

Mason BJ. (2001) Treatment of alcohol-dependent outpatients with acamprosate: a clinical review. J Clin Psychiatry 62/20:42–8.

Mayfield D, McLeod G, Hall P. (1974) The CAGE questionnaire: validation of a new alcoholism instrument. Am J Psychiatry 131:1121–1123.

Mc Grath PJ, Nunes EV, Stewart JW, Goldman D, Agosti V, Ocepek-Welikson K, Quitkin FM. (1996) Imipramine treatment of alcoholics with primary depression: A placebo-controlled clinical trial. Arch Gen Psychiatry 53/3:232–40.

McCartney JS und Fried PA. (1994) Central Auditory Processing in School-Age Children Prenataly Exposed to Cigarette Smoke. Neurotoxicilogy and Teratology 16/3:269–276.

McClelland DC, Davis W, Wanner E, Kalin R. (1972) The Drinking Man, Alcohol and Human Motivation. New York London: The Free Press.

McCord W, McCord J, Gudeman J. (1960) Origins of alcoholism. Stanford University Press.

McLachlan JFC and Stein RL. (1982) Evaluation of a day clinic for alcoholics. Journal of Studies on Alcohol 43:261–272.

McLellan AT, Luborsky I, O'Brien CP, Woody GE. (1980) An improved evaluation instrument for substance abuse patients: The Addiction Severity Index. The Journal of Nervous and Mental Disease 168:26–33.

Medicus G. (1994) Humanethologische Aspekte der Aggression. Ein Beitrag zur den biologischen Grundlagen von Psychotherapie und Psychiatrie. In: Schöny/Rittmannsberger/Guth (Hrsg.) Aggression im Umfeld psychischer Erkrakungen. Ursachen. Folgen. Behandung. Linz-Salzburg: Forum Psychiatrie (Edition Pro Mente).

Melis T, Succu S, Sanna F, Boi A, Argiolas A, Melis MR. (2007) The cannabinoid antagonist SR 141716A (Rimonabant) reduces the increase of extra cellular dopamine release in the rat nucleus accumbens induced by a novel high palatable food. Neurosci Lett 419/3:231–5.

Menninger KA. (1974) Selbstzerstörung. Psychoanalyse des Selbstmords. Frankfurt: Suhrkamp Verlag.

Merrill JC, Kleber HD, Shwartz M, Liu H, Lewis SR. (1999) Cigarettes, alcohol, marijuana, other risk behaviors, and American youth. Drug and Alcohol Depend 56:205–12.

Mihas AA, Hung PD, Heuman DM. (2007) Alcoholic hepatitis. EMedicine from WebMD. www.emedicine.com/med/topic 101.htm

Miller WR and Rollnick S. (2002) Motivational interviewing: Preparing people for chane (2nd edition). New York: Guilfort Press.

Miller WR and Taylor CA. (1980a) Relative effectiveness of bibliotherapy, individual and group self-control training in the treatment of problem drinkers. Addictive Behaviors 5:13–24.

Miller WR, Gribskov CJ, Mortell RL. (1981) Effectiveness of a self-control manual for problem drinkers with and without therapist contact. International Journal of the Addictions 16:1247–1254.
Miller WR, Meyers RJ, Tonigan JS, Grant KA. (2001) Community reinforcement and traditional approaches: Findings of a controlled trial. In Meyers RJ and Miller WR. A community reinforcement approach to addiction treatment. Cambridge, UK, Cambridge University Press:79–103.
Miller WR, Taylor CA, West JC. (1980b) Focused versus broad-spectrum behaviour therapy for problem drinkers. Journal of Consulting and Clinical Psychology 48:590–601.
Miller WR. (1978) Behavioral treatment of problem drinkers: A comparative outcome study of three controlled drinking therapies. Journal of Consulting and Clinical Psychology 46:74–86.
Möller HJ. (1993) Therapie psychiatrischer Erkrankungen. Ferdinand Enke Verlag.
Montgomery SM und Ekbom A. (2002) Smoking during pregnancy and diabetes mellitus in a British longitudinal birth cohort. British Medical Journal 324/7328:26–27.
Monti PM, Abrams DB, Binkoff JA, Zwick WR, Liepman MR, Nirenberg TD, Rohsenow DR. (1990) Communication skills training, communications skills training with family and cognitive behavioural mood management training for alcoholics. Journal of Studies on Alcohol 51:263–270.
Moreno JL. (1960) The social atom and death, Sociometry 10/1947:81–86. Nachdruck: The Sociometry Reader, Free Press, Glencoe.
Morey LC and Blashfield RK. (1981) Empirical classifications of alcoholics. J Stud Alcohol 42:925–37.
Mueller TI, Stout RL, Rudden S, Brown RA, Gordon A, Solomon DA, Recupero PR. (1997) A double-blind, placebo-controlled pilot study of carbamazepine for the treatment of alcohol dependence. Alcohol Clin Exp Res 21/1:86–92.
Mulchowski-Conley P. (1981) The effects of a systematic skills training program for female alcoholics and their significant others on selected rehabilitation outcome. Unpublished doctoral dissertation, Boston University.
Müller L und Petzold H. (2004) Resilienz und protektive Faktoren im Alter und ihre Bedeutung für den Social Support und die Psychotherapie bei älteren Menschen. In: Petzold H. (Hrsg.) Mit alten Menschen arbeiten. Teil 1. Konzepte und Methoden sozialgerontologischer Praxis. Stuttgart: Pfeiffer.
Murphy JK, Edwards NB, Downs AD, Ackerman BJ, Rosenthal TL. (1990) Effects of doxepin on withdrawal symptoms in smoking cessation. Am J Psychiatry 147:1353–1357.
Musshoff F, Daldrup T, Bonte W, Leitner A, Lesch OM. (1996) Formaldehyde-derived tetrahydroisoquinolines and tetrahydro-beta-carbolines in human urine. J Chromatogr B Biomed Appl 683/2:163–76.
Musshoff F, Daldrup T, Bonte W, Leitner A, Lesch OM. (1997) Salsolinol and norsalsolinol in human urine samples. Pharmacol Biochem Behav 58/2:545–50.
Musshoff F, Daldrup T, Bonte W, Leitner A, Nimmerichter A, Walter H, Lesch OM. (1995) Ethanol-independent methanol elimination in chronic alcoholics. Blutalkohol 32/6:317–36.
Musshoff F, Lachenmeier DW, Schmidt P, Dettmeyer R, Madea B. (2005) Systematic regional study of dopamine, norsalsolinol, and (R/S)-salsolinol levels in human brain areas of alcoholics. Alcohol Clin Exp Res 29/1:46–52.

Mutius Ev. (2001) Privates Symposium der Stiftung Kindergesundheit im Dr. v. Haunerschen Kinderspital der Universität München.
Naeye RL und Peters ED. (1984) Mental development of children whose mothers smoked during pregnancy. Am J Obstet Gynecol 64:601–607.
Nagy J. (2004) Renaissance of NMDA receptor antagonists: do they have a role in the pharmacotherapy for alcoholism? IDrugs 7/4:339–50.
Naranjo CA and Knoke DM. (2001) The role of selective serotonin reuptake inhibitors in reducing alcohol consumption. Journal of Clinical Psychiatry 62/20:18–25.
National Institute for Clinical Excellence. (2004) Guidance on the Use of Nicotine Replacement Therapy (NRT) and Bupropion for Smoking Cessation. London, England: National Institute for Clinical Excellence, Reference No. N0082.
National Institutes of Health Consensus Development Conference Statement: management of hepatitis C: 2002-June 10–12. (2002) Hepatology 36(5/1):3–20.
Nelson JE and Howell RJ. (1983) Assertiveness training using rehearsal and modelling with male alcoholics. American Journal of Drug and Alcohol Abuse 9:309–323.
Ness L, Rosekrans DL, Welford JF. (1977) An epidemiologic study of factors affecting extrinsic staining of teeth in an English population. Community Dent Oral Epidemiol 5:55–60.
Nguyen SA, Malcolm R, Middaugh LD. (2007) Topiramate reduces ethanol consumption by C57BL/6 mice. Synapse 61/3:150–6.
Nicolas JM, Fernandez-Sola J, Fatjo F, Casamitjana R, Bataller R, Sacanella E, Tobias E, Badia E, Estruch R. (2001) Increased circulating leptin levels in chronic alcoholism. Alcohol Clin Exp Res 25/1:83–8.
Niederberger JM. (1987) Rauchen als sozial erlerntes Verhalten. Physiologie und Sozialisationstheorie einer alltäglichen Sucht. Stuttgart.
Nimmerrichter A, Grohs-Kellner G, Lesch OM. (1988) Ein Modell für organisch bedingte psychische Störungen -Chronischer Alkoholismus. Wiener Zeitschrift für Suchtforschung, 11/4:3–13.
Nimmerrichter A, Walter H, Gutierrez-Lobos K, Lesch OM. (2002) Double-blind controlled trial of gamma-hydroxybutyrate and clomethiazole in the treatment of alcohol withdrawal. Alcohol & Alcoholism Vol 37/1:67–73.
Nygard O, Nordrehaug JE, Refsum H, Ueland PM, Farstad M, Vollset SE. (1997) Plasma homocysteine levels and mortality in patients with coronary artery disease. The New England Journal of Medicine 337:230–236.
O'Brien CP. (2005) Efficacy and tolerability of long-acting injectable naltrexone for alcohol dependence. Curr Psychiatry Rep 7/5:327–8.
O'Connel JM. (1987) Effectiveness of an alcohol relapse prevention program. Unpublished doctoral dissertation, Fordham University.
Oberländer FA, Mengering F, Platz WE. (1999) Veränderungen des Patientenprofils einer großstädtischen Abteilung für Abhängigkeitskrankheiten in einer Zehnjahresperiode: Struktureller Veränderungsbedarf für die Organisationsziele und den Behandlungsauftrag. Wiener Zeitschrift für Suchtforschung 22/4:35–45.
Oberländer FA, Platz WE, Mengering F. (1998) Studie zur Motivationsarbeit während der qualifizierten Entgiftung in einer Berliner Nervenklinik. Diagnostisches Profil und

Bereitschaft zur Entwöhnungsbehandlung. Wiener Zeitschrift für Suchtforschung 21/4:35–42.

Obernier JA, White AM, Swartzwelder HS, Crews FT. (2002) Cognitive deficits and CNS damage after a 4-day binge ethanol exposure in rats. Pharmacol Biochem Behav 72/3:521–32.

Oei TPS and Jackson PR. (1980) Long-term effects of group and individual social skills training with alcoholics. Addictive Behaviors 5:129–136.

Oei TPS and Jackson PR. (1982) Social skills and cognitive behavioural approaches to the treatment of problem drinking. Journal of Studies on Alcohol 43:532–547.

Ogurtsov PP, Nuzny VP, Garmash IV, Moiseev VS. (2001) Mortality in Russia. The Lancet 358/9282:669–670.

Öjehagen A, Berglund M, Appel CP, Andersson K, Nilsson B, Skjaerris A, Wedlin-Toftnow AM. (1992) A randomized study of long-term out-patient treatment in alcoholics. Alcohol Alcohol 27:649–658.

Olson RP, Ganley R, Devine VT, Dorsey GC Jr. (1981) Long-term effects of behavioural versus insight-oriented therapy with inpatient alcoholics. Journal of Consulting and Clinical Psychology 49:866–877.

O'Malley SS, Cooney JL, Krishnan-Sarin S, Dubin JA, McKee SA, Cooney NL, Blakeslee A, Meandzija B, Romano-Dahlgard D, Wu R, Makuch R, Jatlow P. (2006) A controlled trial of naltrexone augmentation of nicotine replacement therapy for smoking cessation. Arch Intern Med 166/6:667–74.

O'Malley SS, Jaffe AJ, Chang G, Schottenfeld RS, Meyer RE, Rounsaville B. (1992) Naltrexone and coping skills therapy for alcohol dependence. A controlled study. Arch Gen Psychiatry 49/11:881–7.

O'Malley SS, Krishnan-Sarin S, Farren C, Sinha R; Kreek MJ. (2002) Naltrexone decreases craving and alcohol self-administration in alcohol-dependent subjects and activates the hypothalamo-pituitary-adrenocortical axis. Psychopharmacology (Berl) 160:19–29.

O'Malley SS, Sinha R, Grilo CM, Capone C, Farren CK, McKee SA, Rounsaville BJ, Wu R. (2007) Naltrexone and cognitive behavioral coping skills therapy for the treatment of alcohol drinking and eating disorder features in alcohol-dependent women: a randomized controlled trial. Alcohol Clin Exp Res 31/4:625–34.

Oncken C, Gonzales D, Nides M, Rennard S, Watsky E, Billing CB, Anziano R, Reeves K. (2006) Efficacy and Safety of the Novel Selective Nicotinic Acetylcholine Receptor Partial Agonist, Varenicline, for Smoking Cessation. Arch Intern Med 166:1571–1577.

Ooteman W, Koeter MW, Verheul R, Schippers GM, van den Brink W. (2007) The effect of naltrexone and acamprosate on cue-induced craving, autonomic nervous system and neuroendocrine reactions to alcohol-related cues in alcoholics. Eur Neuropsychopharmacol 17/8:558–66.

Passett P. (1981) Gedanken zur Narzissmuskritik: Die Gefahr, das Kind mit dem Bade auszuschütten. In Psychoanalytisches Seminar Zürich 1981. Die neuen Narzissmustheorien: zurück ins Paradies? Frankfurt/Main: Syndikat.

Patton D, Barnes GE, Murray RP. (1997) A personality typology of smokers. Addict Behav 22:269–273.

Pelc I, Verbanck P, Le Bon O, Gavrilovic M, Lion K, Lehert P. (1997) Efficacy and safety of acamprosate in the treatment of detoxified alcohol-dependent patients. A 90-day placebo-controlled dose-finding study. Br J Psychiatry 170:73–77.

Peniston EG and Kulkosky PJ. (1989) Alpha-theta brainwave training and b-endorphin levels in alcoholics. Alcohol Clin Exp Res 13:271–279.

Petrakis IL, O'Malley S, Rounsaville B, Poling J, McHugh-Strong C, Krystal JH; VA Naltrexone Study Collaboration Group. (2004) Naltrexone augmentation of neuroleptic treatment in alcohol abusing patients with schizophrenia. Psychopharmacology (Berl) 172/3:291–7.

Petry J. (1998) Zwangssterilisation von Alkoholikern im Nationalsozialismus (Unter Hinweis auf die Badische Heil- und Pflegeanstalt Wiesloch) (zuerst 1996). In: Petry J. Alkoholismus. Kulturhistorische, psychosoziale und psychotherapeutische Aspekte. Geesthacht:23–32.

Petry W, Heintges T, Hensel F, Erhardt A, Wenning M, Niederau C, Häussinger D. (1997) Hepatozelluläres Karzinom in Deutschland. Epidemiologie, Ätiologie, Klinik und Prognose bei 100 konsekutiven Patienten einer Universitätsklinik. Z Gastroenterologie 35:1059–1069.

Pettinati HM, Oslin DW, Kampmann KM, Dundon WD, Xie H, Gallis TL,Dackis CA, O'Brien CP (2010) A Double-Blind, Placebo-Controlled Trial Combining Sertraline and Naltrexone for Treating Co-Occurring Depression and Alcohol Dependence Am. J. Psychiatry 167: 668–675

Pettinati HM, Kranzler HR, Madaras J. (2003) The status of serotonin-selective pharmacotherapy in the treatment of alcohol dependence. Recent developments in alcoholism: An official publication of the American Medical Society On Alcoholism, the Research Society On Alcoholism and the National Council On Alcoholism 16:247–262.

Pettinati HM, O'Brien CP, Rabinowitz AR, Wortman SP, Oslin DW, Kampman KM, Dackis CA. (2006) The status of naltrexone in the treatment of alcohol dependence: specific effects on heavy drinking. J Clin Psychopharmacol 26/6:610–25.

Pettinati HM, Volpicelli JR, Kranzler HR, Luck G, Rukstalis MR, Cnaan A. (2000) Sertraline treatment for alcohol dependence: Interactive effects of medication and alcoholic subtype. Alcohol Clin Exp Res 24:1041–1049.

Pettinati HM, Volpicelli JR, Luck G, Kranzler HR, Rukstalis MR, Cnaan A. (2001) Double-blind clinical trial of sertraline treatment for alcohol dependence. Journal of Clinical Psychopharmacology 21:143–153.

Pettinati HM. (2001) The use of selective serotonin reuptake inhibitors in treating alcoholic subtypes. Journal of Clinical Psychiatry 62/20:26–31.

Petzold H und Bubolz E. (1979) Psychotherapie mit alten Menschen, Paderborn: Junfermann.

Petzold H. (1985) Mit alten Menschen arbeiten. Bildungsarbeit, Psychotherapie, Soziotherapie. München: Pfeiffer.

Petzold H. (2003) Soziotherapie als methodischer Ansatz in der Integrativen Therapie. In: Integrative Therapie. Modelle, Theorien und Methoden für eine schulenübergreifende Psychotherapie. 3. Klinische Praxeologie. 2. erw. Auflage.

Petzold H. (2004) Mit alten Menschen arbeiten Teil 1. Konzepte und Methoden sozialgerontologischer Praxis. Stuttgart: Pfeiffer bei Klett-Cotta.

Piano MR. (2002) Alcoholic cardiomyopathy: incidence, clinical characteristics, and pathophysiology. Chest 121:1638–1650.

Picchioni MM and Murray RM. (2007) Schizophrenia. BMJ 335:91–95.

Pi-Sunyer FX, Aronne LJ, Heshmati HM, Devin J, Rosenstock J, RIO-North America Study Group. (2006) Effect of rimonabant, a cannabinoid-1 receptor blocker, on weight and cardiometabolic risk factors in overweight or obese patients: RIO-North America: a randomized controlled trial. JAMA 295/7:761–75.

Pittman B, Gueorguieva R, Krupitsky E, Rudenko AA, Flannery BA, Krystal JH. (2007) Multidimensionality of the Alcohol Withdrawal Symptom Checklist: a factor analysis of the Alcohol Withdrawal Symptom Checklist and CIWA-Ar. Alcohol Clin Exp Res 31/4:612–8.

Pittman DJ and Tate RL. (1972) A comparison of two treatment programs for alcoholics. International Journal of Social Psychiatry 18:183–193.

Platz W. (2007) Forensische Psychiatrie. In: Brüssow R, Gatzweiler N, Krekeler W, Mehle V. Strafverteidigung in der Praxis. 4. Auflage. Deutscher Anwalt Verlag.

Plinius Maior Society. (1994) Guidelines on evaluation of treatment of alcohol dependence. Alcoholism 30:315–336.

Plinius Secundus G. (1669) Naturalis Historiae, Tomus Prinus.

Poldrugo F and Lesch OM. (1994) The diagnosis of chronic alcoholism: new perspectives in classification. Alcologia 6/1:11–15.

Pombo S, Barbosa F, Lourenco R, Benkovskaia I, Almeide J, da Costa NF (2009) Cognitive-Behavioral Indicators of Alcoholism Phenotypes in Patients in Opioid Maintainance Treatment. In: Social Drinking: Uses, Abuses and Psychological Factors. Editors: Katherine T Everly and Eva M Cosell, pp.
Nova Science Publishers, Inc.

Pombo S and Lesch OM (2008) The Alcoholic Phenotypes among Different Multidimensional Typologies: Similarities and Their Classification Procedures. Alcohol & Alcoholism, pp. 1–9

Pombo S, Reizinho R, Ismail F, Barbosa A, Figueira LM, Cardoso JMN, Lesch OM. (2008) NETER1 alcoholic 5 subtypes: Validity with Lesch four evolutionary subtypes International Journal of Psychiatry in Clinical Practice 12/1:55–64.

Pomerleau CS, Marks JL, Pomerleau OF. (2000) Who gets what symptom? Effects of psychiatric co-factors and nicotine dependence on patterns of smoking withdrawal symptomatology. Nicotine Tob Res 2:275–280.

Pomerleau O, Pertschuk M, Adkins D, D'Aquili E. (1978) A comparison of behavioural and traditional treatment for middle income problem drinkers. Journal of Behavioral Medicine 1:187–200.

Potamianos G, North WRS, Meade TW, Townsend J, Peters TJ. (1986) Randomized trial of community-based centre versus conventional hospital management in treatment for alcoholism. Lancet 2/8510:797–799.

Powell BJ, Penick EC, Read MR, Ludwig AM. (1985) Comparison of three outpatient treatment interventions: A twelve-month follow-up of men alcoholics. Journal of Studies on Alcohol 46:309–312.

Praschak-Rieder N, Willeit M, Wilson AA, Houle S, Meyer JH. (2008) Seasonal variation in human brain serotonin transporter binding. Arch Gen Psychiatry. Sep;65(9):1072–8.

Preedy VR and Richardson PJ. (1994) Ethanol induced cardiovascular disease. Br Med Bulletin 50:152–163.
Prochaska J, DiClemente C. (1992) Stages of change in modification of problem behaviors. In: Hersen M, Eisler R, Miller P (Eds.) Progress in behavior modification; Newbury Park, Ca: Sage:84–218.
Prochaska JO, DiClemente CC, Norcross JC. (1992) In search of how people change. Amer. Psychol 37:1102–1114.
Prochazka Av, Weaver MJ, Keller RT, Fryer GE, Licari PA, Lofaso D. (1998) A randomized trial of nortriptyline for smoking cessation. Arch Intern Med 158:2035–2039.
Project MATCH Research Group. (1998) Matching Alcoholism Treatments to Client Heterogeneity: Project MATCH Three-Year Drinking Outcomes. Alcohol Clin Exp Res 22/6:1300–1311.
Puddey IB, Beilin LJ, Vandongen R, Rouse IL, Rogers P. (1985) Evidence for a direct effect of alcohol consumption on blood pressure in normotensive men. A randomized controlled trial. Hypertension 7:707–713.
Puls W. (2003) Arbeitsbedingungen, Stress und der Konsum von Alkohol. Theoretische Konzeptionen und empirische Befunde. Forschung Soziologie Bd. 160. Opladen: Leske + Budrich.
Quensel S. (2004) Das Elend der Suchtprävention. Analyse – Kritik – Alternative. Wiesbaden: VS-Verlag für Sozialwissenschaften.
Radó S. (1975, Orig. 1926) Die psychische Wirkung der Rauschgifte. Versuch einer psychoanalytischen Theorie der Süchte. Psyche:29.
Ramskogler K, Brunner M, Hertling I, Dvorak A, Kapusta N, Krenn C, Moser B, Roth G, Lesch OM, Ankersmit HJ, Walter H. (2004) CDT values are not influenced by epithelial cell apoptosis in chronic alcoholic patients – premilinary results. Alcohol Clin Exp Res 28/9:1396–1398.
Ramskogler K, Hertling I, Riegler A, Semler B, Zoghlami A, Walter H, Lesch OM. (2001) Mögliche Interaktionen zwischen Ethanol und Pharmaka und deren Bedeutung für die medikamentöse Therapie im Alter. Wiener Klinische Wochenschrift 113/10:363–370.
Ramskogler K, Hertling I, Riegler A, Semler B, Zoghlami A, Walter H, Lesch OM. (2001) Possible interaction between ethanol and drugs and their significance for drug therapy in the elderly. Wien Klin Wochenschr 113/10:363–70.
Ramskogler K, Hertling I, Riegler A, Walter H, Lesch OM. (2001) Nikotinabhängigkeit – Neue Wege aus der Sucht. Der Mediziner 3:18–20.
Ramskogler K, Riegler A, Lesch OM, Mader R. (2001) Die Alkoholabhängigkeit – und ihre medikamentöse Therapie. In: Brosch R, Mader R. (Hrsg.) Alkohol am Arbeitsplatz 3–13 Orac Verlag.
Ramskogler K, Walter H, Hertling I, Riegler A, Gutierrez K, Lesch OM. (2001) Subgroups of Alcohol Dependence and their Specific Therapeutic Management: A Review and Introduction to the Lesch-Typology. E-journal of the International Society of Addiciton Medicine – International Addiction.
Rathner G and Dunkel D. (1998) Die Häufigkeit von Alkoholismus und Problemtrinken in Österreich. Wiener Klinische Wochenschrift 110/10:356–363.

Rauchfleisch U. (2002) Die ambulante Behandlung von Menschen in psychosozialen Notsituationen. In: Eggebrecht/Pehl (Hrsg.) Chaos und Beziehung. Spielweisen und Begegnungsräume von Sozialtherapie, Psychotherapie und Beratung. Tübingen: edition diskord.
Razum O, Zeeb H, Laaser U. (2006) Globalisierung – Gerechtigkeit – Gesundheit. Bern: Huber.
Reid RD, Quinlan B, Riley DL, Pipe AL. (2007) Smoking cessation: lessons learned from clinical trial evidence (2007) Curr Opin Cardiol 22/4:280–5.
Reinert RE. (1958) A comparison of reserpine and disulfiram in the treatment of alcoholism. Quarterly Journal of Studies on Alcohol 19:617–622.
Reinhardt JD. (2005) Alkohol und Soziale Kontrolle. Gedanken zu einer Soziologie des Alkoholismus. Würzburg: Ergon Velag.
Reker M and Wehn E. (2001) Qualifizierte Hilfen für alkoholabhängige und wohnungslose Menschen. Weiterführende Konzepte an den Schnittstellen von Psychiatrie und Wohnungslosenhilfe. In: Wienberg/Driessen (Hrsg.) Auf dem Weg zur vergessenen Mehrheit. Innovative Konzepte für die Versorgung von Menschen mit Alkoholproblemen. Bonn: Psychiatrieverlag.
Renn H. (1991) Defizite in der Suchtprävention und Notwendigkeiten der Präventionsforschung. In: Projektträger Forschung im Dienste der Gesundheit (FDG). Suchtforschung. Bestandsaufnahme und Analyse des Forschungsbedarfs, Bonn: Wirtschaftsverlag NW:4–13.
Renz-Polster H, Krautzig G, Braun J. (2007) Basislehrbuch Innere Medizin. 3rd. Edt., Urban & Fischer Hamburg.
Reulbach U, Biermann T, Bleich S, Hillemacher T, Kornhuber J, Sperling W. (2007) Alcoholism and homicide with respect to the classification systems of Lesch and Cloninger. Alcohol Alcohol 42/2:103–107.
Rhead JC, Soskin RA, Turek I, Richards WA, Yensen R, Kurlan AA, Ota KY. (1977) Psychedelic drug (DPT) assisted psychotherapy with alcoholics: A controlled study. Journal of Psychedelic Drugs 9:287–300.
Richter M and Hurrelmann K. (2004) Sozioökonomische Unterschiede im Substanzkonsum von Jugendlichen. Sucht 4:258–268.
Riegler A and Lesch OM. (2005) Spezifische therapeutische Strategien bei unterschiedlichen Klassen von Tabakabhängigkeit. Endbericht Mai 2005 (Studiendauer Februar 2004 bis März 2005, mit Unterstützung des Medizinschwissenschaftlichen Fonds des Bürgermeisters der Bundeshauptstadt Wien, Projekt Nr. 2233).
Riegler A, Ramskogler K, Lesch OM. (2002) Patientencharakteristika Alkoholabhängiger und ihre spezifische Psycho- und Pharmakotherapie. In: Peter K. (Hrsg.) Fortschritte in Psychiatrie und Psychotherapie. Interdisziplinäre und integrative Aspekte. Wien New York: Springer: 83–96.
Riley EP, McGee CL. (2005) Fetal Alcohol Spectrum Disorders: An Overview with Emphasis on Changes in Brain and Behavior. Exp Biol Med 230: 357–365
Roache JD, Wang Y, Ait-Daoud N, Johnson BA. (2008) Prediction of serotonergic treatment efficacy using age of onset and Type A/B typologies of alcoholism. Alcohol Clin Exp Res. Aug;32(8):1502–12. Epub 2008 Jun 28.

Robertson I, Heather N, Dzialdowski A, Crawford J, Winton M. (1986) A comparison of minimal versus intensive controlled drinking treatment for problem drinkers. British Journal of Clinical Psychology 25:185–194.

Rodríguez de Fonseca F, Del Arco I, Bermudez-Silva FJ, Bilbao A, Cippitelli A, Navarro M. (2005) The endocannabinoid system: physiology and pharmacology. Alcohol Alcohol 40/1:2–14.

Rogers CR. (1951). Client-centered therapy. Boston: Houghton Mifflin.

Röhrle B and Sommer G. (1998) Zur Effektivität netzwerkorientierter Interventionen. In: Röhrle/Sommer/Nestmann (Hrsg.) Netzwerkintervention. Tübingen.

Röhrle B, Sommer G, Nestmann F. (1998) Netzwerkintervention. Fortschritte der Gemeindepsychologie. Band 2. Tübingen.

Rohsenow DJ, Smith RE, Johnson S. (1985)Stress management training as a prevention program for heavy social drinkers: Cognitive, affect, drinking and individual differences. Addictive Behaviors 10:45–54.

Rollema H, Coe JW, Chambers LK, Hurst RS, Stahl SM, Williams KE. (2007) Rationale, pharmacology and clinical efficacy of partial agonists of alpha(4)beta(2) nACh receptors for smoking cessation. Trends Pharamcol Sci 28/7:316–25.

Rommelspacher H and Schuckit M. (1996) Drugs of Abuse. Elsevier.

Rommelspacher H, May T, Dufeu P, Schmidt LG. (1994) Longitudinal observations of monoamine oxidase B in alcoholics: differentiation of marker characteristics. Alcohol Clin Exp Res 18:1322–1329.

Rommelspacher H. (1992) Das mesolimbische dopaminerge System als Schaltstelle der Entwicklung und Aufrechterhaltung süchtigen Verhaltens. Sucht 38:91–92.

Rommelspacher H. (2007) Rauchen aus der Sicht der Hirnforschung. In: Lesch OM. Raucherentwöhnung – Tipps zur Prävention und Therapie in der Praxis. Uni-Med Verlag.

Rona RJ, Fear NT, Hull L, Greenberg N, Earnshaw M, Hotopf M, Wessely S. (2007) Mental health consequences of overstretch in the UK armed forces: first phase of a cohort study. BMJ 335:203–205.

Rosenqvist M. (1998) Alcohol and cardiac arrhythmias. Alcohol Clin Exp Res 22:318–322.

Rossow I and Amundsen A. (1997) Alcohol abuse and mortality: a 40-year prospective study of norwegian conscripts. Soc Sci Med 44:261–267.

Rounsaville BJ, Dolinsky ZS, Babor TF, Meyer RE. (1987) Psychopathology as a predictor of treatment outcome in alcoholics. Arch Gen Psychiatr 44:505–513.

Roy TS and Sabherwal U. (1994) Effects of Prenatal Nicotine Exposure on the Morphogenesis of Somatosensory Cortex. Neurotoxicology and Teratology 16/4:411–421.

Ruigomez A, Johansson S, Wallander MA, Rodriguez LAG. (2002) Incidence of chronic atrial fibrillation in general practice and its treatment pattern. Journal of Clinical Epidemiology 55:358–363.

Rychtarik RG, Connors GJ, Whitney RB, Mc Gillicuddy NB, Fitterling JM, Wirtz P. (2000) Treatment settings for persons with alcoholism: Evidence for matching clients to inpatient versus outpatient care. Journal of Consulting and Clinical Psychology 68/2:277–289.

Saffroy R, Benyamina A, Pham P, Marill C, Karila L, Reffas M, Debuire B, Reynaud M, Lemoine A. (2008) Protective effect against alcohol dependence of the thermolabile variant of MTHFR. Drug Alcohol Depend. Jul 1; 96(1–2): 30–6

Saffroy R, Pham P, Chiappini F, Gross-Goupil M, Castera L, Azoulay D, Barrier A, Samuel D, Debuire B, Lemoine A. (2004) The MTHFR 677 C>T polymorphism is associated with an increased risk of hepatocellular carcinoma in patients with alcoholic cirrhosis. Carcinogenesis 25/8:1443–1448.

Saint-Exupéry Antoine de (1995) The little Prince. Wordsworth Editions Limited, ISBN 1 85326 1580

Salafia C, Shiverick K. (1999) Cigarette Smoking and Pregnancy I: Ovarian, Uterine and Placental Effects. Placenta 20:265–272.

Salafia C, Shiverick K. (1999) Cigarette Smoking and Pregnancy II: Vascular Effects. Placenta 20:273–279.

Salaspuro VJ and Salaspuro MP. (2004) Synergistic effect of alcohol drinking and smoking on in vivo acetaldehyde concentration in saliva. Int J Cancer 111:480–3.

Salaspuro VJ, Hietala JM, Marvola ML, Salaspuro MP. (2006) Eliminating carcinogenic acetaldehyde by cysteine from saliva during smoking. Cancer Epidemiol Biomarkers Prev 15/1:146–149.

Saletu-Zyhlarz G and Hartl D. (2005) Darstellung des Rauchverhaltens von Schwangeren anhand der European Smoker Classification. Endbericht mit Unterstützung des Medizinisch-wissenschaftlichen Fonds des Bürgermeisters der Bundeshauptstadt Wien, Projekt Nr. 2195, Februar 2005.

Saletu-Zyhlarz GM, Arnold O, Anderer P, Oberndorfer S, Walter H, Lesch OM, Böning J, Saletu B. (2004) Differences in brain function between relasping and abstaining alcohol-dependent patients, evaluated by EEG mapping. Alcohol Alcohol 39:233–240.

Sällström Baum S, Hill R, Rommelspacher H. (1995) Norharmaninduced changes of extracellular concentrations of dopamine in the nucleus accumbens of rats. Life Sci 56:1715–1720.

Sällström Baum S, Hill R, Rommelspacher H. (1996) Harmaninduced changes of extracellular concentrations of neurotransmitters in the nucleus accumbens of rats. Eur J Pharmacol 314:75–82.

Samochowiec J, Kucharska-Mazur J, Grzywacz A, Pelka-Wysiecka J, Mak M, Samochowiec A, Bienkowski P. (2008) Genetics of Lesch's typology of alcoholism. Prog Neuropsychopharmacol Biol Psychiatry 32/2:423–7.

Sanchez-Craig M, Annis HM, Bornet AR, MacDonald KR. (1984) Random assignment to abstinence and controlled drinking: Evaluation of a cognitive-behavioural program for problem drinkers. Journal of Consulting and Clinical Psychology 52:390–403.

Sanchez-Craig M, Leigh G, Spivak K, Lei H. (1989) Superior outcome of females over males after brief treatment for the reduction of heavy drinking. British Journal of Addiction 84:395–404.

Sanchez-Craig M, Spivak K, Davila R. (1991) Superior outcome of females over males after brief treatment for the reduction of heavy drinking: Replication and report of therapist effects. British Journal of Addiction 86:867–876.

Sandahl C and Ronnberg S. (1990) Brief group psychotherapy relapse prevention for alcohol dependent patients. International Journal of Group Psychotherapy 40:453–476.

Sandahl C, Herlitz K, Ahlin G, Roenberg S. (1998) Time-limited group psychotherapy for moderately alcohol dependent patients: A randomized controlled clinical trial. Psychotherapy Research 8/4:361–378.

Sander D, Poppert H, Sander K. (2006) Medikamentöse Prophylaxe des Schlaganfalls. Akt Neurol 33:403–411.

Sannibale C. (1989) A prospective study of treatment outcome with a group of male problem drinkers. Journal of Studies on Alcohol 50:236–244.

Saremi A, Hanson RL, Williams DE, Roumain J, Robin RW, Long JC, Goldman D, Knowler WC. (2001) Validity of the CAGE questionnaire in an American Indian population. Journal of Studies on Alcohol 62:294–300.

Sass H, Soyka M, Mann K, Zieglgänsberger W. (1996) Relapse prevention by acamprosate: results from a placebo-controlled study on alcohol dependence. Arch Gen Psychiatry 53:673–680.

Saß U, Wittichen HU, Zaudig M. (1996) DSM IV. Göttingen : Hogrefe.

Scharf D and Shiffman S. (2004) Are there gender differences in smoking cessation, with and without bupropion? Pooled-and meta-analyses of clinical trials of Bupropion SR. Addiction 99:1462–1469.

Schmid C. (1993) Systemische Therapie im stationären Kontext – Möglichkeiten und Grenzen. In: Deutsche Hauptstelle gegen die Suchtgefahren (Hrsg.): Sucht und Familie. Freiburg im Breisgau:168–175.

Schmidt B, Alte-Teigeler A, Hurrelmann K. (1999) Soziale Bedingungsfaktoren von Drogenkonsum und Drogenmissbrauch. In: Gastpar M, Mann K, Rommelspacher H. (Hrsg.) Lehrbuch der Suchterkrankungen. Stuttgart: Thieme:50–69.

Schmidt G and Heinz A. (2005) Neurobiologie abhängigen Verhaltens. In: Riederer P, Laux G, Pöldinger W (eds.) Neuro-Psychopharmaka Bd. 6, 2. Auflage. Wien New York: Springer:291–311.

Schmidt G. (1992) Sucht-„Krankheit" und/oder Such(t) – Kompetenzen lösungsorientierte systemische Therapiekonzepte für eine gleichrangig-partnerschaftliche Umgestaltung von „Sucht" in Beziehungs- und Lebensressourcen. In: Richelshagen K. Süchte und Systeme. Lambertus-Verlag.

Schmidt G. (2004) Liebesaffären zwischen Problem und Lösung. Hypnosystemisches Arbeiten in schwierigen Kontexten. Carl-Auer Verlag.

Schmitz JM and DeLaune KA. (2003) Psychological foundations. In Johnson B, Ruiz P, Galanter M. Handbook of Clinical Alcoholism Treatment. Lippincott Williams & Wilkins:19–25.

Schneider C. (1927) Über Picksche Krankheit. Monatsschr Psychiatr Neurol 65:230–275.

Schneider C. (1929) Weitere Beiträge zur Lehre von der Pickschen Krankheit. Z Ges Neurol Psychiat 120:340–384.

Schnoll RA and Lerman C. (2006) Current and emerging pharmacotherapies for treating tobacco dependence. Expert Opin Emerg Drugs 11/3:429–44.

Schoberberger R and Kunze M. (1999) Nikotinabhängigkeit. Diagnostik und Therapie. Wien New York: Springer.

Schoberberger R, Bayer P, Groman E, Kunze M. (2002) New Strategies in Smoking Cessation: Experiences with Inpatient Smoking Treatment in Austria. In: Varma AK (Ed.): Tobacco Counters Health 2; Macmillan, New Delhi:177–181.

Schoberberger R. (2006a) Expanding Access to Cessation Treatment as an Important Tobacco Control Measure. In: Varma AK (Ed.). Tobacco Counters Health 4; Northern Book Centre, New Delhi:3–10.

Schoberberger R. (2006b) In-patient smoking cessation treatment. Psychology and Health 21/1:133.

Scholz H. (1996) Syndrombezogene Alkoholismustherapie. Ein verlaufsorientierter Stufenplan für die Praxis. Verlag für Psychologie, Göttingen, Bern, Toronto, Seattle: Hogrefe.

Schöniger-Hekele M, Petermann D, Lesch OM, Müller Ch. (1998) Prevalence of hepatitis G-virus infection in alcohol abusing patients with and without liver cirrhosis. Wiener klinische Wochenschrift 110/19:686–690.

Schoppet M and Maisch B. (2001) Alcohol and the heart. Herz 26:345–352.

Schreckling S. (1999) Ein Wunschtraum wird Gesetz. Kerbe 3/99.

Schuckit M, Smith T, Pierson J, Danko G, Beltran IA. (2006) Relationships among the level of response to alcohol and the number of alcoholic relatives in predicting alcohol-related outcomes. Alcohol Clin Exp Res 30/8:1308–14.

Schuckit MA, Tipp J, Smith TL, Shapiro E, Hesselbrock V, Bucholz K, Reich T, Nurnberger JI Jr. (1995) An evaluation of Type A and Type B alcoholics. Addiction 90:1189–204.

Schuckit MA, Tipp JE, Berman M, Reich W, Hesselbrock VM, Smith TL. (1997) Comparison of induced and independent major depressive disorders in 2945 alcoholics. Am J Psychiatry 154:948–957.

Schuckit MA. (1979) Drug and Alcohol Abuse. A clinical Guide to Diagnosis and Treatment. New York: Plenum.

Schuckit MA. (1985) The clinical implications of primary diatgnostic groups among alcoholics. Arch Gen Psychiatry 42:1043–1049.

Schuckit MA. (1995) Alcohol-related disorders. In: Kaplan HI, Sadock BJ. Comprehensive Textbook of Psychiatry (6th edition, vol 1):775–790.

Schulz W. (1976) Ansatz einer Theorie sozialen Trinkens: In: Antons K, Schulz W. (Hrsg.) Normales Trinken und Suchtentwicklung. Göttingen: Hogrefe:158–166.

Schwendter R. (2000) Einführung in die Soziale Therapie. Tübingen.

Schwoon DR. (1992) Motivation – ein kritischer Begriff in der Behandlung Suchtkranker. In : Wienberg G. (Hrsg.) Die vergessene Mehrheit. Zur Realität der Versorgung alkohol- und medikamentenabhängiger Menschen. Bonn: Psychiatrieverlag.

Seitz HK and Stickel F. (2007) Molecular mechanisms of alcohol-mediated carcinogenesis. Nature Reviews Cancer, Volume 7:599–612.

Shiffman S, Gnys M, Richards TJ, Paty JA, Hickcox M, Kassel JD. (1996) Temptations to smoke after quitting: a comparison of lapsers and maintainers. Health Psychol 15:455–461.

Shiffman S, Johnston JA, Khayrallah M, Elash CA, Gwaltney CJ, Paty JA, Gnys M, Evoniuk G, DeVeaugh-Geiss J. (2000) The effect of bupropion on nicotine craving and withdrawal. Psychopharmacology 148:33–40.

Simiand J, Keane M, Keane PE, Soubrié P. (1998) SR 141716, a CB1 cannabinoid receptor antagonist, selectively reduces sweet food intake in marmoset. Behav Pharmacol 9/2:179–81.

Simon JA, Duncan C, Carmody TP, Hudes ES. (2004) Bupropion for smoking cessation: a randomized trial. Arch Intern Med 164/16:1797–803.

Sinclair JD. (2001) Evidence about the use of naltrexone and for different ways of using it in the treatment of alcoholism. Alcohol Alcohol 36/1:2–10.

Singer MV und Teyssen S. (2005) Alkohol und Folgekrankheiten. 2nd ed. Mannheim: Springer.
Skinner BF. (1938) The behaviour of organism. An experimental analysis. New York: Appleton-Century-Crafts.
Skinner HA. (1982) Statistical approaches to the classification of alcohol and drug addiction. Br J Addict 77:259–73.
Skutle A and Berg G. (1987) Training in controlled drinking for early-stage problem drinkers. British Journal of Addiction 82:493–501.
Smith D, Hart CL, Hole D, MacKinnon P, Gillis C, Watt G, Blane D, Hawthorne V. (1998) Education and occupational social class: which is the more important indicator of mortality risk? J Epidemiol Community Health Mar; 52(3): 153–60.
Smith DI. (1986) Evaluation of a residential AA program. International Journal of the Addictions 21:33–49.
Smith JE, Meyers RJ, Delaney JHD. (1998) The community reinforcement approach with homeless alcohol-dependent individuals. Journal of Consulting and Clinical Psychology 66:541–548.
Smith TL, Volpe FR, Hashima JN, Schukit MA. (1999) Impact of a stimulant-focused enhanced program on the outcome of alcohol- and/or stimulant-dependent men. Alcohol Clin Exp Res 23/11:1772–1779.
Sobell MB and Sobell LC. (1973) Individualized behaviour therapy for alcoholics. Behavior Therapy 4:49–72.
Söderpalm B, Ericson M, Olausson P, Blomqvist O, Engel JA. (2000) Nicotinic mechanisms involved in the dopamine activating and reinforcing properties of ethanol. Behav Brain Res 113:85–96.
Soyka M, Koller G, Schmidt P, Lesch OM, Leweke M, Fehr C, Gann H, Mann K. (2008) Cannabinoid receptor 1 antagonist SR 141716 (Rimonabant) for treatment of alcohol dependence – results fro a placebo-controlled double-blind trial. J Clin Psychopharmacol, 28/3: 317–324
Spanagel R and Hölter SM. (1999) Long-term-alcohol self-administration with repeated alcohol deprivation phases; an animal model of alcoholism? Alcohol Alcohol 34/2:231–43.
Spanagel R and Zieglgansberger W. (1997) Anti-craving compounds for ethanol: new pharmaco-logical tools to study addictive processes.Trends Pharmacol Sci 18/2:54–9.
Sperling W and Lesch OM. (1996) The reduction of alcohol consumption with novel pharmacological intervention. Eur Psychiatry 11:217–226.
Sperling W, Frank H, Lesch OM, Mader R, Ramskogler K, Barocka A. (1999) Untergruppen Alkoholabhängiger und ihre primäre Vulnerabilität – Eine Untersuchung zweier Typologien (Cloninger, Lesch). Wiener Zeitschrift für Suchtforschung 22/4:21–26.
Sperling W, Frank H, Martus B, Mader R, Barocka A, Walter H, Lesch OM. (2000) The Concept of Abnormal Hemispheric Organization in Addiction Pesearch. Alcohol&Alcoholism 35/4:394–399.
Sperling W, Biermann T, Bleich S, Galvin R, Maihöfner C, Kornhuber J, Reulenbach U. (2010) Cognitive and Behavioural Aspechts, Non-right-handedness and Free Serum

Testosterone Levels in Detoxified Patients with Alcohol Dependence. Alcohol&Alcoholism 45/3:237–240.

Spielhofer H und Lesch OM. (1980) Probleme bei der Rehabilitation psychisch Kranker im ländlichen Raum. Bericht über ein Wohn- und Arbeitsheim im Burgenland (Großpetersdorf). In: Finzen A, Koester H, Rose HK (Hrsg.) Psychiatrische Praxis 7/4. Stuttgart New York: Georg Thieme Verlag:247–254.

Spies C. (2000) Anästhesiologische Aspekte bei Alkoholmißbrauch. Therapeutische Umschau 57/4:261–263.

Spivak K, Sanchez-Craig M, Davila R. (1994) Assisting problem drinkers to change on their own: Effects of specific and non-specific advice. Addiction 89:1135–1142.

Springer A. (1995) Jugendkultur und Drogengebrauch. In: Brosch R und Juhnke G. (Hrsg) Jugend und Sucht Wien.

Springer-Kremser M and Ekstein R. (1987) Wahrnehmung-Fantasie-Wirklichkeit. Franz Deuticke Verlag.

Sprung R, Bonte W, Lesch OM. (1988) Methanol, Ein bisher verkannter Bestandteil aller alkoholischen Getränke; Eine neue biochemische Annäherung an das Problem des chronischen Alkoholismus. Wiener klinische Wochenschrift 100/9:282–288.

Stanger O, Hermann W, Pietrzk K, Fowler B, Geisel J, Dierkes J, Weger M. (2003) Konsensuspapier der D.A.CH.-Liga Homocystein über den rationellen klinischen Umgang mit Homocystein, Folsäure und B-Vitaminen bei kardiovaskulären und thrombotischen Erkrankungen – Richtlinien und Empfehlungen. Journal für Kardiologie 10:190–199.

Stanger O, Weger M, Renner W, Konetschny R. (2001) Vascular dysfunction in hyperhomocyst(e)inemia. Implications for atherothrombotic disease. Clin Chem Lab Med 39/8:725–33.

Stark W. (1996) Empowerment: neue Handlungskompetenzen in der psychosozialen Praxis. Freiburg im Breisgau: Lambertus.

Statistik Austria. (2007) Einkommen, Armut und Lebensbedingungen, EU-SILC 2005.

Stead L and Lancaster T. (2007) Interventions to reduce harm from continued tobacco use. Cochrane Database Syst Rev 18/3:CD005231.

Steensland P, Simms JA, Holgate J, Richards JK, Bartlett SE. (2007) Varenicline, an {alpha}4{beta}2 nicotinic acetylcholine receptor partial agonist, selectively decreases ethanol consumption and seeking. Proc Natl Acad Sci U S A 104/30:12518–12523.

Stein LI, Newton JR, Bowman RS. (1975) Duration of hospitalization for alcoholism. Archives of General Psychiatry 32:247–252.

Steingass HP, Bilstein A, Scheiber S. (1998) Frontalhirn, Handlungsplanung und Problemlösen bei chronisch Alkoholabhängigen. Verhaltensmedizin Heute 9:45–50.

Steingass HP. (1994) Kognitive Funktionen Alkoholabhängiger. Geesthacht: Neuland.

Steingass HP. (1998) Neuropsychologie und Sucht. In: Fachverband Sucht e. V., Entscheidungen und Notwendigkeiten. Geesthacht: Neuland.

Steingass HP. (2001) Soziotherapie – mehr oder weniger anders als Psychotherapie? Geesthacht: Neuland.

Steingass HP. (2004) Neuropsychologische Methoden in der Arbeit mit chronisch mehrfach beeinträchtigten Abhängigen. In Steingass HP. (Hrsg.) Geht doch! Soziotherapie chronisch mehrfach beeinträchtigter Abhängiger. Geesthacht: Neuland.

Stibler H and Borg S. (1986) Carbohydrate composition of transferring in alcoholic patients. Alcohol Clin Exp Res 10:61–64.

Stimmel B, Cohen M, Sturiano V, Hanbury R, Korts D, Jackson G. (1983) Is treatment for alcoholism effective in persons on methadone maintenance? American Journal of Psychiatry 140:862–866.

Sting S and Blum C. (2003) Soziale Arbeit in der Suchtprävention (Soziale Arbeit im Gesundheitswesen 2):167 Seiten.

Straus F and Höfer R. (1998) Die Netzwerkperspektive in der Praxis. In: Netzwerkintervention. Fortschritte der Gemeindepsychologie. Band 2. Tübingen.

Streissguth AP, Barr HM, Sampson PD. (1990) Moderate prenatal alcohol exposure: Effects on child IQ and learning problems at age 7 ½ years. Alcohol Clin Exp Res 14:662–669.

Streissguth AP. (1990) Fetal Alcohol Syndrome and the teratogenicity of alcohol: Policy implications. King County Med Soc Bulletin 69:32–39.

Streubel AC. (1998) Errorless Learning – Eine Chance für alkoholabhängige Patienten mit Gedächtnisstörungen? Diplomarbeit. Bergische Universität – Gesamthochschule Wuppertal.

Strotmann J and Ertl G. (2005) Alkohol und Herz-Kreislauf. In: Singer MV und Teyssen S. Alkohol und Alkoholfolgekrankheiten, Grundlagen – Diagnostik – Therapie. 2. vollst. überarb. u. aktualisierte Aufl., Springer:394–409.

Strotzka H. (1971) Die Soziogenese psychischer Erkrankungen. In: Lauter H, Meyer JE. (Hrsg.) Der psychisch Kranke und die Gesellschaft. Stuttgart.

Strotzka H. (1982) Psychotherapie und Tiefenpsychologie. Ein Kurzlehrbuch. Wien New York: Springer.

Stuppaeck CH, Barnas C, Falk M, Guenther V, Hummer M, Oberbauer H, Pycha R, Whitworth AB, Fleischhacker WW. (1994) Assessment of the alcohol withdrawal syndrome--validity and reliability of the translated and modified Clinical Institute Withdrawal Assessment for Alcohol scale (CIWA-A). Addiction 89/10:1287–92.

Sullivan JT, Sykora K, Schneiderman J, Naranjo CA, Sellers EM. (1989) Assessment of alcohol withdrawal: The revised Clinical Institute Withdrawal Assessment for Alcohol scale (CIWA-Ar). British Journal of Addiction 84:1353–1357.

Sullivan J, Baenziger JC, Wagner DL, Rauscher FP, Nurnberger JI, Holmes S. (1990) Platelet MAO in subtypes of alcoholism. Biological Psychiatry 27:911–922.

Sutherland I, Willner P. (1998) Patterns of alcohol, cigarette and illicit drug use in English adolescents. Addiction 93:1199–1208.

Swann AS, Johnson BA, Cloninger CR, Chen YR. (1999) Alcoholism and serotonin: Relationships of plasma tryptophan availibility to course of illness and clinical features. Psychopharmacology 143:380–384.

Sweeney CT, Fant RV, Fagerström KO, McGovern JF, Henningfield JE. (2001) Combination nicotine replacement therapy for smoking cessation: rationale, efficacy and tolerability. CNS Drugs 15:453–467.

Swenson PR, Struckman-Johnson DL, Ellingstad VS, Clay TR, Nichols JL. (1981) Results of a longitudinal evaluation of court-mandated DWI treatment programs in Phoenix, Arizona. Journal of Studies on Alcohol 42:642–653.

Szasz TS. (1984) Das Ritual der Drogen. Baulino Verlag GmbH.

Tabakoff B and Hoffmann PL. (1991) Neurochemical effects of alcohol. In: Frances RJ and Miller SI. Clinical Textbook of Addictive Disorders. New York: Guilford Press:501–525.

Tarter REH, McBride RN, Bounparte N, Schneider DU. (1977) Differentiation of alcoholics. Arch Gen Psychiatr 34:761–768.

Tasseit S. (1994) Problemfelder der Suchttherapie und Suchtforschung: Beiträge aus Soziologie und Sozialpädagogik. Regensburg: Roderer Verlag.

Terry MB, Zhang FF, Kabat G, Britton JA, Teitelbaum SL, Neugut AI, Gammon MD. (2006) Lifetime alcohol intake and breast cancer risk. Ann Epidemiol 16/3:230–40.

Teschke R and Göke R. (2005) Alkohol und Krebs. In: Singer M und Teyssen S. Alkohol und Alkoholfolgekrankheiten, Grundlagen-Diagnostik-Therapie. Berlin Heidelberg: Springer.

Tiefengraber D. (2008) Retrospektive Verlaufskontrollstudie an Alkoholabhängigen unter Berücksichtigung der Typologie nach Lesch.

Tonetti MS, Pini-Prato G, Cortellini P. (1995) Effect of cigarette smoking on periodontal healing following GTR in infrabony defects. A preliminary retrospective study. J Clin Periodontol 22:229–234.

Tonnesen P, Paoletti P, Gustavsson G, Russell MA, Saracci R, Gulsvik A, Rijcken B, Sawe U. (1999) Higher dosage nicotine patches increase one-year smoking cessation rates: results from the European CEASE trial. Collaborative European Anti-Smoking Evaluation. European Respiratory Society. Eur Respir J 13:238–246.

Tonstad S, Tonnesen P, Hajek P, Williams KE, Billing CB, Reeves KR. (2006) Effect of Maintenance Therapy with Varenicline on smoking cessation – A randomized controlled trial. JAMA 296/1:64–71.

Trager JB and Hanrahan JP. (1995) Maternal smoking during pregnancy. American Journal of Respiratory Diseaseand Cutic Care Medicine 152:977–983.

Trent LK. (1996) Evaluation of a four-versus six-week length of stay in the Navy's alcohol treatment program. Journal of Studies on Alcohol:271–279.

Trombelli L, Lee MB, Promsudthi A, Guglielmoni PG, Wikesjö UM. (1999) Periodontal repair in dogs: histologic observations of guided tissue regeneration with a prostaglandin E1 analog/methacrylate composite. J Clin Periodontol 26/6:381–7.

True WR, Heath AC, Scherrer JF, Waterman B, Goldberg J, Lin N, Eisen SA, Lyons MJ, Tsuang MT. (1997) Genetic and environmental contributions to smoking. Addiction 92:1277–1287.

True WR, Xian H, Scherrer JF, Madden PA, Bucholz KK, Heath AC, Eisen SA, Lyons MJ, Goldberg J, Tsuang M. (1999) Common genetic vulnerability for nicotine and alcohol dependence in men. Archives of General Psychiatry 56:655–661.

Uexküll TV. (1996) Psychosomatische Medizin. Hrsg. Adler RH, Hermman JM, Köhle K, Schonecke OW, Uexküll Tv, Wesiack W. 5. Auflage, Urban und Schwarzenberg Verlag.

Uhl A and Springer A. (1996) Studie über den Konsum von Alkohol und psychoaktiven Stoffen in Österreich unter Berücksichtigung problematischer Gebrauchsmuster – Repräsentativerhebung 1993/1994 Datenband. Bericht des LBI Sucht, Wien.

Unachuku CN. (2006) The endocannabinoid system: association with metabolic disorders and tobacco dependence. Niger J Med 15/3:323–4.

Unger JB, Johnson CA, Marks G. (1997) Functional decline in the elderly: evidence for direct and stress-buffering protective effects of social interactions and physical activity. Annuals of Behavioral Medicine 19/2:152–160.

US Department of Health and Human Services. Management of Nicotine Addiction. Reducing Tobacco Use: A Report of the Surgeon General.(2000) Atlanta. GA: Centers for Disease Control and Prevention, National Center for Chronic Disease Prevention and Health Promotion, Office on Smoking and Health

Van den Bree MBM, Svilkis DS, Pickens RW. (1998) Genetic influences in antisocial personality and drug use disorders. Drug Alcohol Depend:177–181.

Van den Brink W, Montgomery SA, Van Ree JM, van Zwieten-Boot BJ. (2006) ECNP Consensus Meeting March 2003 Guidelines fort he investigation of efficacy in substance use disorders. European Neuropsychopharmacology 16, Issue 3: 224–230.

Van Praag HM, Brown SL, Asnis GM, Kahn RS, Korn ML, Harkavy-Friedman JM, Wetzler S. (1991) Beyond serotonin: A multiaminergic perspective on abnormal behavior. In Brown SL and van Praag HM. (eds.) The Role of Serotonin in Psychiatric Disorders. New York: Brunner/Mazel:302–332.

Vasan RS, Beiser A, D'Agostino RB, Levy D, Selhub J, Jaques PF, Rosenberg IH, Wilson PWF. (2003) Plasma homocysteine and risk for congestive heart failure in adults without prior myocardial infarction. JAMA 289:1251–1257.

Verheul R, Lehert P, Geerlings PJ, Koeter MW, van den Brink W. (2005) Predictors of acamprosate efficacy: results from a pooled analysis of seven European trials including 1485 alcohol-dependent patients. Psychopharmacology 178/2–3:167–73.

Virkkunen M and Linnoila M. (1990) Serotonin in early onset male alcoholics with violent behavior. Annals of the New York Academy of Sciences 22:327–331.

Virkkunen M and Linnoila M. (1993) Brain serotonin, type II alcoholism and impulsive violence. Journal of Studies on Alcohol 11:163–169.

Virkkunen M and Linnoila M. (1997) Serotonin on early-onset alcoholism. Recent Developments in Alcoholism 13:173–189.

Virkkunen M, Eggert M, Rawlings R, Linnoila M. (1996) A prospective follow-up study of alcoholic violent offenders and fire setters. Archives of General Psychiatry 53:523–529.

Virkkunen M, Rawlings R, Tokola R, Poland RE, Guidotti A, Nemeroff C, Bissette G, Kalogeras K, Karonen SL, Linnoila M. (1994) CSF biochemistries, glucose metabolism, and diurnal activity rhythms in alcoholic, violent offenders, fire setters, and healthy volunteers. Archives of General Psychiatry 51:20–27.

Vogler E and Revenstorf D. (1978) Alkoholmissbrauch, sozialpsychologische und lerntheoretische Ansätze. Fortschritte der Klinischen Psychologie 13. München-Wien-Baltimor: Urban & Schwarzenberg.

Vogler RE, Weissbach TA, Compton JV, Martin GT. (1977) Integrated behavior change techniques for problem drinkers in the community. Journal of Consulting and Clinical Psychology 45/2:267–279.

Volpicelli JR, Alterman AI, Hayashida M, O'Brien CP. (1992) Naltrexone in the treatment of alcohol dependence. Arch Gen Psychiatry 49/11:876–80.

Volpicelli JR, Pettinati HM, McLellan AT, O'Brien CP. (2001) Combining medication and psychosocial treatments for addictions: The BRENDA method. NY: Guilford Press.

Volpicelli JR, Rhines KC, Rhines JS, Volpicelli LA, Alterman AI, O'Brien CP. (1997) Naltrexone and alcohol dependence. Role of subject compliance. Arch Gen Psychiatry 54/8:737–42.

vom Scheidt J. (1976) Der falsche Weg zum Selbst. Studien zur Drogenkarriere. Erstausgabe. München. Kinler Verlag.

Vutuc C, Waldhoer T, Haidinger G. (2004) Cancer mortality in Austria:1970–2002. Wien Klin Wschr 116/19–20:669–675.

Vyssoki B, Steindl-Munda P, Ferenci P, Walter H, Höfer P, Blüml V, Friedrich F, Kogoj D, Lesch OM 82010) Alcohol Withdrawal Treatment in Patients with Liver Disease-Usefulness of the Lesch Alcoholism Typology. Accepted in Alcohol & Alcoholism

Wakschlag LS, Lahey BB, Loeber R, Green SM, Gordon RA, Leventhal BL. (1997) Maternal smoking during pregnancy and the risk of conduct disorder in boys. Archives General Psychiatry 54: 670–676.

Walker RD, Donovan DM, Kivlahan DR, O'Leary MR. (1983) Length of stay, neuropsychological performance and aftercare: Influences on alcohol treatment outcomes. Journal of Consulting and Clinical Psychology 51:900–911.

Wallerstein RS, Chotlos JW, Friend MB, Hammersley DW, Perlswig EA, Winship GM. (1957) Hospital treatment of alcoholism: A comparative experimental study. New York: Basic Books.

Walsh DC, Hingson RW, Merrigan DM, Morelock Levenson S, Cupples A, Heeren T, Coffman GA, Becker CA, Barker TA, Hamilton SK, McGuire TG, Kelly CA. (1991) A randomized trial of treatment options for alcohol-abusing workers. The New England Journal of Medicine 325:775–782.

Walter H, Berner P, Lesch OM, Rommelspacher H, Bonte W, Werner E. (1994) Typologie de l'alcoolisme dans la perspective du modèle de vulnérabilité. Annales Medico- Psychologiques, 152/1:43–45.

Walter H, Dvorak A, Gutierrez K, Zitterl W, Lesch OM. (2005) Gender differences: Does alcohol affect females more than males? Neuropsychopharmacologia Hungarica VII/2:78–82.

Walter H, Gutierrez K, Lesch OM. (1998) The Role of CDT in Reflecting Alcohol Abuse. Biochemical Markers of Alcohol Problems. Papers presented at the workshop on „Use of Carbohydrate Deficient Transferrin among General Practitioners". 30. August – 4. September 1998, Malta, an ICAA publication:27–40.

Walter H, Gutierrez K, Ramskogler K, Hertling I, Dvorak A, Lesch OM. (2003) Gender-specific differences in alcoholism: Implications for treatment. Archives of Woman's Mental Health 3:253–258.

Walter H, Gutierrez-Lobos K, Skala K, Thau K, Wiesbeck GA, Schlaff WB, Lesch OM. (2008) The role of Dual Acting Antidepressants in Relapse Prevention in Chronic Alcoholism. in press.

Walter H, Hertling I, Benda N, König B, Ramskogler K, Riegler A, Semler B, Zoghlami A, Lesch OM. (2001) Sensitivity and specificity of carbohydrate-deficient transferrin in drinking experiments and different patients. Alcohol 25/3:189–194.

Walter H, Lesch OM, Musalek M. (1990) Psychosozialer Dienst Burgenland: Organisation und Eigenreflexionen. In: Meise, Hafner, Hinterhuber (Hrsg.) Die Versorgung psychisch Kranker in Österreich. Proceedings der Tagung (Innsbruck 8. bis 9.Nov. 1990) Springer Verlag.

Walter H, Ramskogler K, Semler B, Lesch OM, Platz W. (2001) Dopamine and Alcohol Relapse: D1 and D2 Antagonists Increase Relapse Rates in Animal Studies and in Clinical Trials. Journal of Biomedical Science 8:83–88.

Walter H, Ramskogler-Skala K, Dvorak A, Gutierrez-Lobos K, Hartl D, Hertling I, Munda P, Thau K, Lesch OM and De Witte P. (2006) Glutamic acid in withdrawal and weaning in patients classified according to Cloninger's and Lesch's typologies. Alcohol and Alcoholism 41/5:505–511.

Walter H. (2007) Rauchen und Alkohol. In: Raucherentwöhnung – Tipps zur Prävention und Therapie in der Praxis. Uni-Med Verlag:49–51.

Walter H et al. (2008) Breath Alcohol Level and Plasma Amino Acids: A Comparison between Older and Younger Chronic Alcohol-Dependent Patients. Alcohol & Alcoholism, pp 1–5

Walter M. (2004) Was ist Soziotherapie? Versuch einer Begriffsbestimmung und rechtlichen Abgrenzung. In: Therapie Kreativ. Zeitschrift für kreative Sozio- und Psychotherapie. Heft 39/40. Affenkönig. Neunkirchen-Vluyn:131–147.

Wanberg KW, Horn JL, Fairchild D. (1974) Hospital versus community treatment of alcoholism problems. International Journal of Mental Health 3:160–176.

Weinshenker D and Schroeder JP. (2007) There and back again: a tale of norepinephrine and drug addiction. Neuropsychopharmacology 32/7:1433–51.

Wells-Parker E, Anderson BJ, Landrum JW, Snow RW. (1988) Effectiveness of probation, short-term intervention and LAI administration for reducing DUI recidivism. British Journal of Addiction 83:415–422.

Welter-Enderlin R und Hildenbrand B. (2006) Gedeihen – trotz widriger Umstände. Heidelberg: Carl Auer.

Werner EE. (2006) Wenn Menschen trotz widriger Umstände gedeihen – und was man daraus lernen kann. In: Welter-Enderlin/Hildenbrand (Hrsg.) Gedeihen – trotz widriger Umstände. Heidelberg: Carl Auer.

West PT. (1979) Three modes of training alcoholics in interpersonal communications skills: A comparative study. Unpublished doctoral dissertation, University of Western Ontario.

Whitfield JB, Fletcher LM, Murphy TL, Powell LW, Halliday J, Heath AC , Martin NG (1998) Smoking, obesity and hypertension alter the dose-response curve and test sensitivity of carbohydrate-deficient transferring as a merker of alcohol intake. Clin Chem 44:2480–2489.

Whitworth AB, Fischer F, Lesch OM, Nimmerrichter A, Oberbauer H, Platz T, Potgieter A, Walter H, Fleischhacker WW. (1996) Comparison of acamprosate and placebo in long-term treatment of alcohol dependence. Lancet 347/9013:1438–42.

Whyte CR and O'Brien PM. (1974) Disulfiram implant: A controlled trial. British Journal of Psychiatry 124:42–44.

Widiger TA, Frances AJ, Picus HA, First MB, Ross R, Davis W. (1994) DSM-IV Sourcebook. Volume 1. American Psychiatric Association.

Wieck HH. (1956) Zur Klinik der sogenannten symptomatischen Psychosen. Dtsch. med. Wschr. 81

Wieck HH. (1967) Lehrbuch für Psychiatrie. Stuttgart: Schattauer.

Wienberg G. (1992) Die vergessene Mehrheit. Zur Realität der Versorgung alkohol- und medikamentenabhängiger Menschen. Bonn: Psychiatrieverlag.

Wienberg G. (2001) Die „vergessene Mehrheit" heute – Teil II: Zur Situation der traditionellen Suchtkrankenhilfe. In: Wienberg/Driessen (Hrsg.) Auf dem Weg zur vergessenen Mehrheit. Innovative Konzepte für die Versorgung von Menschen mit Alkoholproblemen. Bonn: Psychiatrieverlag.

Wiesbeck G, Weijers HG, Lesch OM, Glaser T, Toennes PJ, Boening J. (2001) Flupenthixol Decanoate and Relapse Prevention in Alcoholics: Results from a Placebo-Controlled Study. Alcohol Alcohol 36/4:329–334.

Wiesbeck GA. (2007) Alkoholismus-Forschung – aktuelle Befunde, künftige Perspektiven. Pabst Science Publisher.

Williams KE, Reeves KR, Billing CB Jr, Pennington AM, Gong J. (2007) A double-blind study evaluating the long-term safety of varenicline for smoking cessation. Current Medical Research and Opinion 23/4:793–801.

Wilson A, Davidson WJ, Blanchard R, White J. (1978) Disulfiram implantation: A placebo-controlled trial with two-year follow-up. Journal of Studies on Alcohol 39:809–819.

Wilson A, Davidson WJ, Blanchard R. (1980) Disulfiram implantation: A trial using placebo implants and two types of controls. Journal of Studies on Alcohol 41:429–436.

Wirnsberger K, Walter H, Lesch OM, Hartl D. (2007) Different degrees of liver damage between subgroups of alcohol-addicted persons. Alcohol Alcohol 42/1:i56.

Wisborg K, Kesmodel U, Henriksen TB, Olsen SF, Secher NJ. (2000) A prospective study of smoking during pregnancy and SIDS. Archives of disease in childhood 83/3:203–206.

Withworth AB, Fischer F, Lesch OM, Nimmerrichter A, Oberbauer H, Platz T, Potgieter A, Walter H, Fleischhacker WW. (1996) Comparison of acamprosate and placebo in long-term treatment of alcohol dependence. The Lancet 347/9013:1438–1442.

Wlassak R. (1922) Grundriss der Alkoholfrage. Leipzig: Hirzel.

Wöber C, Wöber-Bingöl C, Krawautz A, Nimmerrichter A, Deecke L, Lesch OM. (1999) Postural control and lifetime alcohol consumption in alcohol-dependent patients. Acta Neurol Scand 99:48–53.

Wodarz N, Lange K, Laufkötter R, Johann M. (2004) ADHS und Alkoholabhängigkeit: Gemeinsame genetische Grundlagen? Psychiatr Prax 31/1:111–113.

Wolf PA, D'Agostino RB, Kannel WB, Bonita R, Belanger AJ. (1988) Cigarette smoking as a risk factor or stroke: the Framingham Study. JAMA 259:1025–1029.

World Health Organization. Policy Recommendations for Smoking Cessation and Treatment of Tobacco Dependence. Geneva. Switzerland: World Health Organization 2003.

Wurst FM, Bechtel G, Forster S, Wolfersdorf M, Huber P, Scholer A, Pridzun L, Alt A, Seidl S, Dierkes J, Dammann G. (2003) Leptin levels of alcohol abstainers and detoxification patients are not different. Alcohol Alcohol 38/4:364–8.

Wurst FM. (2001) New and upcoming markers of alcohol consumption. Steinkopff Verlag Darmstadt.

Wurst FM, Vogel R, Jachau K, Varga A, Alling Ch, Alt A, Skipper GE. (2003) Ethyl Glucuronide Discloses Recent Covert Alcohol Use Not Detected by Standard Testing in Forensic Psychiatric Inpatients. Alcohol Clin Exp Res, Vol 27, No 3:471–476

Wurst FM, Thon N, Aradottir S, Hartmann S, Wiesbeck G, Lesch OM, Skala K, Wolfsdorfer M, Weinmann W, Alling C (2010) Phoshatidylethanol: Normalisation during detoxification, gender aspects and correlation with other biomarkers and self-reports. Addiction Biology, 15: 88–95

Wynne J and Braunwald E. (2005) Cardiomyopathy and myocarditis. Harrison's Principles of Internal Medicine. Vol. 16.

Xie S, Furjanic MA, Ferrara JJ, McAndrew NR, Ardino EL, Ngondara A, Bernstein Y, Thomas KJ, Kim E, Walker JM, Nagar S, Ward SJ, Raffa RB. (2007) The endocannabinoid system and rimonabant: a new drug with a novel mechanism of action involving cannabinoid CB1 receptor antagonism – or inverse agonism – as potential obesity treatment and other therapeutic use. J Clin Pharm Ther 32/3:209–31.

Yalom ID. (1999) Theorie und Praxis der Gruppenpsychotherapie. Ein Lehrbuch. München: Pfeiffer-Verlag.

Yates GL, MacKenzie R, Pennbridge J, Cohen E. (1988) A risk profile comparison of runaway and non-runaway youth. American Journal of Public Health 78:820–821.

Yusuf S, Hawken S, Ounpuu S, Dans T, Avezum A, Lanas F, McQueen M, Budaj A, Pais P, Varigos J, Lisheng L, INTERHEART Study Investigators. (2004) Effect of potentially modifiable risk factors associated with myocardial infarction in 52 countries (the INTERHEART study): case-control study. Lancet 364:937–952.

Zacny JP. (1990) Behavioral aspects of alcohol-tobacco interactions. Recent Developments in Alcoholism 8:205–219.

Zago-Gomes MdP and Nakamura-Palacidos EM. (2009) Cognitive Components of Frontal Lobe Function in Alcoholocs Classified According to Lesch´s Typology. Alcohol & Alcoholism Vol. 44, No. 5: 449–457

Zander M, Hartwig L., Jansen I. (2006) Geschlecht Nebensache? Zur Aktualität einer Genderperspektive in der sozialen Arbeit. Wiesbaden: VS-Verlag für Sozialwissenschaften.

Ziegler H. (1992) Der Bedarf: Welche Hilfen brauchen Abhängigkeitskranke? Fachliche Standards für die 90er-Jahre. In: Wienberg (Hrsg.) Die vergessene Mehrheit. Zur Realität der Versorgung alkohol- und medikamentenabhängiger Menschen. Bonn: Psychiatrie-Verlag.

Zierler-Brown S and Kyle JA. (2007) Oral Varenicline for Smoking Cessation. The Annals of Pharmacotherapy 41:95–99.

Zimberg S. (1974) Evaluation of alcoholism treatment in Harlem. Quarterly Journal of Studies on Alcohol 35:550–557.

Zimmermann P, Wittchen HU, Höfler M, Pfister H, Kessler RC, Lieb R. (2003) Primary anxiety disorders and the development of subsequent alcohol use disorders: a 4-year community study of adolescents and young adults. Psychological Medicine 33:1211–1222.

Zingerle H. (1994) Psychologische Hintergründe des Alkoholismus. Update, Internationale Zeitschrift für ärztliche Fortbildung 43, Konsensusstatement, November 94. Wien: Update Europe – Gesellschaft für ärztliche Fortbildung GmbH.

Zingerle H. (1997) Motivation und Gesprächsführung. In Fleisch/Haller/Heckmann (Hrsg.) Suchtkrankenhilfe. Lehrbuch zur Vorbeugung, Beratung und Therapie. Weinheim und Basel: Beltz Edition Sozial:237–248.

Index

About the Authors

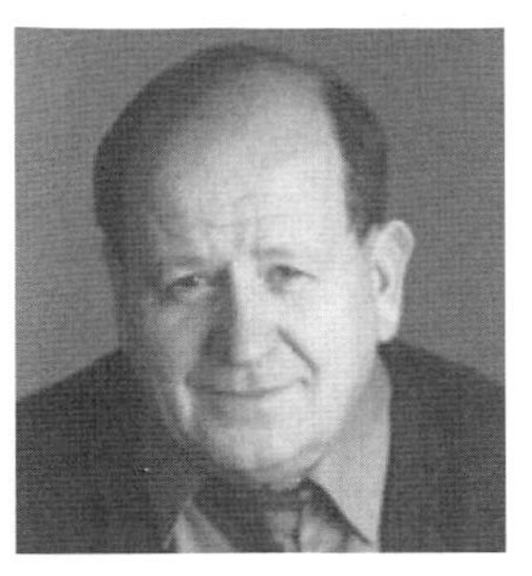

Otto Michael Lesch, MD,
is currently President of the Austrian Society of Addiction Medicine, Head of the Alcohol Research Group of the Medical University of Vienna, Department of Psychiatry and Psychotherapy. Since 1972 he is responsible for longterm studies in alcohol dependence. He organized many international clinical trials and basic research in alcohol and tobacco dependence. He served 12 years as secretary of ESBRA and organized European networks for alcohol research. He always bridged the gap between basic and clinical research and developed clinical used tools to define subgroups of addiction for better treatment approaches. His assessment tools are now available in many different languages (www.LAT-online.at).

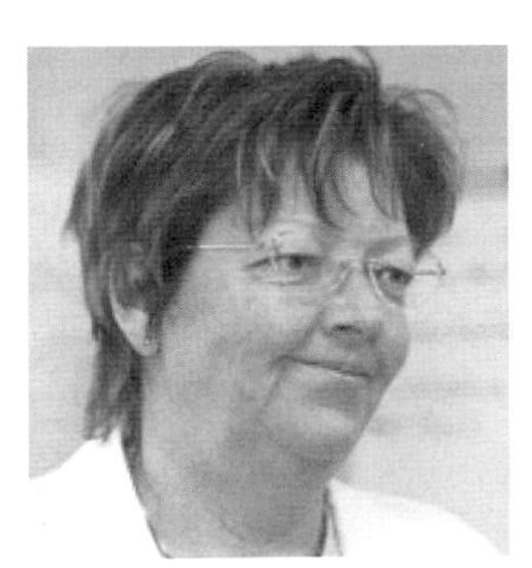

Henriette Walter, MD,
is University Professor at the Dept. of Psychiatry and Psychotherapy. She is a member of the Senate and of many commissions of the Medical University, Vienna. Dr. Walter is working in the field of alcoholism since more than 20 years, both, practically and scientifically, with over 200 publications. She is secretary of the 'AUSAM', the Austrian Society of Addiction Medicine and an ESBRA board member. She is associate editor of the Journal "Hypnose", a field in which she takes an active scientific interest since 1982. With the "theory of frontalisation" as the neuro-equivalent for the hypnotic state, she contributed to the neuroimaging research in this field. She gives regular training courses in medical hypnosis.

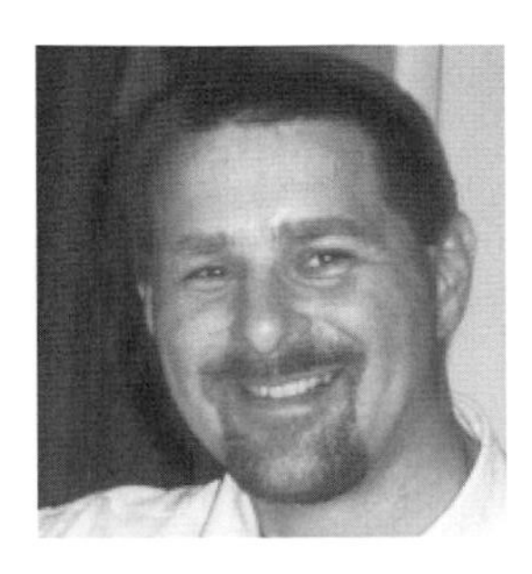

Christian Wetschka, PhD,
is socialpedagogue, working in diverse socialtherapeutic and pastoral fields, supervisor, founder of Verein Struktur, Vienna, which provides commune-flats for alcohol dependent persons.

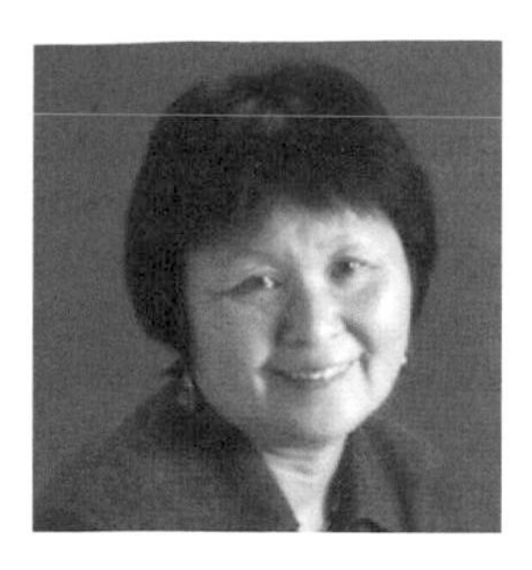

Michie N Hesselbrock, PhD,
is Professor Emeritus at the School of Social Work, and Professor of Psychiatry at the School of Medicine, University of Connecticut. She held the Zach's Chair, and was the founder and director of the PhD program at the School of Social Work before her retirement. She has served on several NIH study sections and VA Merit review committees as a regular member and as an ad hoc reviewer. Her research interests include epidemiology, behavior genetics, and health disparities of alcoholism and treatment.

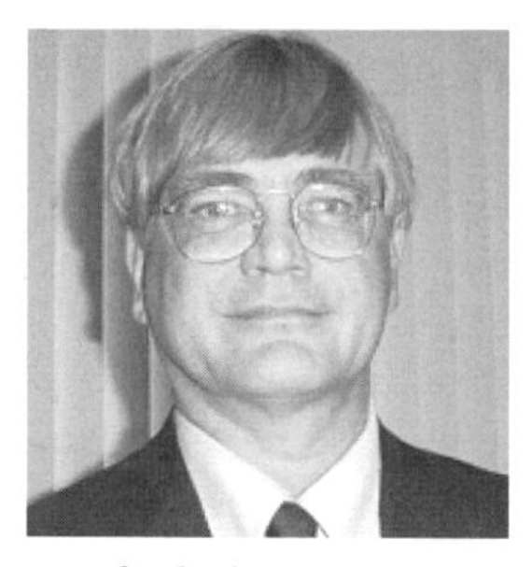

Victor Hesselbrock, PhD,
is currently Professor and Interim Chairman, Department of Psychiatry, University of Connecticut School of Medicine. He holds the Physicians Health Services endowed chair in Addiction Studies. Dr. Hesselbrock is the Principal Investigator and Scientific Director of the University of Connecticut's NIH/NIAAA funded Alcohol Research Center and is co-PI of the NIH funded national Collaborative Study on the Genetics of Alcoholism (COGA). He is a past President of the Research Society on Alcoholism (RSA). Dr. Hesselbrock is Associate Editor of *Alcoholism: Clinical and Experimental Research,* a Review Editor for *Addiction,* and a member of the editorial board of the *Journal of Studies on Alcohol and Drugs.* His research interests include: the genetic epidemiology of alcoholism; co-morbid psychiatric conditions and substance dependence; and psychosocial, cognitive, and genetic risk factors for developing alcohol dependence and alcohol-related problems.